METABOLIC TRAINING

The Ultimate Guide to the Ultimate Workout

John Graham
ACSM EP-C, CSCS*D, RSCC*E, FNSCA

Michael Barnes
CSCS*D, NSCA-CPT*D

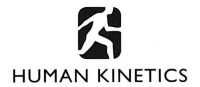

HUMAN KINETICS

Library of Congress Cataloging-in-Publication Data

Names: Graham, John, 1962- author. | Barnes, Michael, 1966- author.
Title: Metabolic training : the ultimate guide to the ultimate workout /
  John Graham, Michael Barnes.
Description: Champaign, IL : Human Kinetics, 2023. | Includes
  bibliographical references.
Identifiers: LCCN 2023021123 (print) | LCCN 2023021124 (ebook) | ISBN
  9781718212466 (paperback) | ISBN 9781718212473 (epub) | ISBN
  9781718212480 (pdf)
Subjects: LCSH: Physical fitness. | Exercise--Physiological aspects. |
  Energy metabolism. | BISAC: SPORTS & RECREATION / Training | HEALTH &
  FITNESS / Exercise / General
Classification: LCC GV481 .G69 2023 (print) | LCC GV481 (ebook) | DDC
  613.7--dc23/eng/20230629
LC record available at https://lccn.loc.gov/2023021123
LC ebook record available at https://lccn.loc.gov/2023021124

ISBN: 978-1-7182-1246-6 (print)

Senior Acquisitions Editor: Michelle Earle; **Developmental Editor:** Amy Stahl; **Copyeditor:** Jeffrey D. Castle; **Proofreader:** Lyric Dodson; **Permissions Manager:** Laurel Mitchell; **Senior Graphic Designer:** Joe Buck; **Cover Designer:** Keri Evans; **Cover Design Specialist:** Susan Rothermel Allen; **Photographs (cover and interior):** Thomas Volk Photography/© Human Kinetics; photo on page 204 © Human Kinetics; **Photo Asset Manager:** Laura Fitch; **Photo Production Specialist:** Amy M. Rose; **Photo Production Manager:** Jason Allen; **Senior Art Manager:** Kelly Hendren; **Illustrations:** © Human Kinetics; **Printer:** Versa Press

We thank St. Luke's Fitness & Sports Performance Center in Allentown, Pennsylvania, for assistance in providing the location for the photo shoot for this book.

Human Kinetics books are available at special discounts for bulk purchase. Special editions or book excerpts can also be created to specification. For details, contact the Special Sales Manager at Human Kinetics.

Printed in the United States of America

10 9 8 7 6 5 4 3 2 1

The paper in this book is certified under a sustainable forestry program.

Human Kinetics
1607 N. Market Street
Champaign, IL 61820
USA

United States and International
Website: **US.HumanKinetics.com**
Email: info@hkusa.com
Phone: 1-800-747-4457

Canada
Website: **Canada.HumanKinetics.com**
Email: info@hkcanada.com

E8580

METABOLIC
TRAINING

Contents

Acknowledgments

I would like to thank my family, Lindsey, Lexi, Kelley, and Ryan; my parents, Ruth and Ed; and our extended family for their incredible support—not only with this book but throughout my life. Thank you to Rick Anderson and Bob Martin from St. Luke's University Health Network for your incredible leadership and support in supporting community health and fitness within health care. Thank you, Dr. Tom Meade, for your vision in Medical Fitness. Thank you to Chris Poirier, Rob and Erin Milani, Perform Better, National Strength and Conditioning Association, and others for always ensuring that we have not only the tools but the knowledge to provide evidence-based fitness and sports performance programs.

Thank you to the amazing team of people who enabled this book to become a reality: Mike Barnes, an incredible coauthor and even better friend; the Human Kinetics staff, including Michelle Earle, Amy Stahl, and Jim Bowling; our incredible photographer, Tom Volk; and exercise models Rosemarie Bencivenni Hulbert, Seth Sommer, Lexi Quilty, and Isabelle Colaiezzi. Last, but certainly not least, thank you to the incredible fitness professionals and participants I have had the unique privilege to work with over the past 40 years. You have made this journey we call a career into more than I could ever have hoped for. I am truly blessed.

John Graham

For my wife Sue and my two wonderful children, Zach and Sydney.

A special thank you to John Graham. John's unwavering support over the years have been a blessing in more ways than he'll ever know. Thank you, my friend.

Mike Barnes

Introduction

If you are looking for an evidence-based workout that will help you increase lean body mass, burn fat, and stimulate your metabolism, then *Metabolic Training* is your guide.

Metabolic Training combines higher-intensity strength and metabolic segments with aerobic (and anaerobic) training intervals to catapult your training efficiency and increase measurable fitness results. You have the option to use a variety of equipment, assorted implements, or your own body weight to produce maximum gains in muscle development, strength, and fat burning. Combining exercises in a purposeful order and with a focus on metabolism ensures reaching your fitness goals quickly.

This type of training works for a wide range of athletes and exercise enthusiasts, regardless of experience level. Whether you're a college athlete, weekend warrior, age-group competitor in your sport, or mature adult, you can incorporate these training methods into your overall program with ease. Throughout this book, you'll find programming guidelines and options to optimize your workouts for cutting-edge improvements in strength, endurance, muscle development, and fat burning.

Metabolic Training has three interrelated and interdependent parts. Part I establishes the fundamental theory of metabolic training in easy-to-understand language. Part II describes the fundamental exercises—including technique instruction for each exercise—and associated tools for training such as dumbbells, kettlebells, resistance bands, and weighted sleds. Each chapter in part II includes its own exercise finder at the beginning. Part III provides four sample metabolic workouts within each of the five chapters—for a total of 20 sample workouts—that you can use immediately to jump-start your way to optimal results, whether you are a beginner, intermediate, or advanced athlete.

Whether your goal is to shape your body; increase sport, fitness, or tactical performance; or just improve your overall health and well-being, this book's programs and step-by-step guidance—for dumbbell, kettlebell, heavy rope, medicine ball, bodyweight, and suspension training exercises—will maximize your goal achievement.

PART I

Foundations of Metabolic Training

1

Why Metabolic Training?

In recent years, high-intensity interval training has increased in popularity. Personal trainers, online workout sessions, and group exercise classes offer this style of training, sometimes referred to as *metabolic training*. Metabolic training combines higher intensity strength and metabolic intervals with cardiovascular training to produce maximum gains in muscle development, strength, and cardiovascular improvement. Program format is designed to provide supreme improvements in body composition and fitness. Posture, proper form, and technique are regularly stressed and reinforced throughout the class, though the tempo is quick.

Metabolic training is becoming more and more common and heavily utilized. Metabolic-training programs can be designed to achieve goals such as losing weight, increasing endurance, and building muscle. A properly designed training program minimizes the risk of injury and maximizes training effectiveness. Training programs may include a wide range of exercises as well as variations in sets, reps, and rest intervals, keeping you engaged and motivated. Whether you're looking to improve your performance, change your body composition, add variety to your current program, or simply try something new and enjoyable, we encourage you to explore the world of metabolic training, using this book as your guide.

What Is Metabolic Training?

Metabolic training can be defined as the efficient use of training methods, specifically strength training, to elicit a metabolic response, with consideration given to intended effect, rest or relief intervals, fatigue management, progressive overload, and adaptations to suit each individual. In broad terms, metabolic training is a form of interval training. For the sake of clarity, distinctions should be made between the commonly used terms in sport science and fitness that relate to metabolic training.

- *Interval training.* Repeated bouts or exercise periods varying in intensity, duration, and rest.
- *Maximum interval training (MIT).* "MIT uses short, intense exercise periods with a variety of exercise modes [or specific type of activity or implement used for exercise] combined with brief bouts of recovery to improve performance and body image" (Cissik and Dawes 2015).

- *High-intensity interval training (HIIT).* HIIT consists of repeated bouts of exercise performed in one's red zone, or at an intensity above the anaerobic threshold, separated by relief bouts of easy exercise or complete rest (Laursen and Buchheit 2019).

- *As many reps as possible (AMRAP).* A selected group of exercises is performed for a designated period of time with the goal of executing as many reps as possible.

- *Every minute on minute (EMOM).* A single exercise is performed for a set number of reps every minute on the minute for a designated period of time.

- *Repetition in reserve (RIR).* This refers to the difference between how many repetitions were performed and how many repetitions could actually be performed before failure.

- *Steady-state training.* Cyclical aerobic exercise performed for longer durations. Steady-state intervals are performed at a modified intensity and are generally longer in duration.

- *Tempo or pace training.* A pace that is at one's training rate. Training pace is typically determined by heart rate, power output, or perceived exertion. Training pace workouts are predominately aerobic and performed at or near lactate threshold.

- *Lactate threshold.* The exercise intensity at which lactate production exceeds absorption. Lactate threshold can be expressed as a percentage of maximal oxygen capacity. Untrained individuals have a comparatively lower lactate threshold, while highly trained athletes can push their lactate thresholds to higher than 90 percent of maximal oxygen capacity.

- $\dot{V}O_2max$. The maximum rate oxygen can be used by the body. This measure is often used as a measure of cardiorespiratory fitness.

Metabolic-Training Goals and Objectives

Metabolic training can be implemented to achieve a variety of goals. These goals include, but are not limited to, eliciting a certain training effect, exercising in a time-efficient manner, bringing about general and specific adaptations of metabolic processes, improving maximal aerobic and anaerobic capacity, and improving general health and fitness.

Metabolic training can be adapted to a wide variety of populations, from serious athletes to fitness enthusiasts to those interested in weight control. The training complies with all the fundamental principles (frequency, intensity, type of exercises, and volume of exercise) of training and program design. Training sessions can vary from short to long in duration, from low to high intensity, and from low to high volume or frequency. The most standard approach is to implement higher intensities and lower volume.

It is a common belief among sport scientists, practitioners, and athletes that metabolic training is one of the most time-effective and impactful training methods (Nuñez et al. 2020).

Training cycles can be arranged to elicit a desired outcome. For instance, a four-week block or cycle (also known as a *mesocycle*) can specifically target neuromuscular endurance (the ability of muscles to produce a sustained response to signals aimed at maintaining joint stability), hypertrophy (the enlargement of the cross-sectional area of muscle fibers following training), or power (explosive strength). Exercise selection may take into consideration contraction dynamics (which is the strength exhibited, or the force generated, when a muscle contracts) and motor patterns (three-dimensional sequential arrangements of signals in the nervous system that bring about musculoskeletal movement) that lend themselves to a particular sport, also known as sport-specific training. Training blocks or cycles may build up to or potentiate a subsequent block. For instance, a four-week strength cycle can be followed by a four-week power cycle.

Metabolic training can be used to either complement or supplement an existing training program. For instance, athletes who wish to improve lactate threshold can employ metabolic-training methods intermittently to that end. Activities that are cyclical in nature may lead to overuse injuries, and complementing such activities with metabolic training can prove beneficial.

Metabolic training primarily targets aerobic and anaerobic metabolism; however, neuromuscular impact should not be overlooked.

Who Is Metabolic Training For?

As stated earlier, metabolic training can be implemented by a wide variety of individuals. When it comes to designing a training program, the only limit is creativity! Below are a few different groups who could successfully implement a metabolic-training program.

- *Serious athletes.* Serious or competitive athletes may choose to complement their training with metabolic training for a number of reasons. These reasons include, but are not limited to, improving $\dot{V}O_2$max, increasing exercise tolerance, adding variety to the training regimen, avoiding overtraining, improving fitness level, improving sport-specific performance, and increasing work capacity.

- *Individuals trying to lose weight.* Anyone focused on weight loss can take advantage of the benefits of metabolic-training routines. Metabolic training is time efficient and can elicit a high metabolic response, which can persist for an extended time after workout completion. If you are deconditioned, select exercises or equipment to accommodate your fitness level. For instance, dumbbells, medicine balls, and exercise bands can be used. These pieces of equipment are both inexpensive and space efficient, making them perfect for at-home workouts.

- *Multisport athletes.* Multisport athletes deal with movements and metabolic changes specific to the demands of multiple disciplines. Multisport training is inherently varied, and cross-training is common. Specific and non-specific metabolic training would be a logical complement to any multisport regimen. Multisport athletes could adapt the principles of metabolic training to an array of sport-specific movements, like simulating contraction velocities, loading of anatomical regions, and work-rest ratios, to name a few.

- *Fitness enthusiasts.* Fitness enthusiasts aren't necessarily interested in improving competitively. Instead, they enjoy non-competitive activities aimed at improving one or more physical characteristics, such as agility, balance, coordination, strength, power, speed, or endurance. Metabolic training could be the perfect addition to their training routine. In this context, workouts could be used as a means and an end. In other words, the purpose of the workout is to do the workout. What's more, the possibilities for varying exercises, workloads, intensity ranges, and work-rest ratios are endless.

- *Adaptive enthusiasts.* Individuals with physical disabilities may want to consider metabolic training as an addition to their existing training programs. Due to the wide range of physical limitations among individuals, it does not make sense to make specific recommendations. However, some considerations for program design should be taken into account. These include participants' physical safety, the physical space used as the exercise area, and the support required to perform a given exercise routine. Cables and dumbbells may offer advantages over barbell and machine exercises. Additionally, upper-body ergometers, ropes, and medicine balls used in the three planes of motion—sagittal (front to back), frontal (side to side), and transverse (rotational)—present viable options for alternative exercises.

In sum, metabolic training lends itself well to a number of different exercise situations. Exercise combinations, exercise order, rest intervals, workout duration, exercise intensity, and individual goals can be adapted to suit an individual's needs and fitness goals. Metabolic training can be used to educate, motivate, and inspire individuals looking to push the boundaries of their fitness.

Basic Principles of Metabolic Training

The following principles of exercise are particularly applicable to metabolic training and should always be considered when designing and implementing metabolic-training programs. Adhering to these principles will optimize training results. Measures such as heart rate and rating of perceived exertion (RPE) can be used to objectively evaluate how the body responds to the exercise stimuli associated with these training approaches.

1. *Overload.* The principle of overload refers to the application of a greater amount of stress than an individual has previously experienced. Increased intensity, duration, frequency volume, as well as new types of exercise, can all overload an athlete. For instance, adding a fourth day of running per week from three days is an overload of training.

2. *Specificity.* According to the principle of specificity, a specific method of train-ing produces a specific outcome. As an example, someone who consistently runs long distances will adapt physiologically to long-distance running.

3. *FITT.* FITT stands for "frequency, intensity, time, and type." Frequency refers to how often you exercise. Intensity is the effort exerted to perform a specific exercise. Time is the duration of an exercise session. Type indicates the kind of exercise (cardiorespiratory, strength, or a combination of the two, as well as the exercise modality).

4. *Rest/recovery.* Rest or recovery describes breaks taken during an exercise session—between exercises or between exercise sets—as well as between one exercise session and the next.

Training intensity can be evaluated using heart-rate monitoring. The higher the heart rate, the more intense the training, and vice versa. You should know your resting heart rate and your average heart rate during light to heavy (or very heavy) exercise. Maximal heart rates can be reached during metabolic training. It is important to understand that each individual has his own maximal heart rate (and associated training intensities), and a higher heart rate during the train-ing session does not mean a greater effort or more intense training. World-class athletes can have low or high maximal heart rates; neither is a predictor of car-diorespiratory fitness.

Rating of perceived exertion (RPE) is a subjective measure of how difficult an exercise is. The RPE scale is typically 1-10, with 1 being the lowest level of exer-tion and 10 being the highest. The RPE scale is a simple and effective tool that can be used to determine exercise intensity or the physical demands associated with a particular exercise.

Workout Structure

The following general guidelines should be followed when designing a workout or series of workouts over days, weeks, and months. Doing so will ensure a higher-quality workout and will optimize training.

- *Fatigue management.* Properly managing fatigue during a workout involves close monitoring of exercise selection, rest intervals, exercise order, exercise grouping, training tempo, and workout length. As fatigue accumulates during the workout, biomechanics and exercise technique can be compromised, which can present safety issues.

- *Speed before strength exercises.* Exercises that require higher velocity of move-ment, like plyometrics or jump squats, should be performed before slower move-ments. High-velocity movements can tax the nervous system to an extent that compromises subsequent exercises. In these scenarios, it is advisable to alternate ground-based speed exercises with upper-body exercises. Split-squat jumps, for example, could be followed by push-ups.

- *Technical before gross motor exercises.* Metabolic training involves exercises ranging from low to high demand. Biceps dumbbell curls or jumping jacks, for example, are exercises that have low technical demands. On the other end of the spectrum, a power snatch from the floor or a burpee would present high technical demands. Exercises with higher technical demands, like power movements, should be performed when fatigue is low. This can mean performing them earlier in the training session or after exercises that don't bring about excessive fatigue. In the context of metabolic training, gross motor exercises should be performed after technical exercises. For instance, a hang power clean should be performed after back extensions.

- *Multijoint before single-joint exercises.* Generally speaking, multijoint exercises should be performed before single-joint exercises. Multijoint exercises require more muscle mass and a higher degree of technique, and are more fatiguing, than single-joint exercises. A sequence of exercises might include a landmine squat to press followed by a supine triceps extension.

- *Exercise grouping.* Exercises can be paired or combined to achieve various objectives, including, but not limited to, managing fatigue, promoting muscle growth, improving athletic performance, developing power, developing strength, and calibrating metabolic demand. Participant safety, available equipment, training goals, and individual limitations are also important considerations when grouping exercises.

- *Exercise demand.* Keep in mind that different exercises will have different levels of metabolic demand. Generally speaking, multijoint ground-based movements will have higher levels of metabolic demand than single-joint, isolated, machine-based exercises. Exercises that utilize more muscle mass, like squats and lunges, will have a greater metabolic demand than biceps curls or dumbbell side raises. For a training program to be successful, demand needs to be carefully calibrated.

- *Unstable and stable surfaces.* The efficacy of unstable surfaces in developing athletic performance is debatable, and the primary goal of metabolic training is to improve metabolic efficiency and capacity. With that said, medicine balls, stability balls, balance pads, and balance boards are popular fitness tools. Should you choose to incorporate unstable surfaces into metabolic training, be aware of your surroundings and any safety issues they might present. Careful consideration should also be given to exercise selection. For instance, pre-fatiguing the lower body before performing one-leg squats on a balance pad will increase the difficulty of the exercise.

- *Rest intervals.* Although metabolic training can be demanding, there are times when perceived effort is lower than expected. This is because neuromuscular fatigue is distributed through different areas of the body, not confined to one area or muscle group. One way to manage workout intensity or perceived effort is by changing the rest interval. Longer rest intervals may be warranted after high metabolic efforts, and shorter rest periods after reduced metabolic efforts. Keep in mind that metabolic training will tax nearly every major muscle group during each exercise session. A drawback of this approach is the high demand associated with metabolizing lactate and hydrogen ions and the subsequent high systemic acidity, especially among untrained individuals. Close monitoring of fatigue levels and technique is advised.

• *Ambient conditions.* Ambient conditions—specifically, humidity and temperature—can affect fatigue. The body strives to sustain an internal temperature of about 98.6 degrees Fahrenheit. The mechanical work of exercise generates heat. As body temperature rises, sweat is produced to cool the skin, which helps to maintain body temperature. An indoor-gym temperature ranging from the low to high 60s, with moderate airflow, will assist in fatigue moderation. Additionally, lower humidity will assist in sweat evaporation, which lowers the body's temperature. For these reasons, it is recommended that gyms be kept cool and well circulated.

• *Safety.* Safety considerations for metabolic training include exercise frequency, intensity, duration, and type, all of which should be determined based on each participant's fitness level, as well as appropriate gear selection and proper hydration. Additionally, adequate time and attention must be devoted to warming up and cooling down to ensure that the body transitions in and out of periods of activity safely.

This chapter has covered the fundamental tenets of metabolic training, terms frequently associated with this style of exercise, and factors that must be considered when designing an appropriate training program. The most important aspect of any training program is safety. Though safety is affected by many interrelated and interdependent factors, we recommend paying particular attention to whether a training program is appropriate for you and whether your physical environment is appropriate for exercise. Understanding the topics addressed in this chapter will help you utilize metabolic training to meet your goals and get the most out of your exercise program.

2

Physiological Adaptations to Metabolic Training

Physiological adaptation refers to how the body responds to, accommodates, or adjusts to exercise. To give an over-simplified example, if you lift heavy weights, your muscles get bigger. But there are actually a number of adaptations taking place in response to such a stimulus. These adaptations include a more coordinated neural signal to the activated muscles, uptake of nutrients, and the release of muscle-building hormones.

Learning about the process of physiological adaptation will help you design more effective workouts, understand how your body will respond to training, and know what to expect with consistent and focused training. Two of the most common fitness goals are burning fat and enhancing muscular development. This chapter takes a deeper dive into some of the physiological adaptations to training that can turn these goals into realities.

Adapting to Demands

As discussed in chapter 1, in reference to the specificity principle, adaptations are specific to imposed demands. Adaptions can be morphological (related to muscle size), biomechanical (related to strength and power), anatomical (related to muscle, bone, or fat volumes), neurological (related to motor control), or metabolic (related to aerobic or anaerobic energy pathways) in nature. Workout parameters such as intensity level and rest duration can be set to elicit specific adaptations. For instance, short, high-intensity exercise intervals (up to six seconds in duration, focusing on quick movement with maximal intensity) paired with longer rest intervals (1:1 to 1:4 work:rest ratio) can target the short-duration phosphagen metabolic pathway. Conversely, lower-intensity activity paired with shorter-duration rest intervals can target the aerobic metabolic pathway. Also, keep in mind that exercises targeting multiple joints and muscle groups at one time are more metabolically challenging than exercises targeting individual joints and muscle groups.

It should be pointed out that metabolic training utilizes both aerobic and anaerobic metabolic pathways, while also placing demand on the neuromuscular system by way of strength and power exercises. In other situations, metabolic training can elicit more of an aerobic metabolic (endurance) response—for example, when lighter weights are used. This de-emphasizes the neuromuscular system. These two examples represent the various ways in which metabolic training can be programmed. Neither approach is superior to the other; the optimal program is best determined by the goals of the program and the individual. With this concept in mind, both aerobic and anaerobic adaptations can be observed.

Some metabolic-training programs implement strength-power and aerobic (endurance) methodologies together. This approach is called concurrent training. Research on the effects of concurrent training has yielded the following conclusions:

- Concurrent training does not appear to compromise gains in aerobic capacity.
- The incorporation of resistance training may have a beneficial effect on short-term endurance.
- The incorporation of aerobic training may compromise maximal strength in experienced, resistance-trained individuals.

Consider the intensity of training: Short bursts of high-intensity training target the anaerobic pathway. Longer-duration efforts, lasting more than three minutes, start to emphasize the aerobic pathway. Metabolic activity is elevated by anaerobic efforts of shorter duration if these efforts are performed at high intensity, which includes heavy resistance training exercise (Herda & Cramer 2016). This idea constitutes a fundamental element and benefit of metabolic training.

The Role of Excess Postexercise Oxygen Consumption

It is also worth considering the impact of excess postexercise oxygen consumption (or EPOC). EPOC refers to the prolonged increase in $\dot{V}O_2$ that may be observed for hours after exercise. A comprehensive study conducted by Borsheim and Bahr (2003) determined that heavy resistance training produces greater EPOC than circuit weight training. In other words, EPOC is intensity dependent in response to resistance training. This study also found that EPOC is intensity dependent in relation to aerobic training, with the greatest EPOC values occurring when duration and intensity were high, and that individuals vary in their response. The greatest EPOC values were recorded when the intensity of aerobic exercise was greater than 50 to 60 percent of $\dot{V}O_2$max and the duration was equal to or greater than 40 minutes. It would stand to reason that maximal effort toward the end of a metabolic-training session could optimize EPOC. The benefit of EPOC in the context of metabolic training is its tendency to increase caloric expenditure and fat burning above resting levels following the completion of a workout.

The following physiological factors, among others, are responsible for EPOC (Herda and Cramer 2016):

1. Restoring oxygen in the blood and muscles, which enables the body to return to its pre-exercise state

2. Resynthesizing energy in the form of ATP, enabling the body to perform at an optimal level during a subsequent metabolic-training session

3. Elevating body temperature, circulation, and respiration, which aids in recovery and reduces muscle soreness and fatigue

4. Increasing protein turnover, which enables the body to increase lean body mass as a training effect.

Short-Term Adaptations to Metabolic Training

Short-term adaptations are those that occur within one to four weeks and are specifically related to the composition of the training program. For example, heavy strength training will yield greater increases in strength than low-intensity, high-rep training programs. Short-term adaptations are relatively transient compared to long-term adaptions, meaning that if you stop training after one to four weeks, there is a relatively quick return to pre-training status. In practical terms, this means that you should remain consistent in your training if you want to continue to develop strength. It should be noted that nervous-system adaptations occur faster than structural changes in skeletal muscle. This has led researchers and practitioners to conclude that initial strength improvement is the result of neurological changes. Even if you can't see changes in your muscle size or composition early on in your program, know that your body is adapting and building a foundation for strength. Stick to your program, and the changes will be noticeable over time.

There are some adaptations that you may notice soon after beginning a metabolic-training program. Immediate cardiorespiratory responses to metabolic training include increases in heart rate, oxygen uptake, systolic blood pressure, blood flow to active muscles, the heart's stroke volume, and cardiac output (French 2016). Ventilation rate increases significantly during resistance training (Statler and Dubois 2016), and especially metabolic training, when short rest intervals are employed. These improvements to your cardiorespiratory system will allow you to breathe easier and work harder as you take on more-challenging workouts.

Long-Term Adaptations to Metabolic Training

Following are several adaptions and outcomes that can be achieved when performing metabolic training.

Performance Adaptations

- Increased strength
- Increased endurance
- Increased anaerobic power
- Increased rate of force production
- Increased vertical jump
- Increased aerobic power

Adaptations in Muscle Fiber

- Increased cross-sectional area, also known as hypertrophy
- Increases in type I, IIA, or IIB muscle fiber composition
- Increased capillary density
- Increased mitochondrial density

Adaptations in Enzyme Activity

- Increases in enzymes that contribute to strength and power production

Adaptations in Metabolic Energy Stores

- Increased glycogen stores
- Increased creatine phosphate
- Increased ATP storage
- Increased capacity to buffer hydrogen-ion production

Adaptations in Connective Tissue

- Increased ligament strength
- Increased tendon strength
- Possible increases in collagen content
- Possible increases in bone density

The physiological adaptations to metabolic training can be seen in the restoration of oxygen to blood and muscle; the resynthesizing of energy in the form of ATP; the elevation of body temperature, circulation, and respiration; and increased protein turnover. These adaptations lead to increased strength, endurance, anaerobic power, force production, and explosive power, as well as a higher aerobic threshold. Muscular improvements include increased hypertrophy of Type I, IIA, or IIB muscle fibers and capillary and mitochondrial density. Additional benefits include improvements to metabolic-energy stores in all energy systems, improved connective-tissue strength, and greater resistance to injury.

3

Metabolic-Training Tools

The purpose of this chapter is to introduce the nine training tools utilized in our metabolic workouts. They are

1. bodyweight,
2. dumbbell,
3. kettlebell,
4. resistance band,
5. medicine ball,
6. heavy rope,
7. suspension,
8. weighted sled, and
9. sandbag.

Bodyweight training denotes strength-training exercises in which you move your body against the resistance of gravity. Dumbbell training utilizes round, hexagonal, or square weights connected by a short bar, which you lift or swing in your hand, often in pairs. Kettlebell training provides strength- and cardio-based exercise using a primitive piece of equipment that looks like a cannonball with a handle attached. Resistance-band training is a form of strength training that uses rubber bands of different levels of elasticity. Medicine ball training involves exercising with a weighted ball to increase muscular strength and endurance. Heavy-rope training uses ropes of varying lengths and weights, challenging both cardiorespiratory fitness and muscle strength and endurance. Suspension training uses ropes and straps to increase the difficulty of bodyweight movements. Weighted-sled training uses a piece of equipment resembling a sled with rails or wheels; weight can be added to the sled to increase resistance and emphasize strength, speed, and power development. Sandbag training is a form of resistance training that uses a not-quite-full sandbag to improve functional strength, balance, and cardiorespiratory endurance.

Bodyweight Training

When it comes to enhancing functional strength, your own body can provide you with not only the most accessible and cost-effective training tool but in many ways the most beneficial. Bodyweight-training exercises do not require a gym or specialized equipment to deliver an effective workout—they can be performed virtually anywhere. This training style provides you with a functionally based approach to increasing power, strength, endurance, and flexibility in the pursuit of muscle development and fat metabolism. Most importantly, bodyweight training can be done by anyone, regardless of fitness level.

The simplicity of bodyweight training allows you to quickly transfer from one exercise to another without having to adjust equipment or resistance. This significantly reduces rest time while keeping your heart rate in a target training zone and increasing caloric expenditure per unit of time. Bodyweight training is an excellent way to burn body fat and increase metabolic rate, not only during exercise but after exercise.

Bodyweight training allows for natural progressions in intensity. Progressions commonly involve simply adding repetitions or time to an exercise for increased fitness or changing the movement pattern to increase the demand on strength. Focusing on volume eliminates the risk of utilizing resistances that may potentially result in injury while simultaneously improving flexibility by involving a full range of movement. The engagement of the core musculature required to perform bodyweight exercises naturally develops core strength and stability, which, in turn, appears to reduce injury risk (Haff, Berninger, and Caulfield 2016).

In summary, the benefits of bodyweight training can be tied to the use of functional exercises that are adaptable to all levels of fitness. The use of these exercises in a workout provides a low-cost training method that increases muscle strength in several muscle groups at once, develops relative strength, and improves balance and coordination (Harrison 2011).

Dumbbell Training

Developed over 2,500 years ago, no single piece of fitness equipment has stood the test of time like the dumbbell. Dumbbells can be found in almost any exercise environment, be it a high-tech fitness center, boutique fitness center, hard-core gym, school, hotel, or home gym. Dumbbells offer you the ability to train your entire body and can be utilized regardless of your level of experience, level of fitness, age, or training proficiency. They remain a staple for adults looking to get in shape, youth and professional athletes, tactical professionals, elite fitness participants, and bodybuilders.

Believed to date back to the ancient Greeks, dumbbells (*halteres* or *alteres*, as they were termed) came in various shapes and sizes and were made from materials that could be molded in different ways. Other ancient cultures, including the Indians, Egyptians, and Chinese, are believed to have utilized dumbbell-like objects as well, although the Greeks are recognized as their creators.

The ancient Greek physician Galen is regarded as the first person to write a text (ca. 200 AD) on the benefits of exercising with dumbbells (Ford 1955; Berryman 2012). Other significant exercise-associated works, such as *Dialogues des Gymnastica* in 1544 (Todd 2003) and *De Arte Gymnastica Aput Ancientes* in 1569 (Ford 1955; Todd 2003), discuss dumbbell training as well. The term *dumbbell* was believed to have been coined in England during the 16th century, when athletes trained with handheld bells from which the clappers had been removed. Once the clappers were removed, the bells became silent, which gave rise to the name "dumbbells." In 1864, with the release of John Blundell's book *The Muscles and Their Story* (Todd 2003), dumbbells became even more popular. Ranging from 3 to 100 pounds (1.4 to 45.4 kilograms), they became increasingly commonplace among fitness enthusiasts everywhere and established themselves as standard pieces of gym equipment.

On February 14, 1865, the first plate-loaded dumbbell was patented. Today, there are three different types of dumbbells, each of which offers benefits. Adjustable dumbbells consist of a short metal bar that is slightly knurled in the middle to improve hand grip. Weight plates can be slid onto each end and secured with collars. Adjustable dumbbells are quickly adaptable to weight changes and can be utilized to exercise all muscle groups. Fixed-weight dumbbells are often referred to as gym-style dumbbells because they are most often found in gyms. While they do not offer the versatility of adjustable dumbbells, a complete set of fixed dumbbells allows you to change weights quickly. Selectorized dumbbells are designed to maximize your training time by offering a single pair of dumbbells that can be quickly adjusted using a selector pin or dial to set the desired weight.

Training with dumbbells produces favorable alterations in the muscular, nervous, endocrine, and cardiorespiratory systems, as well as connective-tissue improvements (Ratames and Izquierdo 2008).

- Muscular-system adaptations involve increases in muscle-fiber angle and length, muscle size, muscle fiber type transition (Type I to Type II), pre-exercise energy-substrate levels, protein concentration, fiber number, oxidative capacity (with higher-volume training), and fatigue resistance.

- Neural alterations include increased muscle-fiber recruitment and potentiation, as well as fatigue resistance, which leads to a higher training capacity.

- Benefits to connective tissue include increases in bone-mineral density, tendon and ligament size, and tendon and ligament strength.

- Cardiorespiratory improvements encompass acute cardiac output and stroke volume increases.

- Metabolic alterations are tied to three energy systems:
    1. *Phosphagen energy system.* Provides energy for short-term, high-intensity exercise of 0 to 30 seconds
    2. *Glycolytic energy system.* Provides energy for exercise of 30 seconds to 2 minutes

Training Safely with Dumbbells

When training with dumbbells, safety precautions should be taken to reduce the potential for injury. Complete adequate movement preparation and a dynamic warm-up prior to a training session. Start with lighter weights and progress to heavier weights when performing multiple sets. Select a weight that will provide maximum training benefits without forcing you to sacrifice correct technique and risk getting injured.

Maintain an erect, firm torso and lift the dumbbells from a rack or the floor using your legs, bending at the knees and maintaining a flat back. Enlist the assistance of a spotter when needed to ensure correct form and lift safety. Consult with a medical professional (physician or physical therapist) if you experience persistent or recurring pain or any pain prior to or after starting a lifting program.

3. *Oxidative energy system.* Provides energy for exercise of 2 minutes or greater (Herda and Cramer 2016).

Dumbbells offer an operative means to focus on major muscle groups of the entire body. They can be utilized in a gym, at home, or outdoors with no required installation or setup. Exercising with dumbbells necessitates greater stabilization, recruiting a greater number of secondary muscle groups than machine exercises and forcing limbs to work individually, which helps to prevent imbalances.

Kettlebell Training

Just about any gym, regardless of the population it serves, has kettlebells in its strength-training or group-exercise areas. While the use of kettlebells in the United States is new, training for strength and fitness with kettlebells can be traced back centuries to their Eastern European roots (Harrison, Schoenfeld, and Schoenfeld 2011). A kettlebell consists of an iron handle attached to an iron ball (Cotter 2022). Kettlebell training offers a safer alternative to heavy-load lifting, targeting weaknesses and imbalances and correcting them through short, high-intensity workouts that increase hormonal production for muscle development and keep cortisol levels low.

Kettlebells have been studied more recently by strength and conditioning researchers interested in these tools' ability to enhance strength, power, and cardiorespiratory fitness in individuals ranging from novice exercisers to elite-level athletes and fitness enthusiasts (Beardsley and Contreras 2014). The benefits of kettlebell training are numerous. Kettlebell training has been shown to increase overall strength and power production (Jay et al. 2011); improve core strength by emphasizing power, acceleration, and multiplanar and unilateral movement patterns (Lake and Lauder 2012); encourage the production of force and speed through the hips (Otto et al. 2012); and promote the development of lean body mass through high-repetition sets combined with short rest periods. Often-neglected muscles of the back of the body (core, shoulders, hips) are targeted, which improves posture and posterior-chain function (Jay et al. 2011). Kettlebell training has also been shown to improve grip strength, which enables other strength gains (Manocchia et al. 2013).

Because of its emphasis on higher volume and shorter rest periods, kettlebell training is associated with increased caloric expenditure per unit of time (20 calories per minute), resulting in increased metabolism during and after training, increased fat metabolism, increased muscular endurance, and better cardiorespiratory function (Jay et al. 2011). Kettlebells provide the user with one piece of exercise equipment to train the entire body (Jay et al. 2011). If you are limited with space at home or want to minimize your movement around the gym, kettlebells are the perfect tools to simplify your workout. Kettlebell training uses dynamic movement patterns that increase mobility, proprioception, flexibility, and body awareness by forcing the user to move through all three planes of motion in a controlled, fluid manner. With kettlebells, stabilizing muscle groups are trained in combination with primary muscles, leading to improved joint stability, coordination, and balance (Manocchia et al. 2013). Finally, kettlebells offer a fun and exciting way to train because the exercises are based on movement patterns and require you to be more engaged (Jay et al. 2011).

When performing kettlebell exercises, use the grip position (neutral grip, with palms facing in; supinated grip, with palms facing up; or pronated grip, with palms facing down) and hold position (at your side, between your palms, in your palm, or upside down) that best suits each exercise (Cotter 2022). When performing an exercise in a standing position, place your feet slightly wider than shoulder-width apart. With training resistances between 80 and 100 percent of your repetition maximum (the maximum resistance you can utilize with a given volume and intensity), avoid holding your breath—you should continue to inhale and exhale throughout the movement (Haff, Berninger, and Caulfield 2016).

Resistance-Band Training

Resistance bands have become a staple of just about every fitness environment. Resistance bands come in three basic forms: tube, loop, and mini. Each of the three types provides unique benefits. Resistance bands come in a variety of colors often with handles. The color of a resistance band designates its tension level. What makes resistance-band training unique is that tension increases as the bands are stretched, meaning that resistance increases as more muscle groups are incorporated in a movement pattern (Haff, Berninger, and Caulfield 2016).

Resistance bands can be used at any fitness level and any age. Youth, adults, seniors, competitive athletes, tactical professionals, and individuals with chronic conditions or disorders can all benefit from resistance-band training. Additionally, resistance bands are among the most inexpensive pieces of equipment and can easily be packed in a suitcase and utilized anywhere.

Resistance bands are beneficial for metabolic training because they can be used safely and effectively at higher volumes with shorter rest periods. Training with resistance bands is an excellent way to reduce body fat and simultaneously develop muscle. In conjunction with dietary changes, resistance bands can bring about significant physiological changes when used three to five times per week.

Resistance bands are frequently used while warming up and cooling down. In this context, they serve as an excellent primer, increasing heart rate and joint mobility through dynamic range-of-motion movements at reduced resistances. Following this approach ensures that there is adequate blood flow to the exercising muscles and the heart before higher-resistance exercise commences. The use of resistance bands as part of the postworkout cool-down can improve blood flow, reduce muscle soreness, and prevent injuries by enhancing stretches and flexibility exercises (Page and Ellenbecker 2020).

Resistance bands are excellent tools for increasing muscle strength and endurance, and they can be used to simulate many of the same exercises performed with barbells and dumbbells. They also lend themselves well to developing explosive power, through multijoint exercises as well as exercises that target specific muscle groups. The unstable, elastic nature of resistance bands means that users will recruit secondary and stabilizing muscle groups when working with them. Resistance bands also allow exercisers to increase range of motion in a manner that is safe for the joints and the spine.

Resistance bands can serve as an excellent tool to assist with bodyweight movements and other strength-training exercises. When utilized with bodyweight exercises, they can decrease bodyweight, for movements such as the pull-up, or increase resistance, for movements like the bodyweight squat. Adding bands to traditional strength-training exercises, such as the bench press or the squat, can increase the demands on muscle stabilization and power throughout the lift.

Resistance bands are effective in targeting all three planes of movement utilized in sports and other fitness activities. Please refer to chapter 1 for a review of planes of motion. Sagittal-plane movements are movements that occur forward and backward. Frontal-plane movements are movements that occur side to side. One of the most important planes for functional movement is the transverse plane. Movement in the transverse plane is rotational in nature and can vary in speed. Developing power, muscle strength, and endurance in the transverse plane not only increases power for functional movement but also reduces injury risk from rotational movements.

By following the FITT principle and adjusting training frequency (number of sessions per week), intensity (band resistance), type (exercise selection), and time (pace of the exercise, including movement speed, exercise volume, and recovery between sets or exercises), exercisers can use resistance bands to reach physiological and athletic goals, such as developing lean body mass, losing fat, increasing strength and conditioning levels, and enhancing sports performance. For example, performing higher-repetition sets with shorter rest periods can be effective in increasing lean body mass and burning body fat, while lower-repetition sets paired with longer rest periods can be effective in increasing strength, power, and technical skill. Based on the goals of the program, training loads and recovery periods can be assigned based on the repetition maximum (the maximum amount of resistance that can be used to perform a given number of repetitions and sets with structured recovery periods) (Sheppard and Triplett 2016).

Medicine Ball Training

Medicine balls can be traced back to ancient Persia, Greece, and Rome, where they were used by athletes to increase strength, power, and athletic performance. It is believed that the ancient Greeks stuffed animal skins for patients to toss for medicinal purposes. A similar type of ball is believed to have been used in Persia in the 1700s. The term *medicine ball* can be dated back to 1876 (Roberts 2020). Hippocrates believed them to be an essential tool for helping people regain normal body movement after injury, as well as a means for enhancing and maintaining overall health. Few, if any, pieces of equipment are versatile in the way that medicine balls are: not only can they be lifted, but they can also be thrown and slammed. The adaptability of medicine balls enables users to utilize nontraditional methods to expand training goals and objectives. In addition, nearly every medicine ball exercise can be combined with other exercises to create a continuous flow with minimal rest. This is beneficial for two reasons:

1. It mimics functional movements used in everyday life.
2. It enables users to program any number of exercise combinations and variations.

Today, medicine balls are used to develop power, strength, anaerobic endurance, and cardiorespiratory fitness.

Medicine balls can be soft or firm, can come with or without handles, and can vary in weight from 2 to 100 pounds (0.9 to 45.4 kilograms). Medicine ball training has a wide spectrum of applications, ranging from injury rehabilitation to strength and sports-performance enhancement (Faigenbaum et al. 2006; Hagberg et al. 2009). Its ability to recruit a significant number of muscle groups and to develop explosive power through functional movement makes medicine ball training an essential tool in fitness, rehabilitation, and sports performance (Vincent, Traywick, and Washburn 2013). When training with a medicine ball, perform 10 to 15 reps or perform reps for a designated time, provided that you can do so with good form (Faigenbaum et al. 2006). When selecting a medicine ball, it is important to choose one heavy enough to reduce movement speed but not so heavy that technique, form, and range of motion will be negatively impacted. Medicine balls weighing between 4 and 15 pounds (1.8 to 6.8 kilograms) are generally recommended as a starting point (Faigenbaum et al. 2006; Vincent, Traywick, and Washburn 2013).

Medicine ball training can be effective as a fat-burning exercise when periods of high-intensity, high-volume training are implemented to maximize caloric expenditure. This results in an increased postexercise metabolic effect as well. Training with medicine balls allows exercisers to utilize their full range of movement, which is important for developing total-body strength. Medicine balls also lend themselves to developing strength in the context of sports that require rotational movement.

This is accomplished through an increased focus on acceleration. Along with general strength, increased levels of explosive strength and power can be developed when performing functional movements using medicine balls. Cardiorespiratory fitness is another important benefit of utilizing medicine balls in a workout. Performing total-body medicine ball exercises such as slams for 30 to 45 seconds provides a strong cardiorespiratory stimulus, along with helping to develop power and strength (Faigenbaum et al. 2018).

Emphasizing medicine ball exercises that link upper and lower extremities can help to develop core strength and enhance postural alignment (Haff, Berninger, and Caulfield 2016). Unlike other training methods (barbells, dumbbells, exercise machines), medicine ball training enhances functional performance through movements that combine multiple patterns and planes of motion. For individuals experiencing lower-back pain or other orthopedic issues, medicine balls can aid rehabilitation by promoting proper alignment, which, in turn, reduces stress to muscles and connective tissue.

Medicine balls are a safe, simple, and effective fitness tool for rehabilitative as well as fitness- and performance-based exercises, allowing users to focus on strength, endurance, and recovery with minimal risk for injury. In addition to their training benefits, medicine ball exercises, which can often be done with a partner or in a group, provide an opportunity for socialization that is sometimes lacking from resistance-based exercise.

Heavy Rope, Suspension, Weighted Sleds, and Sandbag Training

When developing metabolic-training programs, heavy ropes, suspension trainers, weighted sleds, and sandbags can be valuable additions to traditional training tools. These alternative pieces of equipment have grown rapidly in popularity and become staples in metabolic-training programs, alongside traditional training tools (Cissik and Dawes 2015; Haff, Berninger, and Caulfield 2016). When selecting these implements for training, consider the advantages and disadvantages of each piece of equipment, along with your level of fitness. As with all exercise modalities, proper technique and appropriate assistance are necessary aspects of safe and effective training. Let's look at each of these pieces of equipment and consider how they can be used to vary your training.

Heavy ropes, also known as battle ropes, are thick ropes of varying lengths and weights that can be linked together, anchored, or wrapped around a pole or training rack. Heavy ropes are a fun alternative to traditional strength training and conditioning, and can be used by people of all ages and fitness levels. The benefits of using heavy ropes include the following:

- Expend calories and burn fat through continuous moderate- to high-intensity exercise.
- Get a total-body workout by combining the upper-body focus of the ropes with lower-body lunging, jumping, and squatting while performing rope exercises.
- Participate in a lower-impact cardiorespiratory activity that greatly reduces the impact to joints associated with some traditional cardiorespiratory activities.

- Increase grip strength, upper-extremity strength and power, and triple-extension strength and power from the hip, knee, and ankle.
- Increase or decrease the resistance used by standing closer or farther away from the anchoring point, respectively.
- Correct muscle imbalances through the independent movement of the ropes with each hand, using alternating grips and varying movement directions.
- Improve dynamic and static flexibility through constant motion and stretch, and improve stability by maintaining a stable base.
- Develop stability and balance by working against gravity and overcoming the force of the ropes.

Suspension training involves the use of two sets of adjustable bands, buckles, and handles that can be attached overhead to a stable rack or training bar. Suspension training provides a limitless variety of exercises, helping to prevent boredom and lack of motivation. The benefits of using a suspension trainer include the following:

- Train all the muscles of the body in a functional manner and easily adjust resistance by changing the angle between the body and the floor.
- Correct muscle imbalances by providing a unilateral approach to training.
- Enhance cardiorespiratory fitness by enabling quick transition from one exercise to another while keeping heart rate elevated.
- Get an effective moderate- to high-intensity workout with minimal stress and impact on the joints.
- Aid in recovery from injury by improving range of motion, functional movement, and flexibility while minimizing stress and further injury to the affected body part.
- Enhance the balance, flexibility, coordination, and stability of muscles of the upper extremity, the pelvis, the lower back, and the abdomen, making the suspension trainer an excellent training implement for the core.
- Ramp up bodyweight training by placing the feet instead of the hands in the handles for specific movements.

Weighted-sled training can be traced back to ancient logging communities that used sleds to transport heavy trees from forests. Today, weighted sleds allow athletes in a variety of sports and fitness programs to increase power, muscle strength and endurance, and cardiorespiratory fitness. Weighted-sled training involves the use of a multifunctional exercise tool that can be loaded with weight to increase resistance. Weighted sleds come in a variety of shapes and sizes and can be pushed, pulled, or dragged. The benefits of using a weighted sled include the following:

- Increase functional fitness by incorporating numerous muscles and joints in a multijoint format to increase upper-body, lower-body, and core strength and power.
- Improve both anaerobic and aerobic conditioning by using heavier or lighter resistances for various distances or periods of time.

- Because weighted-sled training only involves the concentric movement (shortening) of muscles against resistance, and not eccentric movement (lengthening), it's an excellent form of training for injury prevention.
- The enhanced muscle stimulation provided by constant resistance with each push, pull, or drag enhances acceleration capability for athletic, tactical, functional, and fitness performance.

Sandbags have been a popular training option for tactical professionals and strongmen for many years. More recently, sandbags have become popular in fitness, metabolic, and sports training programs. Sandbags offer several training benefits, including the following:

- Achieve maximum muscle recruitment when performing multijoint exercises (cleans, squats, rows, etc.).
- Train for strength, power, muscle development, or endurance by using sandbags of different weights.
- Develop strength and reduce the risk of injury by training in all three planes of motion: sagittal (movement forward and backward), frontal (movement side to side), and transverse (rotational). Please refer to chapter 1 for a review of planes of motion.
- Improve balanced strength and muscle development in all muscle groups as well as increase grip strength through the challenge of shifting weight in sandbags. This is particularly beneficial for learning to control awkward movements in daily life, professional activities, and athletics.
- Enjoy the convenience and value of sandbags: An adjustment in weight requires nothing more than inexpensive sand to be added or removed; sandbag training can be done anywhere with a limited amount of space; sandbags are easy to empty to travel with and reload when traveling; and sandbags provide a challenging workout to increase strength and metabolic fitness with minimal equipment.

Conclusion

Metabolic training employs a variety of training modalities. In order to understand your options in full, you need to understand the benefits offered by bodyweight, dumbbells, kettlebells, resistance bands, medicine balls, heavy ropes, suspension, weighted sleds, and sandbags. Consider your level of fitness to determine which training modalities to use in your program. As an example, bodyweight and dumbbell exercises may be more appropriate for beginners. Conversely, an exerciser with a higher level of fitness may receive additional benefits from a metabolic-training program incorporating kettlebells, medicine balls, suspension trainer, sandbags, weighted sleds, and heavy ropes. No matter the implement used, frequency, intensity, and volume of training should be adjusted to suit each individual's fitness level.

4

Periodization for Metabolic Training

Periodization is the variation of training over a period of time in order to achieve an optimal outcome. Or, in more detailed terms, "Periodization is a theoretical and practical construct that allows for the systematic, sequential, and integrative programing of training interventions into mutually dependent periods of time in order to induce specific physiological adaptations that underpin performance outcomes" (Haff 2016). Another way to think of it is that periodization is the concept, and programming (sets, reps, exercises, weight used, days per week, etc.) is the application.

Components of Periodization

There are three concepts central to understanding periodization: general adaptation syndrome, stimulus–fatigue–recovery–adaptation (SFRA) theory, and the fitness–fatigue paradigm. In the following, we explain what they are and how they fit into metabolic training.

General Adaptation Syndrome

This theory is the most fundamental to physical training. When you perform a training session that takes your body beyond its current state, you're applying a stress to your systems. The body initially responds to the stress in an alarm stage where fatigue is experienced possibly in the form of soreness or stiffness in, generally, the first 24 to 48 hours following your training session. After this alarm stage the body transitions into the resistance stage and the body further adapts to the stress. In the final stage, the body experiences what is known as supercompensation. Upon reaching the supercompensation stage, the body is at a higher level of adaptation which means you are becoming stronger or fitter than you were before the training.

Stimulus–Fatigue–Recovery–Adaptation Theory

The SFRA theory suggests that training stimuli produce a general response (Haff 2016). The greater the magnitude of the stimulus or workload, the greater the fatigue response. In other words, there is a direct positive correlation between training workload and fatigue. As you adapt to the training workload, however, your fatigue will lessen. When a new training stimulus is introduced, the adaptation cycle continues. The SFRA theory emphasizes timing or scheduling of interventions and is essential to optimizing training effects. Keep in mind that if you stop training after a single intervention, you will return to your untrained state. Consistency is key to maximizing your results.

Complete recovery is often not reached after training interventions. However, partial recovery does often occur, and training programs should have the frequency, intensity, and volume of training adjusted in such a manner to optimize results. The general trend is to gradually decrease volume of training while increasing intensity. This concept is central to periodization.

Fitness–Fatigue Paradigm

The fitness–fatigue paradigm posits a relationship between fitness and fatigue known as the "state of readiness" (Haff 2016; see figure 4.1). This model was first proposed by the sport scientist Vladimir Zatsiorsky (Zatsiorsky & Kraemer 2006). There is a direct positive relationship between volume load of training and fatigue, where *volume load* refers to amount of weight times the number of repetitions assigned to an exercise. As an example, 10 reps at 100 pounds (45.4 kilograms) performed for three sets results in a volume load of 3,000 pounds (1,360.7 kilograms) for that exercise. The volume load of an exercise for a specific period of time (a day, a week, a month, etc.) can be quickly calculated by multiplying reps by weight by sets. The importance of accumulated fatigue as a result of volume load cannot be overstated.

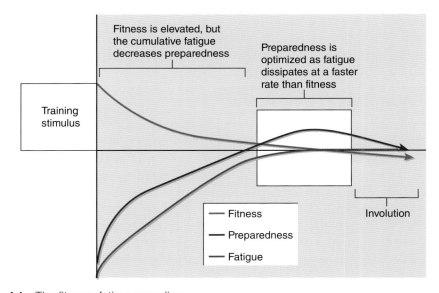

Figure 4.1 The fitness–fatigue paradigm.
Adapted by permission from G.G. Haff and E.E. Haff, "Training Integration and Periodization," in *NSCA's Guide to Program Design*, edited by J. Hoffman (Champaign, IL: Human Kinetics, 2012), 219.

Accumulated fatigue recedes more quickly than fitness. A reduction in volume load, or perhaps cessation of training, can potentiate a peak in fitness. This concept is also central to periodization.

Training Principles of a Periodization Model

There are several models of periodization that can be applied to metabolic training programs For the purpose of this book we will focus on block, linear, and undulating periodization. These models adjust training volume and intensity over a period of time in an effort to avoid mental and physical stagnation. It is important to remember that proper fatigue management during the training session and between training sessions is a central element of metabolic training. For the purposes of metabolic training, we will provide frequency, intensity, and volume guidelines to ensure fatigue management in very general terms.

Block Periodization

The general approach to block periodization involves the sequencing of three different training blocks (Issurin 2008). The three different training blocks are accumulation, transmutation, and realization. During each block of training, there is a targeted physical characteristic to be improved. Those characteristics include strength, power, endurance, agility, or speed to name a few.

During the accumulation phase, training volume is emphasized. As stated, there is a specific focus on one aspect of fitness (e.g., power, speed, or endurance). During transmutation, workload is decreased, allowing the body to adapt fully to the stresses introduced during accumulation. Workouts become shorter and more goal specific. During realization, workload is decreased even further, allowing fitness adaptations to peak. The training intensities associated with these phases are 50 to 75 percent for accumulation, 75 to 90 percent for transmutation, and 90 percent and higher for realization. The salient point to remember is intensity starts low and volume starts high, progressing to high intensity to low volume. Each block lasts about two to four weeks. Progressions from more repetitions at lower weight to fewer repetitions at higher weight over two- to four-week blocks are the most applicable to metabolic training (see table 4.1).

Table 4.1   Example of Block Periodization for Selected Exercises

	Weight	Sets	Repetitions	Volume load (Weight × sets × repetitions)
Block 1: weeks 1-4	100 lb	3	12	3,600 lb
Block 2: weeks 5-8	105 lb	3	10	1,050 lb
Block 3: weeks 9-12	110 lb	3	8	880 lb

Another concept of block periodization is training a physical characteristic over a duration of time. For instance, a training block could last three months. Each month, a different physical characteristic could be the focus. As an example, the focus of month 1 is muscle endurance, the focus of month 2 is strength, and the focus of month 3 is power. Sets, reps, and weights are adjusted to achieve a desired effect. Block periodization modeling is flexible to accommodate changes in training focus. However, there should be thought to the sequencing of blocks, such as endurance followed by strength followed by power.

There is much more that could be said about the nuances of block periodization—especially about its scientific foundations. Such discussions, however, would exceed the scope of this book, which is focused on providing immediately applicable concepts and programs.

Linear and Undulating Periodization

Linear periodization describes programs that progress in a straight, or nearly straight, line. Exercise programming according to this model is characterized by gradual increases in intensity and gradual decreases in volume.

Undulating periodization describes programs that rise and fall on a scheduled timeframe—most often weekly. At its most fundamental, undulating periodization involves scheduling high-repetition, low-volume days in close proximity to low-repetition, high-volume days. (Of course, there are many different applied models, but we will keep the fundamental variables of undulating periodization simple.) For instance, when training twice a week, Monday's exercises are performed with three sets of 10 repetitions, and Thursday's exercises are performed for three sets of six repetitions. A corresponding increase in weight is used when there is a decrease in repetitions.

Periodization's Value to Metabolic Training

A central purpose of periodization is to avoid stagnation and maximize improvement. Periodization is achieved through the manipulation of variables such as frequency, intensity, and duration, among other loading parameters. There have been a multitude of scientific studies validating the use of periodized training models to improve performance and fitness (Bompa, 2009; Bondarchuk, 1988; Bondarchuk, 1994; Foster, 1998; Stone, 1982; Stone, 2007).

Besides being a more effective method of training, periodization offers benefits to the participant by way of

- *Psychological mitigation.* Varying training through sets, reps, and exercises can offer a psychological or mental break.
- *Goal setting.* Periodization offers the participant the opportunity to set both short-term and long-term goals. These goals can be set in accordance with individual desires. Performance goals could be to improve endurance, add muscle mass, or increase strength/power or $\dot{V}O_2$max. Health and fitness goals could be to improve body composition, weight loss, blood profile, blood pres-

sure, or muscle strength and endurance, to name a few. Another goal could be to consistently perform a number of workouts or consecutive workouts. Regardless of what the goal is, it can be measured using the acronym SMART.

- **S**pecific: Focus on one or two specific goals.
- **M**easurable: Use quantifiable metrics.
- **A**ttainable: High but attainable goals are recommended.
- **R**ealistic: Use reference points to help set realistic goals.
- **T**ime sensitive: Have a timeline and monitor progress along the way.

Organizational Methods

There are several methods that can be used to implement periodization strategies. Any one of these strategies can be effective; which strategy is most effective depends on the individual, with factors such as training history, response to training, age, and others playing a determining role. In an effort to simplify and possibly demystify the application of periodization, the following training model is offered as a guide.

"Phases" of training simply refer to time periods. These time periods can be short (lasting only one day) or quite long (lasting weeks or even months). There are many reasons why you may want to stay in a particular training period. It is essential for exercisers to change the phase of training, however, and the frequency, intensity, type, and duration of training on a consistent basis (phases should generally not last longer than two to four weeks). Let's further discuss some of the most common phases of training and how they are characterized.

Hypertrophy Phase

The hypertrophy phase is performed with the intention of increasing muscle mass. Traditionally, the hypertrophy phase is characterized by multiple sets, relatively light weight, and high repetitions. For instance, if you wanted to increase the muscle mass of your thighs, you would perform, squats, lunges, leg extensions, and leg curls, completing three to four sets per exercise and anywhere from 8 to 12 repetitions per set. It should be noted that a one-size-fits-all approach is rarely advisable when considering individual training strategies—a certain level of flexibility is required to achieve optimal results.

Strength Phase

The goal of the strength phase is to increase the amount of force that a muscle or action can produce. Linear periodization models often move immediately from a hypertrophy phase to a strength phase. The strength phase utilizes lower repetitions and heavier weights than the hypertrophy phase. Strength work, therefore, is characterized by a higher level of intensity paired with lower volume. For example, a strength workout might incorporate four sets of five to eight repetitions of squats.

Power Phase

The goal of the power phase of training, which often follows the strength phase, is to improve the body's ability to move weight quickly. Power is defined as work (force times distance) divided by time. The faster you do the work, the higher the power output. During the power phase, your goal is to move the weight as fast as possible against gravity. While lowering the weight, focus on slow and controlled movements. With the power phase comes a further increase in intensity and a further reduction in volume. Using our example of the squat exercise, the loading parameters would be four sets of three to six repetitions.

Competition Phase

The competition phase, which follows the power phase for competitive athletes, represents, as the name suggests, the part of the season during which competition takes place. Individuals who do not compete do not need to concern themselves with this phase of training. This phase is characterized by the highest intensities and the lowest volumes. There is some variation in the ranges of weight and repetitions used. Repetitions per set might range from three to five, and sets per exercise might range from three to four. Typically, auxiliary exercises—such as single-joint isolated movements (biceps and hamstring curls or triceps extensions)—are eliminated during this phase.

Peaking Phase

The peaking phase is used to bring you to the absolute height of your abilities, and it is incorporated into the competition phase. If you are performing metabolic-training exercises for general health and fitness, there is little applicability to the peaking phase. This phase is characterized by low volume and high intensity and prioritizes sport-specific exercises. If you do decide to implement a peaking phase, it will last for a short time.

Transition Phase

The transition phase is the last phase of training following a peaking or competition phase. The purpose is to recover from a period of stressful training both mentally and physically. Very light activities are used, and the emphasis is on low volume and intensity. The transition phase lasts for one to two weeks.

Measurable Outcomes

Periodic assessment of fitness is advisable for various reasons. Assessment can show improvement over time, can be measured against population norms, can be used for goal setting, and can indicate the effectiveness of a training program. There are a number of physical aspects that can be measured to aid in determining personal fitness goals. These include bodyweight, body fat, muscle endurance, muscle strength or power, flexibility, agility, cardiorespiratory endurance or capacity, speed, agility, and balance.

Field and Clinical Tests

There is a difference between field tests and clinical tests. A field test is conducted in the environment in which the activity is normally performed—a gym for weightlifting or a track for running. For instance, using a pull-up bar in the gym for max reps is a field test for upper body muscular endurance. Field tests are often more convenient than clinical tests. A clinical test is performed in a laboratory, with the goal of maximizing accuracy and precision. For instance, it may be desirable to measure three-dimensional peak power while performing a countermovement depth jump. This can be done using a force platform. Additionally, two independent platforms could be used to measure discrepancies between the test subject's legs. Clinical tests can be used to shed light on training interventions and injury-prevention techniques.

It should be noted that in order to accurately measure fitness, tests must be both reliable and valid. Reliability refers to how consistent the test is. For instance, a reliable running test could be performed on a quarter-mile (400-meter) track, under unchanged conditions (weather), at the same time of the day, and with an accurate timer. Validity describes the accuracy of the test—in other words, does the test measure what it was designed to measure? A valid measure of sprint speed, for instance, would be a 60-meter dash. An invalid measure of sprint speed would be a 10-kilometer race.

As you determine and work toward your goals, you may want to assess yourself at regular intervals. Be sure to conduct an assessment before you begin a new training program so that you know where you're starting from. The tests shown in table 4.2 can be used to assess different areas of fitness and performance. You can find more information on assessing these areas in Jay Hoffman's *Norms for Fitness, Performance, and Health* (Human Kinetics, 2006).

Table 4.2 Fitness and Performance Tests

Physical characteristics	Tests
Muscular endurance	Push-ups, pull-ups, bent-knee sit-ups, parallel bar dips, bench press for reps
Muscular strength	Bench press (1 rep), squat (1 rep), chest press (1 rep), leg press (1 rep)
Anaerobic power	Wingate power test, standing long jump, vertical jump, 300-yard (274.3-meter) shuttle run
Aerobic power and endurance	Maximal oxygen consumption tests, 1.5-mile (2.4-kilometer) run for time, 12-minute run for distance
Body composition	Comparing height and weight against population norms, calculating body mass index, hydrostatic weighing, DEXA (dual X-ray absorptiometry), skinfold measurements
Flexibility	Sit-and-reach test, joint-angle measurement via goniometer
Speed and agility	40-yard (36.6-meter) dash, 30-yard (27.4-meter) dash, pro agility test, T-test

Physiological Optimization

To optimize your physiology, you must consider your daily activities and your goals. The optimal physiology of a competitive road cyclist (see table 4.3) is vastly different from that of a college offensive lineman (see table 4.4) and equally different from that of a 40-year-old recreational exerciser (see table 4.5). Let's look at these three individuals and what could be optimal physiological attributes for each and how these attributes are attained.

Table 4.3   Optimal Physiological Composition for a Road Cyclist

Physiological ideal	Training intervention
High $\dot{V}O_2$max	Long-duration aerobic efforts, high-intensity intervals of varying duration
High anaerobic threshold	Training slightly below, at, and above anaerobic threshold
Relatively low strength and power capabilities	A function of an endurance athlete's muscle composition and endurance training
Lower body-fat percentages	Controlled diet and long-duration training
High power-to-weight ratio	Variable-interval training
Generally lower bodyweight	A function of genetics, diet, and training
High peak power output	Anaerobic training

Road cyclists perform best with certain physical characteristics. They typically have an efficient cardiorespiratory system with good endurance capabilities, they can process or metabolize high levels of lactate quickly, and their strength is good but not compared to strength and power athletes. To keep their energy expenditure low, it is optimal to keep a low body composition.

Table 4.4   Optimal Physiological Composition for a Collegiate Football Lineman

Physiological ideal	Training intervention
High bodyweight	A function of strength and power training, genetics, and diet
High relative speed and agility	Speed and agility training, emphasis on changing directions
Low endurance capabilities	A function of genetics, diet, and training
High anaerobic capability	Variable anaerobic interval training
High absolute strength and power	Strength and power training, specifically resistance training

Football lineman are relatively taller, bigger, and stronger than all other football positions. Larger athletes are generally more effective than smaller players at the same position. They possess efficient anaerobic capabilities, they demonstrate speed and agility in a small area, and they have high strength and power capabilities. To overcome and absorb the forces of line play, these athletes generally have the greatest amount of mass.

Table 4.5   Optimal Physiological Composition for a Recreational Exerciser

Physiological ideal	Training intervention
Moderate to high relative strength	2-3 times per week low-volume, high-intensity resistance training
Moderate to high power	2 times per week power training
Moderate flexibility	Incorporation of flexibility exercises
Low to moderate body composition	Controlled diet
Moderate muscle endurance	2-3 times per week high-repetition, low-volume resistance training
Moderate anaerobic capabilities	2-3 times per week anaerobic interval training
Moderate aerobic capabilities	2-3 times per week aerobic interval training

Recreational exercisers should concentrate their training efforts on maintaining general health and fitness. This would include maintaining an ideal body composition, adequate muscle strength and endurance, and optimal whole-body flexibility.

The physiological systems of the human body are trainable. Metabolic conditioning can be programmed to improve or complement the activities that comprise your daily life. From the casual exerciser to the competitive athlete, metabolic training can benefit anyone.

Where Metabolic Conditioning Fits within Your Training

Metabolic training is integrated into training programs with the goal of optimizing results by way of targeting specific metabolic systems. The frequency with which this style of training is implemented can range from once a week to multiple times per week. Adaptive capabilities, training history, the ability to manage fatigue, the nature of the training session, and fitness goals should all be carefully considered when selecting the best times to perform metabolic training.

It is wise to gradually progress into a metabolic-training routine. This could be achieved by manipulating the following variables:

- Training frequency: measured in times per week
- Training duration: measured in the amount of time spent in the training session
- Combination of training frequency and duration

Implementing a single training session per week could be the most manageable method to progress into a more concentrated metabolic-training program. Once you have made an initial adaptation or accommodation to the metabolic training, a second session can be added. A third session can be added if signs of fatigue and maladaptation are absent. As a general guideline, engaging in high-intensity or long-duration (longer than one hour) metabolic training more than three times per week will exceed the adaptive capabilities of most people. It is important to carefully monitor your training program as well as your reactions to it.

Shorter-duration metabolic training—lasting 20 to 30 minutes per session—places less physiological stress on the body than longer-duration sessions do. Metabolic-training sessions can be implemented more frequently if the duration of each session is shorter. It may be wise to first start with shorter-duration metabolic-training sessions to avoid exhaustion and to ensure an optimal training load.

In this chapter, we addressed the concept of periodization and some of the theory and evidence that periodization is founded on. Because of the multitude of variables of each person, we gave some general guidelines on how to apply periodization and specifics were intentionally left out. We presented three different periodization models (block, linear, and undulating), and they all may have some application to your training program. The chapter also included three different individual activities to illuminate their specific needs and how metabolic training could be targeted to improve the athletes' fitness.

PART II

Metabolic-Training Exercises

5

Warm-Up Exercises

A structured warm-up is essential for proper preparation for a metabolic training workout. Its value in preventing injury and enhancing performance should not be underestimated. The primary goal of a warm-up is to prepare the body for more strenuous exercise by increasing the body's core and muscle temperature. This change in temperature makes the muscles and the core pliable and adaptable for movement. Additionally, cardiovascular output improves through an increased heart rate resulting in adequate delivery of oxygen and nutrients to the muscles being exercised.

In this chapter, we will discuss three different types of warm-up exercises in: movement preparation, dynamic warm-up, and calisthenics. Movement preparation uses low-intensity movements to increase the muscular, circulatory, respiratory, and nervous systems' functions to enhance workout performance. Dynamic warm-up involves a series of active movements to increase movement and flexibility in muscles, connective tissues, and joints and enhances muscle performance. Calisthenic exercises prepare the body for more intense muscular strength, endurance, and power exercises through movements that incorporate bodyweight for resistance. Calisthenics can also provide increased muscular and aerobic conditioning, in addition to increased coordination, agility, and balance. Table 5.1 provides a list of warm-up exercises.

Table 5.1   Warm-Up and Calisthenic Exercises

Exercise name	Muscles used	Page number
Hand walk	Hamstrings, calves, and lower-back and core muscles	39
Knee-hug lunge	Hamstrings and glute muscles in the front leg and hip flexors in back leg and core muscles	40
Front lunge with forearm to instep	Groin, glute muscles, and hamstrings in the front leg and groin and hip flexor in back leg	41
Lateral lunge	Hip adductors (inner thigh)	42
Backward lunge and twist	Hip flexors, quadriceps, latissimus dorsi, and core muscles	43
High knees (including High knees with lower-leg extension and Lateral high knees variations)	Quadriceps, hamstrings, glute muscles, hip flexors, and hip extensors	44
Heel-up	Quadriceps, hamstrings, glute muscles, hip flexors, and hip extensors	46
Power skip	Quadriceps, hamstrings, glute muscles, hip flexors, and hip extensors	47
Jumping jacks	Deltoids, latissimus dorsi, quadriceps, hamstrings, glute muscles, hip flexors, hip extensors, and hip abductors	48
Mountain climbers	Quadriceps, hamstrings, glute muscles, hip flexors, hip extensors, and hip abductors	49
Burpee	Deltoids, pectoralis major and minor, latissimus dorsi, quadriceps, hamstrings, glute muscles, hip flexors, hip extensors, and hip abductors	50
Groiner	Quadriceps, hamstrings, glute muscles, hip flexors, hip extensors, and hip abductors	51
Single-leg squat	Quadriceps, glute muscles, and hamstrings	52

HAND WALK

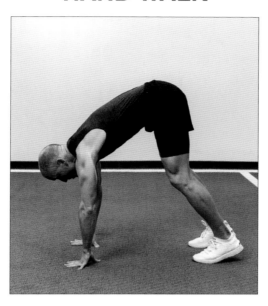

Fundamentals

- Functional range of motion and flexibility in the hamstrings, calves, and lower-back muscles, and core stability

Movement

- Bend forward at the waist and walk your hands forward into a push-up position (to increase difficulty, walk your hands out farther to a point past your head).
- Keep your abdominals pulled in.
- Keeping your legs straight, walk your feet forward toward your hands.
- Once you begin to feel the stretch in the first leg, repeat the movement on the other leg.
- Perform the movement for 10 yards (9.1 meters), turn around, and return to the initial starting position performing the movement.

KNEE-HUG LUNGE

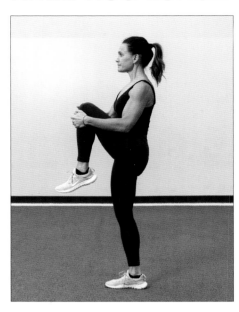

Fundamentals

- Improves functional range of motion and flexibility by increasing extensibility of the hamstrings and glute muscles in the front leg and hip flexors in the back leg

Movement

- Keeping your chest up, step forward with your right leg into a lunge.
- Lift your left knee to your chest and grab below the knee with both hands.
- Pull your left knee to your chest while contracting your right glute.
- Step forward with the left leg into a lunge.
- Lift your right knee to your chest and grab below the knee with both hands.
- Pull your right knee to your chest while contracting your left glute.
- Perform the movement for 10 yards (9.1 meters), turn around, and return to the starting position.

FRONT LUNGE WITH FOREARM TO INSTEP

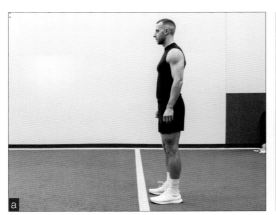
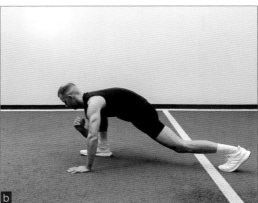

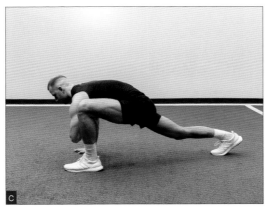

Fundamentals

- Functional range of motion and flexibility in the groin, glutes, and hamstrings in the front leg and the groin and hip flexors in the back leg

Movement

- Step forward into a lunge position with your right leg.
- Place your left hand on the ground and your right elbow to the inside of your right ankle.
- Lift your left leg off the ground and hold the stretch for 1 to 2 seconds.
- Keeping your right elbow as close to your ankle as possible, push your hips upward and straighten your right leg.
- Step forward into a lunge position with your left leg.
- Place your right hand on the ground and your left elbow to the inside of your left ankle. Lift your right leg off the ground and hold the stretch for 1 to 2 seconds.
- Keeping your left elbow as close to your ankle as possible, push your hips upward and straighten your left leg.
- Perform the movement for 10 yards (9.1 meters), turn around, and return to the starting position performing the movement.

LATERAL LUNGE

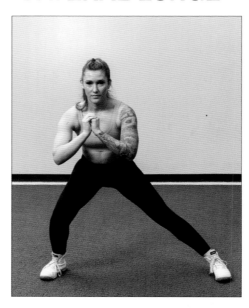

Fundamentals

- Functional range of motion and flexibility in the hip adductors (inner thigh)

Movement

- Step to the side with your right foot, keeping your toes pointing forward and both feet flat on the ground.
- Lower yourself into a squat position on your right side while keeping your left leg straight.
- Bring your left foot into a squat position and repeat the lunge.
- Perform the movement for 10 yards (9.1 meters), and return to the starting position by stepping to the left with the left foot.

BACKWARD LUNGE AND TWIST

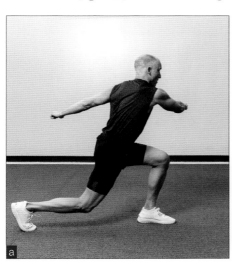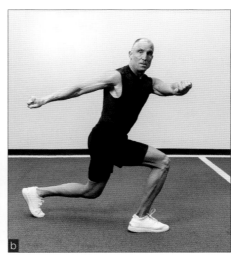

Fundamentals

- Functional range of motion and flexibility in the hip flexors, quadriceps, latissimus dorsi, and core

Movement

- Step backward with your right leg into a lunge.
- Twist your torso over your left (front) leg.
- Step backward with your left leg into a lunge.
- Twist your torso over your right (front) leg. Perform the movement for 10 yards (9.1 meters), turn around, and return to the initial starting position, stepping backward with your left leg first.

HIGH KNEES

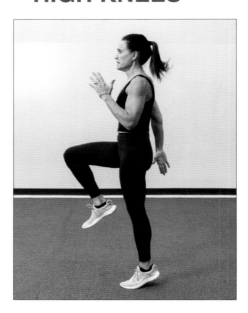

Fundamentals

- Functional range of motion and flexibility in the lower extremity

Movement

- Taking short, quick steps, sprint for 10 yards (9.1 meters), lifting your knees up high so they are parallel to the ground.
- When one leg is lifted, be certain that the opposite leg is fully extended toward the ground.
- Lean forward slightly at your waist and keep your back straight.
- Your shoulders should be as relaxed as possible, with the swing coming from your shoulder joint.
- Pivot your arms at your shoulders, with your elbows locked at 90 degrees.
- Keep your elbows close to your body. Your arms should move from shoulder to hip.
- Move your hands from "cheek to cheek" (from your face to your buttocks).
- Keep your thumbs on top of your hands, with your hands relaxed.
- Keep your face and neck relaxed.
- After a short recovery (15 to 20 seconds), repeat the exercise, moving back to your starting position.

Variations in Movement

High Knees With Lower-Leg Extension

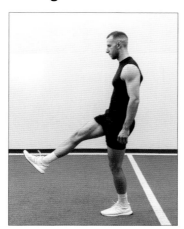

- Lifting your front knee high as high as possible, skip with your back leg when your front knee reaches its highest point.
- As the skip is performed lift your front lower leg until it is parallel to the ground.
- Repeat on the other side.

Lateral High Knees

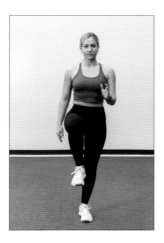

- Taking short quick steps without crossing your feet laterally, sprint 10 yards (9.1 meters), lifting your knees up so they are parallel to the ground.
- When one leg is lifted, be certain that the opposite leg is fully extended toward the ground.
- Lean forward slightly at your waist and keep your back straight.
- Return to the starting position performing the movement.

HEEL-UP

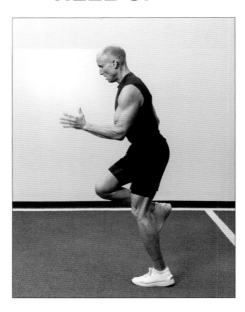

Fundamentals

- Functional range of motion and flexibility in the lower extremity

Movement

- Keeping your knees pointed down at ground and your body leaned slightly forward, run for 10 yards (9.1 meters) on your toes, alternately swinging the heel of each foot up to your buttocks.
- Keep the movement quick and smooth, swinging your lower leg at the knee.
- Avoid moving forward too fast or lifting your knees by flexing at your hips.
- Your shoulders should be as relaxed as possible, with the swing coming from your shoulder joint.
- Your arms should pivot at your shoulders, with your elbows locked at 90 degrees.
- Keep your elbows close to your body.
- Your arms should move from shoulder to hip. Your hands should move from "cheek to cheek" (face to buttocks).
- Keep your thumbs on top of your hands, and keep your hands relaxed.
- Keep your face and neck relaxed.
- After a short recovery (15 to 20 seconds), repeat the exercise, heading back to the original starting position.

POWER SKIP

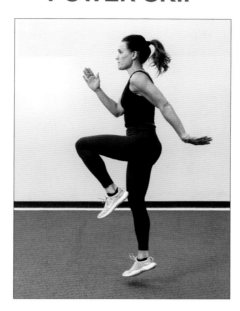

Fundamentals

- Functional range of motion and flexibility in lower extremity

Movement

- Using your arms to help propel you forward and upward by reaching up with your hands, skip explosively with triple extension of your back leg, driving your front leg up as high as possible and trying to elevate your body as high as possible off the ground.
- Prepare for ground contact and repeat the motion with the opposite leg immediately upon landing.
- Continue skipping for 20 yards (18.2 meters). Keep your face and neck relaxed. After a short recovery (15 to 20 seconds), repeat the exercise, heading back to the original starting position.

JUMPING JACKS

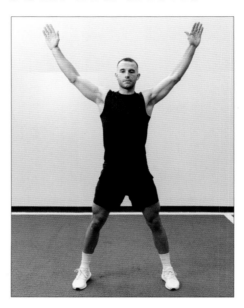

Fundamentals

- Functional movement in the shoulder and lower extremity. This exercise can be used as a warm-up as well as a way to improve coordination and metabolic fitness.

Movement

- Initiate the movement with your feet together and your hands at your sides.
- Explosively move your feet laterally to about shoulder-width apart and raise your arms in an arc fashion overhead, tapping your hands together.
- Return to the starting position.
- Repeat the exercise for the desired length of time or number of repetitions.

MOUNTAIN CLIMBERS

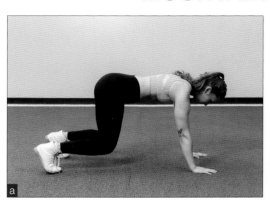
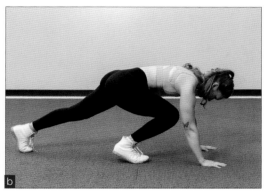

Fundamentals

- Functional movement in the shoulder and lower extremity. This exercise can be used as a warm-up as well as a way to improve coordination and metabolic fitness.
- Ability to hold plank position

Movement

- Begin in a plank position by facing downward while positioned on your toes and hands. Maintain a flat back, your arms straight and aligned directly below your shoulders, and your knees relaxed below your hips.
- Explosively move one leg forward toward your chest and then return that leg to the starting position as your opposite leg moves forward toward your chest.
- Repeat the exercise for the desired length of time or number of repetitions.

BURPEE

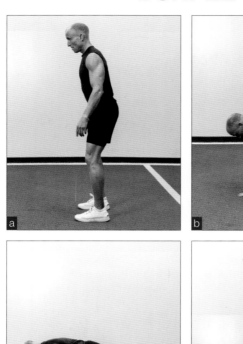
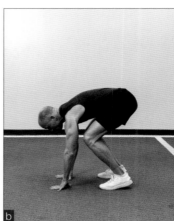
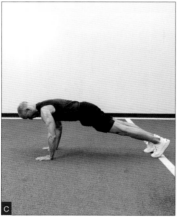
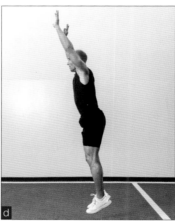

Fundamentals

- Functional movement in the shoulder and lower extremity. This exercise can be used as a warm-up as well as a way to improve coordination and metabolic fitness.
- Core stability
- Ability to perform a squat with full range of motion through the balls of the feet

Movement

- Begin in a standing position with your feet shoulder-width apart.
- Explosively descend into a squat position, with your hands placed on the ground in front of you, and thrust your legs backward, arriving in a plank or push-up position.
- Return your legs to a squat position, with your hands touching the ground, and explosively jump upward, straightening your legs and reaching high with the hands while maintaining straight arms.
- Return to the starting position.
- Repeat the exercise for the desired length of time or number of repetitions.

GROINER

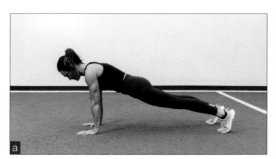 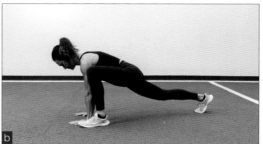

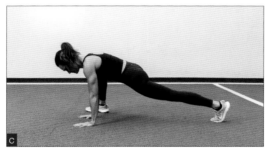

Fundamentals

- A functional movement that can be used as a warm-up or to improve coordination and metabolic fitness
- Hip and hamstring flexibility
- Core strength and endurance

Movement

- Begin in a plank position by facing downward while positioned on your toes and hands. Maintain a flat back, your arms straight and aligned directly below your shoulders, and your knees relaxed below your hips.
- Move one leg outward and forward and plant your heel near or slightly beyond your shoulder on the same side of your body.
- Return your leg to the starting position and repeat with the opposite leg.
- Repeat the exercise for the desired length of time or number of repetitions.

SINGLE-LEG SQUAT

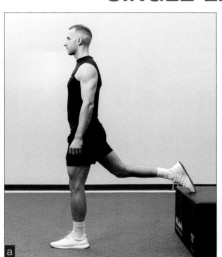
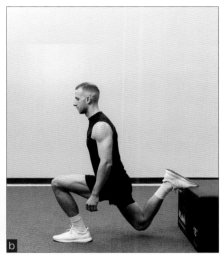

Fundamentals

- Capability to perform a dumbbell squat for 10 repetitions

Setup

- Place the top of your foot on top of a bench or box positioned directly behind you. Position your front leg in front of the bench or box, with your knee aligned above your ankle.
- Keep your torso erect.
- Before beginning the downward movement, inhale.

Downward Movement

- Lower your hips and flex your front leg in a controlled manner.
- Keep your front knee above your ankle throughout the downward movement.
- Maintain a flat back.
- Continue the downward movement until the thigh of your front leg is parallel to the floor and your back knee nearly reaches the floor.
- When you reach the bottom of the downward movement, avoid bouncing or increasing the rate of movement before beginning the upward movement.

Upward Movement

- Extend your front knee and hip.
- Keep your back flat.
- Continue the upward movement by extending the lower-body joints at a consistent rate, until you reach the initial starting position.
- Exhale at the completion of the upward movement.
- Repeat the exercise for the desired length of time or number of repetitions on both legs.

6

Total-Body Exercises

Total-body exercises are exercises that impact the upper-body, lower-body, and core muscles, and that incorporate two or three movement planes (sagittal [forward and backward], frontal [side to side], and transverse [rotational]).

Total-body exercises offer a higher-intensity workout and enable the body to burn more calories per unit of time than using single-joint or isolated muscle group training. Total-body training offers the opportunity to link strength training with cardiorespiratory training, resulting in greater metabolic benefits. Total-body exercises can be incorporated into any fitness routine, generally with minimal or no equipment, using bodyweight, free weights, or other implements. Implementing total-body exercises reduces the need for additional lower-body, upper-body, and core exercises, which, in turn, reduces total workout time. Total-body exercises also allow for intensity adjustments, which can be beneficial when returning to exercise after a break. Table 6.1 provides a list of total-body exercises.

Table 6.1   Total-Body Exercises

Exercise name	Muscles used	Page number
Dumbbell hang clean (including sandbag hang clean variation)	Gluteus maximus, hamstrings, quadriceps, soleus, gastrocnemius, trapezius, deltoids	56
Dumbbell one-arm snatch (including kettlebell one-arm snatch variation)	Gluteus maximus, hamstrings, quadriceps, soleus, gastrocnemius, trapezius, deltoids, triceps brachii	58
Dumbbell push press (including kettlebell push press and sandbag push press variations)	Gluteus maximus, hamstrings, quadriceps, soleus, gastrocnemius, erector spinae, trapezius, deltoids	60
Kettlebell two-hand swing (novice to intermediate)	Gluteus maximus; hamstrings; quadriceps; latissimus dorsi; rectus abdominis; transverse abdominis; pectoralis major; pectoralis minor; anterior, medial, and posterior deltoid; trapezius	62
Kettlebell one-hand swing (intermediate to advanced)	Gluteus maximus; hamstrings; quadriceps; latissimus dorsi; erector spinae; quadratus lumborum; rectus abdominis; transverse abdominis; pectoralis major; pectoralis minor; anterior, medial, and posterior deltoid; trapezius	62
Kettlebell one-arm clean (novice to intermediate; including kettlebell two-arm clean variation [intermediate to advanced])	Gluteus maximus, hamstrings, quadriceps, soleus, gastrocnemius, trapezius, deltoids	63
Resistance band pull-through	Gluteus maximus, hamstrings, erector spinae, latissimus dorsi, serratus anterior	65
Medicine ball slam (including medicine ball rotational slam variation)	Quadriceps; hamstrings; erector spinae; quadratus lumborum; rectus abdominis; transverse abdominis; anterior, medial, and posterior deltoid; trapezius; serratus anterior (for rotational slam); internal and external oblique (for rotational slam)	66
Medicine ball side slam	Quadriceps; hamstrings; erector spinae; quadratus lumborum; rectus abdominis; transverse abdominis; internal and external oblique; anterior, medial and posterior deltoid; trapezius; serratus anterior	67
Medicine ball upward throw	Quadriceps; hamstrings; erector spinae; quadratus lumborum; transverse abdominis; anterior, medial, and posterior deltoid; trapezius	68

Exercise name	Muscles used	Page number
Medicine ball backward throw	Quadriceps; hamstrings; erector spinae; quadratus lumborum; transverse abdominis; anterior, medial, and posterior deltoid; trapezius	69
Medicine ball burpee	Quadriceps; hamstrings; erector spinae; quadratus lumborum; rectus abdominis; transverse abdominis; pectoralis major; anterior, medial, and posterior deltoid; trapezius; triceps brachii	70
Medicine ball squat and jump	Quadriceps; hamstrings; anterior, medial, and posterior deltoid; trapezius; triceps brachii	71
Medicine ball chop (including medicine ball woodchop and medicine ball side chop variations)	Quadriceps; hamstrings; erector spinae; quadratus lumborum; rectus abdominis; transverse abdominis; internal and external oblique; anterior, medial and posterior deltoid; trapezius	72
Weighted sled push	Gluteus maximus and minimus, quadriceps, hamstring, core	74
Weighted sled pull and push	Gluteus maximus and minimus, quadriceps, hamstring, rectus abdominis; transverse abdominis; pectoralis major; pectoralis minor; anterior, medial, and posterior deltoid; trapezius; serratus anterior	75
Weighted sled drag	Gluteus maximus and minimus, quadriceps, hamstring, core	76

DUMBBELL HANG CLEAN

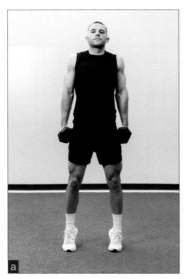 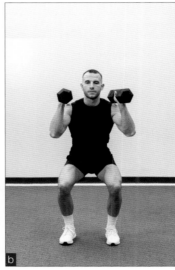

Fundamentals

- Capability to perform a squat with full range of motion, driving through the balls of the feet
- Sufficient core stability (hold a front, side plank, and Superman for 30 seconds)

Setup

- Select two dumbbells of equal weight and hold one in each hand.
- Keeping your arms straight and holding the dumbbells with a neutral grip, push your hips back until the dumbbells are adjacent to the outsides of your knees.
- Position your shoulders forward, in front of your lower body.
- Look straight ahead, keeping your head and neck straight.
- Shift your bodyweight onto balls of your feet.

Upward Movement

- Inhale and explosively extend the hips, knees, and ankles, and perform a slight jump while keeping your arms straight.
- Lift your shoulders forcefully and pull the dumbbells upward without bending the elbows, bringing the dumbbells as high as possible.
- Keep your head and neck straight and your eyes looking straight ahead.
- Once the dumbbells have reached maximum height (ideally chest level) drop below them into a squat position while simultaneously bringing your elbows up and around the dumbbells. The dumbbells should come to a rest on your shoulders.
- You should reach the squat position at the same time that the dumbbells reach your shoulders.
- Keep your elbows and chest up, extend your hips and knees from the squat position, and stand up straight.
- Exhale at the completion of the upward movement.

Downward Movement

- Maintaining a flat back, flex your hips and knees and lower the dumbbells in a controlled manner back to their starting position, beside the knees.
- Repeat for the desired length of time or number of repetitions.

Variations in Fundamentals, Setup, and Movements

Sandbag Hang Clean

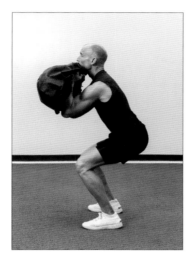

Fundamentals

The same fundamentals listed for the dumbbell hang clean apply here as well, in addition to enough strength and flexibility to hold a sandbag on your shoulder.

Setup

- Place the sandbag on the floor and stand above it, with your feet shoulder-width apart.
- Stabilize your core utilizing correct body alignment.
- Keeping your weight on the balls of your feet, squat and grab the sandbag with a neutral grip.
- Stand while keeping your arms straight.
- Keeping your arms straight and continuing to hold the sandbag, push your hips back until the sand is touching the tops of your knees.
- Position your shoulders forward in front of your lower body.
- Look straight ahead, keeping your head and neck straight.

Upward and Downward Movements

- Use the same cues as for the dumbbell hang clean.
- Repeat for the desired length of time or number of repetitions.

DUMBBELL ONE-ARM SNATCH

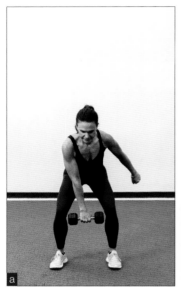 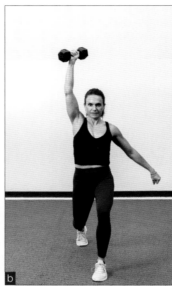 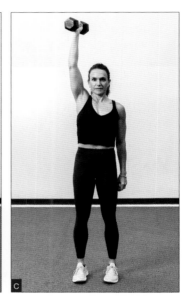

Fundamentals

- Capability to perform a squat with full range of motion, driving through the balls of the feet
- Ability to lift and control resistance overhead
- Sufficient core stability

Setup

- Select a dumbbell and hold it in one hand.
- Keeping your arm straight and holding the dumbbell with a neutral grip, push your hips back until the dumbbell is evenly between your legs at knee level.
- Position your shoulders forward in front of your lower body.
- Look straight ahead, keeping your head and neck straight.
- Shift your bodyweight onto balls of your feet.

Upward Movement

- Inhale and explosively extend your hips, knees, and ankles and perform a slight jump while keeping the arm holding the dumbbell straight.
- Lift both shoulders forcefully and pull the weight upward without bending your elbow. Bring the dumbbell as high as possible.
- Continue the movement until your elbow is below dumbbell, and then push the weight up.
- Keep your head and neck straight and your eyes looking straight ahead.
- Once the weight has reached its maximum height (above your head with arm straight), drop under the dumbbell by moving one foot forward (the foot that is on the opposite side as the dumbbell) and one foot backward (the foot that is on the same side as the dumbbell).

- Your front foot should be flat on the ground, and your thigh should be parallel to the ground.
- The ball of your rear foot should be planted on the ground, with your knee flexed.
- During the split movement, explosively raise the dumbbell over your shoulder and turn your arm over until the dumbbell is locked overhead, with your arm straight.
- Next, step back with your front foot and move your rear foot forward until your feet are parallel.
- Keep your elbow locked and the dumbbell over your hips.

Downward Movement

- Maintaining a flat back, flex your hips and knees, stabilize the dumbbell with the free hand, and return the dumbbell in a controlled manner to its starting position, between the knees.
- After completing the desired number of repetitions on one side, switch and repeat on the opposite side.

Variation in Setup

Kettlebell One-Arm Snatch

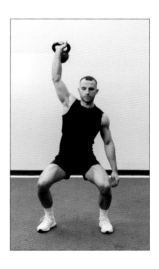

Setup

- Place a kettlebell on the floor and stand above it, with your feet shoulder-width apart.
- Keeping your weight on the balls of your feet, squat and grab the kettlebell with a one-handed pronated grip.
- Stand while keeping your arm straight.
- Keeping your arm straight and holding the kettlebell with a pronated grip, push your hips back until the kettlebell is between your knees.
- Position your shoulders forward, in front of your lower body.
- Look straight ahead, keeping your head and neck straight.
- Shift your bodyweight onto balls of your feet.

Upward Movement

- Once the kettlebell has reached its maximum height overhead, drop below the kettlebell into a squat position.
- The squat position should be reached at the same time that the kettlebell is overhead, with your arm straight.
- Extend your hips and knees from the squat position until you are standing straight, with your arm overhead.
- Exhale at the completion of the upward movement.

Downward Movement

- The downward movement is the same for both the dumbbell and kettlebell one-arm snatch.
- After completing the desired number of repetitions on one side, switch and repeat on the opposite side

DUMBBELL PUSH PRESS

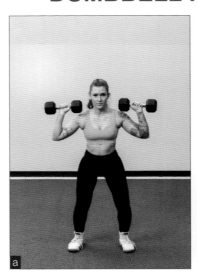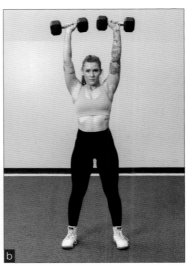

Fundamentals

- Capability to perform a squat with full range of motion, driving through the balls of the feet. Enough strength and flexibility to lift and control resistance on your shoulders and overhead.
- Sufficient core stability

Setup

- Select two dumbbells of equal weight and hold one in each hand.
- Grab the dumbbells with a neutral grip.
- Lift the dumbbells onto your shoulders.
- Keep your elbows under the dumbbells.
- Your feet should be hip-width apart.

Upward Movement

- Keeping your weight on the balls of your feet and the weight of the dumbbells on the shoulders, explosively drop into a quarter squat by pushing your hips back and flexing your knees.
- Without pausing at the bottom of the squat, explosively reverse directions and drive up with your legs by pushing from the balls of your feet.
- Use the leg explosion to push the weights up off of your shoulders.
- At the completion of the drive, press the weights over your shoulders until your arms are fully extended.
- At the completion of the upward movement, the weights should be in line with your hips (slightly behind your head).

Downward Movement

- Maintaining a flat back, flex your hips and knees and lower the weights in a controlled manner to their starting position, on your shoulders.
- Repeat the exercise for a designated number of repetitions or time.

Variations in Setup

Use the same movement cues for these variations as you did for the dumbbell push press.

Kettlebell Push Press

- Select two kettlebells of equal weight and hold one in each hand, using a pronated grip.
- Lift the kettlebells onto your shoulders.
- Keep your elbows under the kettlebells.
- Your feet should be hip-width apart.
- Repeat the exercise for a designated number of repetitions or time.

Sandbag Push Press

- Select a sandbag of an appropriate weight.
- Lift the sandbag onto your shoulder.
- Hold the sandbag with a neutral grip.
- Keep your elbows under the sandbag.
- Your feet should be hip-width apart.
- Repeat the exercise for a designated number of repetitions or time.

KETTLEBELL TWO-HAND SWING

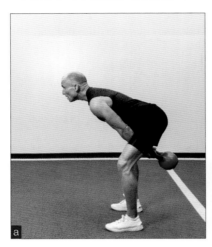 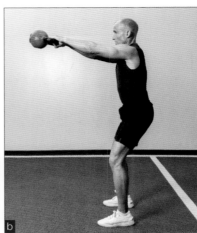

Fundamentals

- Capability to perform a squat with full range of motion, driving through the balls of the feet
- Sufficient core stability

Setup

- Place a kettlebell on the floor and stand above it, with your feet shoulder-width apart.
- Stabilize your core utilizing correct body alignment.
- Keeping your weight on the balls of your feet, squat and grab the kettlebell with a two-handed pronated grip.
- Stand while keeping your arms straight.

Upward Movement

- Flex at the hips (push the hips back) and let the kettlebell swing back between your knees.
- Keeping your weight on the balls of your feet and utilizing a triple-extension movement (hips, knees, and ankles) explosively swing the kettlebell forward until your straightened arms reach a position parallel to the floor.

Downward Movement

- Return to the starting position by reversing the swinging motion.
- Repeat the exercise for a designated number of repetitions or time.

Variations in Fundamentals, Setup, and Movements

Kettlebell One-Hand Swing

Fundamentals

- Capability to perform a full-range-of-motion two-hand swing with a weight equal to 15 percent of your bodyweight for at least eight repetitions
- Sufficient core stability

Setup

- Place a kettlebell on the floor and stand above it, with your feet shoulder-width apart.
- Stabilize your core utilizing correct body alignment.
- Keeping your weight on the balls of your feet, squat and grab the kettlebell with a one-handed pronated grip.
- Stand while keeping your arms straight.

Upward Movement

- The upward movement for the one-arm swing is the same as for the two-arm swing.

Downward Movement

- Return to the starting position by reversing the swinging motion.
- After completing the desired number of repetitions on one side, switch and repeat on the opposite side.

KETTLEBELL ONE-ARM CLEAN

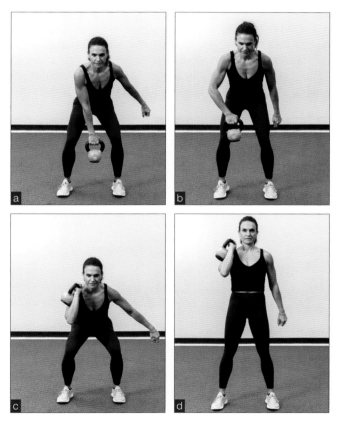

Fundamentals

- Capability to perform a squat with full range of motion driving through the balls of the feet
- Sufficient core stability
- Enough strength and flexibility to hold a kettlebell on your shoulder

Setup

- Place a kettlebell on the floor and stand above it, with your feet shoulder-width apart.
- Stabilize your core utilizing correct body alignment.
- Keeping your weight on the balls of your feet, squat and grab the kettlebell with a one-handed pronated grip.
- Stand while keeping your arm straight.
- Keeping your arm straight and continuing to hold the kettlebell with a pronated grip, push your hips back until the kettlebell is adjacent to the outside of your knee.
- Position your shoulders forward in front of your lower body.
- Look straight ahead, keeping your head and neck straight.
- Shift your bodyweight onto balls of your feet.

Upward Movement

- Inhale and explosively extend your hips, knees, and ankles and perform a slight jump while keeping your arm straight.
- Lift your shoulders forcefully and pull the kettlebell upward, without bending your elbow, as high as possible.
- Keep your head and neck straight and your eyes looking straight ahead.
- Once the kettlebell has reached its maximum height (ideally chest level), drop below kettlebell into a squat position while simultaneously moving your elbow up and around the kettlebell. The kettlebell should come to rest on your shoulder.
- The squat position should be reached at the same time that the kettlebell reaches your shoulder.
- Keep your elbows and chest up extend your hips and knees from the squat position until you are standing straight.
- Exhale at the completion of the upward movement.

Downward Movement

- Maintaining a flat back, flex your hips and knees and lower the kettlebell in a controlled manner to its starting position, beside your knee.
- After completing the desired number of repetitions on one side, switch and repeat on the opposite side.

Variations in Fundamentals and Movements

Kettlebell Two-Arm Clean

Fundamentals

- At least three months of being able to perform a full-range of motion one-handed clean
- Sufficient core stability
- Enough strength and flexibility to hold a kettlebell on your shoulder

Setup

- The setup for this exercise is the same as for the one-arm clean, except that one kettlebell is held in each hand.

Upward Movement

- The upward movement is the same as for the one-arm clean with the following exception: Once the kettlebells have reached their maximum height (ideally chest level) drop below kettlebells into a squat position while simultaneously moving your elbows up and around the kettlebells. The kettlebells should come to rest on your shoulder.

Downward Movement

- The downward movement for the two-arm clean is the same as for the one-arm clean.
- Repeat the exercise for a designated number of repetitions or time.

RESISTANCE BAND PULL-THROUGH

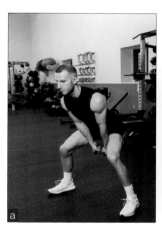 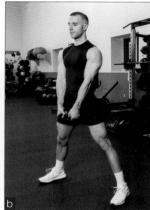 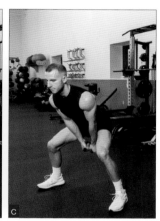

Fundamentals

- Capability to perform 10 one-leg hip thrusts on each leg

Setup

- Attach a resistance band to a sturdy anchor point, such as a stable rack, bench, or resistance machine.
- Hold the end of the resistance band that is not attached to the anchor point and walk forward, with your back to the anchor point.
- Position your feet about hip-width apart and have the resistance band run between your legs.
- Hinge by pushing your hips back and leaning forward at your upper torso, bringing your upper body to almost parallel with the floor.
- Allow your hands to be pulled through your legs toward the anchor point, while maintaining a firm torso.
- Before beginning the upward movement, inhale.

Upward Movement

- With tension on your hamstrings, extend your hips forward and into an erect position.
- Keep your arms straight and maintain a neutral grip throughout the movement. Avoid pulling or using your arms.
- Exhale at the completion of the upward movement.

Downward Movement

- Return to the starting position by keeping your knees slightly flexed and your back flat, allowing your hands to be pulled back through your legs.
- Repeat the exercise for a designated number of repetitions or time.

MEDICINE BALL SLAM

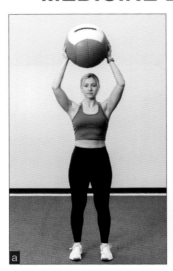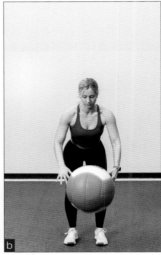

Fundamentals

- Sufficient core stability
- No current shoulder or lower-back injuries

Setup

- Hold the medicine ball overhead with both hands.
- Maintain an erect posture, with the ball overhead.
- Position your feet shoulder-width apart.
- Your bodyweight should be on the balls of your feet, and your back should be straight.

Movement

- Drop into an athletic position—bend the knees, keeping weight on the balls of the feet and the chest—by pushing your hips back while simultaneously pushing your hands down below your knees and explosively driving the medicine ball to the floor.
- Catch the medicine ball as it bounces up from the floor and stand up, lifting your arms overhead.
- Without pausing at the top, return to an athletic position explosively, driving the medicine ball to the ground again.
- Repeat this movement pattern continuously for the desired number of repetitions or length of time.

Variation in Movement

For this variation, use the following cues:

- Drop into an athletic position by pushing your hips back while simultaneously pushing your hands down and to your right side, explosively driving the medicine ball to the floor.
- Catch the medicine ball as it bounces from the floor and stand up, lifting your arms overhead.

Medicine Ball Rotational Slam

- Without pausing at the top, drop back into an athletic position by pushing your hips back while pushing the hands down and to your left side, explosively driving the medicine ball to the floor.
- Catch the medicine ball as it bounces from the floor and stand up, lifting your arms overhead.
- Repeat this movement pattern continuously, alternating sides, for the desired number of repetitions or length of time.

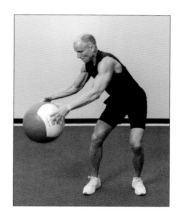

MEDICINE BALL SIDE SLAM

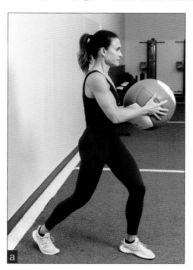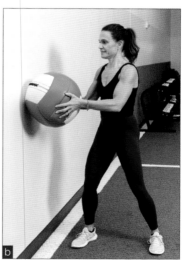

Fundamentals

- Sufficient core stability
- No current shoulder or lower-back injuries

Setup

- Grab the medicine ball with both hands.
- Maintain an erect posture, with the ball waist level.
- Stand three feet from a solid wall. Turn sideways, with your right side facing the wall.
- Stand in an athletic position. Your bodyweight should be on the balls of your feet, and your back should be straight.
- Hold the medicine ball straight out in front of your chest.
- Keep your arms straight and your palms facing each other, with one hand on each side of the medicine ball.

Movement

- Explosively twist your torso to the left, away from the wall.
- Reverse directions quickly, twisting your body to the right (toward the wall), and throw the ball against the wall as hard as possible.
- Catch the ball as it bounces off the wall and repeat the movement as quickly as possible.
- Perform for the desired number of repetitions or continue for the desired length of time.
- Perform the movement on the opposite side (with your left side facing the wall).

MEDICINE BALL UPWARD THROW

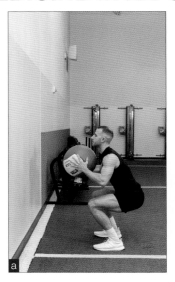 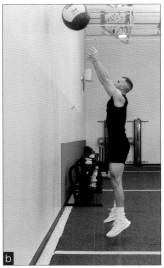

Fundamentals

- Sufficient core stability
- Capability to perform a squat with full range of motion, driving through the balls of the feet
- No current shoulder or lower-back injuries

Setup

- Grab the medicine ball with both hands.
- Maintain an erect posture and hold the ball at shoulder level.
- Position your feet shoulder-width apart.
- Your bodyweight should be on the balls of your feet, and your back should be kept straight.
- Stand three feet from a solid wall.

Movement

- Perform a squat with full range of motion.
- Explosively ascend and release the ball, jumping as you reach the end of the upward movement.
- Catch the ball as it comes back down, and then repeat the movement pattern.
- Perform for the desired number of repetitions or continue for the desired length of time.

MEDICINE BALL BACKWARD OVERHEAD THROW

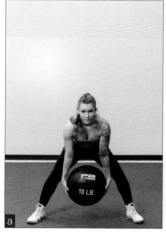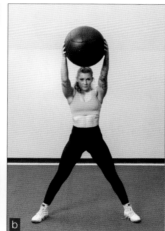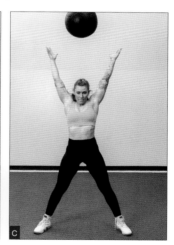

Fundamentals

- Sufficient core stability
- Capability to perform a squat with full range of motion, driving through the balls of the feet
- No current shoulder or lower-back injuries

Setup

- Stand six to nine feet from a solid, high wall.
- Grab the medicine ball with both hands.
- Stand with your feet wider than shoulder-width apart.
- Hold the medicine ball overhead, with your hands on either side of the ball.

Movement

- Lower the ball, with your arms slightly flexed, in an arc fashion.
- Squat down into athletic position and swing the ball down between both legs.
- Immediately lean back slightly.
- Swing the ball forward, flexing your arms slightly and extending your body and legs.
- Throw the ball backward and upward.
- Walk backward a few steps to reestablish your balance.
- Perform for the desired number of repetitions or for the desired length of time.

MEDICINE BALL BURPEE

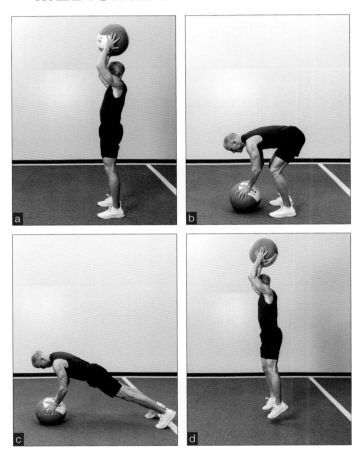

Fundamentals

- Capability to perform a bodyweight burpee
- Core stability and capability to perform a squat with full range of motion, driving through the balls of the feet

Movement

- Begin in a standing position, with your feet shoulder-width apart, holding a medicine ball at chest level with your hands on either side.
- Explosively descend into a squat position, plant the medicine ball on the ground in front of your feet, and thrust your legs back to a plank/push-up position.
- Return your legs to a squat position while keeping the medicine ball planted on the ground.
- Explosively jump upward, straightening your legs and reaching high with the medicine ball.
- Return to the starting position.
- Repeat the exercise for the desired number of repetitions or for the desired length of time.

MEDICINE BALL SQUAT AND JUMP

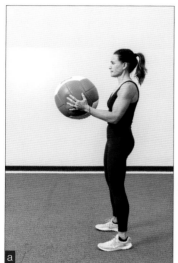 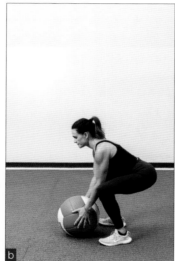 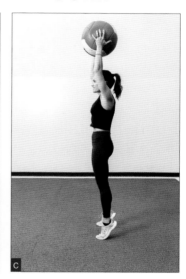

Fundamentals

- Capability to perform a squat with full range of motion, driving through the balls of the feet

Setup

- Grab the medicine ball with both hands.
- Maintain an erect posture, with the ball at chest level.
- Position your feet shoulder-width apart.
- Your bodyweight should be on the balls of your feet, and your back should be straight.

Movement

- Perform a squat with full range of motion.
- Touch the medicine ball to the ground between your feet.
- Explosively jump upward and press the medicine ball overhead.
- Perform the exercise for the desired number of repetitions or for the desired length of time.

MEDICINE BALL CHOP

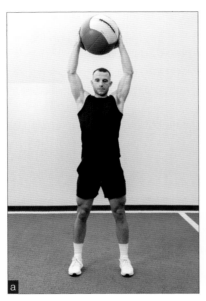
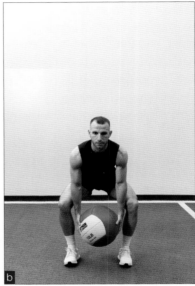

Fundamentals

- Sufficient core stability
- No current shoulder or lower-back injuries

Setup

- Grab the medicine ball with both hands.
- Maintain an erect posture, with the ball overhead.
- Stand in an athletic stance, with your feet shoulder-width apart.
- Your bodyweight should be on the balls of your feet, and your back should be straight.

Movement

- Keep your arms straight and move the ball downward to knee level between your legs. The ball should move downward in an arc. At the completion of the movement, return in a reverse-arc pattern to the starting position.
- Perform the exercise for the desired number of repetitions or for the desired length of time.

Variations in Movement

Use the same setup for these variations as you did for the chop exercise.

Medicine Ball Woodchop

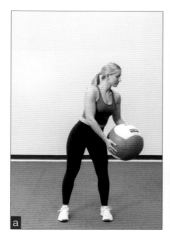 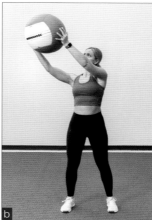

Movement

- Rotating from the waist, explosively lift the ball up above your shoulder to one side.
- Control the movement at the top and bring the ball back down to waist height on the opposite side.
- Perform on one side for the desired number of repetitions or length of time.
- Switch to the opposite side and perform for the desired number of repetitions.

Medicine Ball Side Chop

Movement

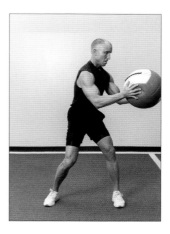

- Hold the medicine ball in front of your chest, with your palms facing each other on either side of the medicine ball.
- Twist your torso to one side by rotating at the waist, while keeping the medicine ball in line with your chest.
- Reverse directions and rotate to the opposite side, keeping the medicine ball in line with your chest throughout.
- Perform for the desired number of repetitions or for the desired length of time.

WEIGHTED SLED PUSH

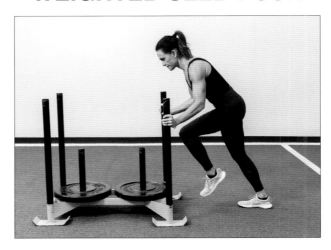

Fundamentals

- Caution with preexisting injuries to your lower back and lower extremity.
- Excellent exercise for sports and professions that require moving or pushing an opponent or weighted object

Setup

- Place a load equivalent to 20 to 30 percent of your bodyweight onto a weighted sled. If the sled has multiple loading locations, attempt to distribute the load evenly.
- Grab the handlebars at a high position, keeping your arms fairly straight, your torso firm, your shoulders back and upright, and your head up, looking in front of the sled.

Movement

- Drive the sled forward by pushing off the ball of one foot and performing a triple extension of the ankle, knee, and hip. Repeat with your second foot, and then continue to alternate.
- Push the sled for a specified distance in one direction, and then in the opposite direction.
- Repeat the movement for a specified number of repetitions or a specified length of time.

WEIGHTED SLED PULL AND PUSH

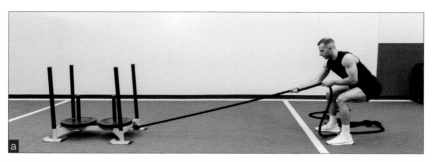

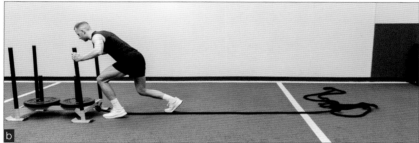

Fundamentals

- Caution with preexisting injuries to your shoulders, upper and lower back, and lower extremity.
- Excellent exercise for sports and professions that require pulling and pushing an opponent or weighted object.

Setup

- Attach a 30- to 50-foot rope (10 to 15 yards, or about 9 to 13 meters) to the weighted sled and stand at the opposite end of the rope.
- Place a load equivalent to 20 to 30 percent of your bodyweight onto the sled. If the sled has multiple loading locations, attempt to distribute the load evenly.
- Pull the rope tight before initiating the exercise.
- Position your body in an athletic stance, keeping your torso firm and upright and your hips, knees, and ankles bent.

Movement

- Using an overhand grip (palms facing toward the body), pull the sled toward you, moving one hand over the other as you progress.
- Allow the rope to fall between your feet.
- Once the sled has been pulled all the way in, drive the sled back toward the starting position by pushing off the ball of your foot and performing a triple extension of your ankle, knee, and hip, and then repeating with your other foot. Alternate feet as you go. When you reach the starting position, the rope should be fully lengthened.
- Repeat the movement for a specified number of repetitions or a specified length of time.

WEIGHTED SLED DRAG

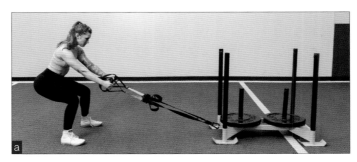

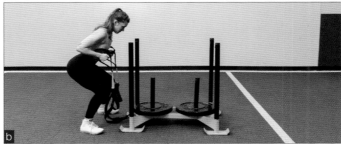

Fundamentals

- Caution with preexisting injuries to your shoulder, upper and lower back, and lower extremity.
- Excellent exercise for sports and professions that require dragging an opponent or weighted object.

Setup

- Attach a suspension training device to the training sled.
- Place a load equivalent to 20 to 30 percent of your bodyweight onto a weighted sled. If the sled has multiple loading locations, attempt to distribute the load evenly.
- Pull the suspension trainer tight before initiating the exercise.
- Position your body in an athletic stance, keeping your torso firm and upright and your hips, knees, and ankles bent.

Movement

- Grab the suspension trainer handles, and fully extend your arms.
- Pull the sled toward your feet with an explosive pull.
- Once the sled has been pulled to your feet, walk back a few steps until the suspension trainer is tight, and then repeat.
- Repeat the movement for a specified number of repetitions or length of time.

7

Lower-Body Exercises

Lower-body exercises increase muscle strength, endurance, and power in the glutes, the quadriceps, the hamstrings, the hip abductors and adductors, the calves, and the stabilizing muscles of the hip. Lower-body exercises enable us to strengthen the muscles responsible for everyday movement and function (sitting, standing, squatting, walking, running, climbing stairs, etc.).

Without lower-body strength, endurance, and power, performing everyday movements, even at a basic level, would be difficult. In the context of metabolic training, lower-body exercises not only improve functional movement but also increase fat burning and overall fitness—these are the muscles with the highest metabolic demand, due to their size, and the highest potential for power output. Table 7.1 provides a list of lower-body exercises.

Table 7.1 Lower-Body Exercises

Exercise name	Muscle(s) used	Page number
Dumbbell squat (with resistance band squat, kettlebell goblet squat, suspension squat, and sandbag front squat variations)	Gluteus maximus, quadriceps, hamstrings	80
Dumbbell split squat	Gluteus maximus, quadriceps, hamstrings, hip flexors	82
Kettlebell overhead squat (with resistance band overhead squat, medicine ball overhead squat, and sandbag overhead squat variations)	**Kettlebell overhead squat, resistance band overhead squat, and sandbag overhead squat:** Gluteus maximus, hamstrings, quadriceps, soleus, gastrocnemius, erector spinae, trapezius, deltoids **Medicine ball overhead squat:** Gluteus maximus, hamstrings, quadriceps, erector spinae, trapezius, deltoids	83
Dumbbell box step-up (with medicine ball overhead box step-up variation)	**Dumbbell box step-up:** Gluteus maximus, quadriceps, hamstrings; **Medicine ball overhead box step-up:** Gluteus maximus, hamstrings, quadriceps, erector spinae, trapezius, deltoids	86
Dumbbell front lunge (with kettlebell overhead lunge, medicine ball overhead lunge, and sandbag overhead lunge variations)	**Dumbbell front lunge:** Gluteus maximus, quadriceps, hamstrings, soleus, gastrocnemius **Kettlebell and sandbag overhead lunge:** Gluteus maximus, hamstrings, quadriceps, soleus, gastrocnemius, erector spinae, trapezius, deltoids **Medicine ball overhead lunge:** Gluteus maximus, hamstrings, quadriceps, erector spinae, trapezius, deltoids	87
Dumbbell lateral lunge (with medicine ball overhead lateral lunge variation)	**Dumbbell lateral lunge:** Gluteus maximus and medius, quadriceps, hamstrings, soleus, gastrocnemius **Medicine ball overhead lateral lunge:** Gluteus maximus, hamstrings, quadriceps, gluteus minimus, erector spinae, trapezius, deltoids	90
Dumbbell backward lunge (with medicine ball overhead backward lunge variation)	**Dumbbell backward lunge:** Gluteus maximus, quadriceps, hamstrings, soleus, gastrocnemius **Medicine ball overhead backward lunge:** Gluteus maximus, hamstrings, quadriceps, erector spinae, trapezius, deltoids	92
Kettlebell deadlift (with sandbag deadlift variation)	Gluteus maximus, quadriceps, hamstrings, erector spinae, quadratus lumborum	94
Kettlebell straight-leg deadlift (with resistance band straight-leg deadlift and sandbag straight-leg deadlift variations)	Gluteus maximus, erector spinae, hamstrings	95

Exercise name	Muscle(s) used	Page number
Dumbbell one-leg straight-leg deadlift (with kettlebell one-leg straight-leg deadlift variation)	Gluteus maximus, erector spinae, hamstrings	97
Farmer's walk (with sandbag farmer's walk variation)	Gluteus maximus, quadriceps, hamstrings, grip strength, core	98
Dumbbell hip thrust	Gluteus maximus, gluteus medius, hamstrings	100
Resistance band forward walk	Gluteus medius, gluteus minimus, tensor fasciae latae	101
Resistance band lateral walk	Gluteus maximus, gluteus medius, gluteus minimus	102
Suspension one-leg squat	Gluteus maximus, gluteus medius, gluteus minimus, quadriceps, hamstrings, core	103
Suspension hip bridge	Gluteus maximus, hamstrings, core	104
Suspension backward lunge	Gluteus maximus, quadriceps, hamstrings, core	105
Suspension leg curl	Gluteus maximus, quadriceps, hamstrings, core	106

DUMBBELL SQUAT

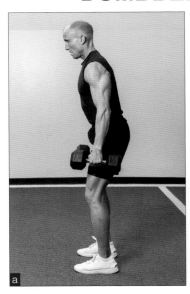 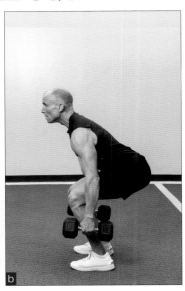

Fundamentals

- Capability to perform a squat with full range of motion, driving through the balls of the feet
- Sufficient core stability

Setup

- Select two dumbbells of equal weight, holding them with a neutral grip (palms facing in).
- Position your feet between hip- and shoulder-width apart, pointing forward or just slightly outward.
- Hang the dumbbells at your sides with your arms straight.
- Maintain an erect torso, with the chest up, shoulders back, head and neck straight, and eyes looking straight ahead.
- Before beginning the initial descent, inhale.

Downward Movement

- Maintain a flat back; flex your knees and hips in a controlled manner while keeping your bodyweight on the balls of the feet.
- Keep your knees aligned above or slightly in front of your ankles, but behind the tips of your toes, throughout the downward movement.
- Continue the downward movement until the backs of your thighs are parallel to the floor, or when your heels begin to lift off the floor.
- When you reach the bottom position, avoid bouncing or increasing the rate of the downward movement before beginning the upward movement.

Upward Movement

- Lift the dumbbells forcefully and with control by pushing through the balls of your feet and extending your knees and hips. Keep your back flat, your arms at your sides, your head and neck erect, and your eyes looking straight ahead.
- Keep your knees aligned above or slightly in front of your ankles.
- Continue the upward movement by extending your lower-body joints at a consistent rate until you reach the starting position.
- Exhale at the completion of the upward movement.
- Repeat for the desired length of time or number of repetitions.

Variations in Setup

For all of these variations, keep the following cues in mind:

- Maintain an erect torso with your chest up, your shoulders back, your head and neck straight, and your eyes looking straight ahead.
- Before beginning the initial descent, inhale.

Resistance Band Squat

- Stand in the middle of a large band, placing the balls of the your securely on the band and keeping your feet between hip- and shoulder-width apart and pointing forward or just slightly outward.
- Bring the band around the outsides of your feet.
- Lift the band up over the top of both shoulders and hold in a front-squat position.

Kettlebell Goblet Squat

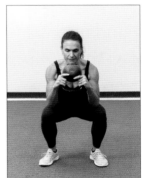

- Position your feet shoulder-width apart.
- Grip the kettlebell between your palms (with one hand on each side of kettlebell or the handle).
- Hold the kettlebell against your chest, with your elbows pointing down.
- Keep your weight on the balls of your feet.

Suspension Squat

- Adjust the suspension straps to a height at which your knee forms a 90-degree angle with the floor when you are in the bottom position, with your arms fully extended.
- Grasp the handles with a neutral or pronated grip.
- Step back to a point at which your arms are fully extended at shoulder level.
- Position your feet hip-width apart with a neutral spine, neck straight, and knees above the ankles.

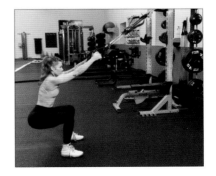

Sandbag Front Squat

- Position your feet shoulder-width apart.
- Grip the sandbag with a neutral grip.
- Hold the sandbag against your chest, with your elbows up.
- Keep your weight on the balls of your feet.

DUMBBELL SPLIT SQUAT

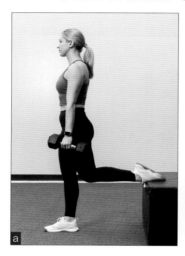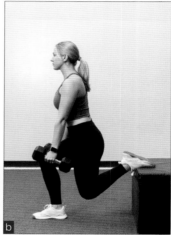

Fundamentals

- Capability to perform a squat with full range of motion, driving through the balls of the feet
- Sufficient core stability

Setup

- Standing in front of a bench or box, place the top of your back foot on top of it.
- Position your lead leg in front of the bench, with your knee aligned above your ankle.
- Keeping your arms straight, hold the dumbbells firmly at your sides.
- Your torso should remain erect.
- Before beginning the downward movement, inhale.

Downward Movement

- Lower your hips and flex your lead leg in a controlled manner.
- Keep your leading knee aligned above your ankle throughout the downward movement.
- Maintain a flat back.
- Continue the downward movement until the thigh of your lead leg is parallel to the floor and the knee of your back leg nearly reaches the floor.
- When you reach the bottom position of the downward movement, avoid bouncing or increasing the rate of movement before beginning the upward movement.

Upward Movement

- Extend the knee and hip of your lead leg.
- Keep your back flat.
- Continue the upward movement by extending your lower-body joints at a consistent rate until you reach the initial starting position.
- Exhale at the top of the upward movement.
- Repeat for the desired length of time or number of repetitions on each leg.

KETTLEBELL OVERHEAD SQUAT

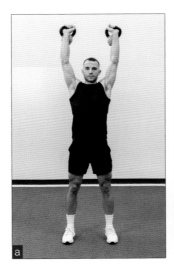
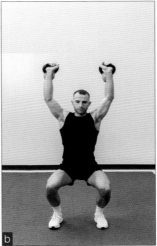

Fundamentals

- Capability to perform a squat with full range of motion, driving through the balls of the feet Sufficient core stability
- Enough strength and flexibility to hold two kettlebells, a resistance band, a medicine ball, or a sandbag overhead

Setup

- Select two kettlebells of equal weight and hold their handles with a neutral grip.
- Position your feet between hip- and shoulder-width apart, pointing forward or just slightly outward.
- Lift the kettlebells overhead, keeping your arms straight.
- Maintain an erect torso, with your chest up, your shoulders back, your head and neck straight, and your eyes looking straight ahead.
- Before beginning the initial descent, inhale.

Downward Movement

- Maintain a flat back, flex your knees and hips in a controlled manner while keeping your bodyweight on the balls of your feet.
- Keep your knees aligned above or slightly in front of your ankles throughout the downward movement.
- Continue the downward movement until the backs of your thighs are parallel to the floor, or until your heels begin to lift off the floor.
- When you reach the bottom position of the downward movement, avoid bouncing or increasing the rate of downward movement before beginning the upward movement.

Upward Movement

- Lift the kettlebells forcefully and with control by pushing through the balls of your feet, extending your knees and hips while keeping your back flat, your arms overhead, your head and neck erect, and your eyes looking straight ahead.
- Keep your knees aligned above or slightly in front of your ankles.
- Continue the upward movement by extending your lower-body joints at a consistent rate until you reach the starting position.
- Exhale at the top of the upward movement.
- Repeat for the desired length of time or number of repetitions.

Variations in Setup and Movement

For all of these variations, keep the following cues in mind:

- Maintain an erect torso, with your chest up, your shoulders back, your head and neck straight, and your eyes looking straight ahead.
- Before beginning the initial descent, inhale.
- Keep your knees above or slightly in front of your ankles throughout the downward movement.
- Continue the downward movement until the backs of your thighs are parallel to the floor, or until your heels begin to lift off the floor.
- When you reach the bottom position of the downward movement, avoid bouncing or increasing the rate of downward movement before beginning the upward movement.
- During the upward movement, keep your knees positioned above or slightly in front of your ankles.
- Continue the upward movement by extending your lower-body joints at a consistent rate until you reach the starting position.
- Exhale at the top of the upward movement.
- Repeat for the desired length of time or number of repetitions.

Resistance Band Overhead Squat

- Stand in the middle of a large band by placing the balls of your feet securely on the band, keeping your feet between hip- and shoulder-width apart and pointing forward or just slightly outward.
- Bring the band around the outsides of your feet.
- Lift the band up over the tops of both shoulders and hold the sides of the band three feet apart above your head.

- Keep the band in line with your upper back and traps. Ideally, the band should form a perfect 90-degree angle with the floor.
- During the downward movement, maintain a flat back, flex your knees and hips in a controlled manner, and keep your bodyweight on the balls of your feet and securely on the band.
- Ensure that your arms do not move forward and that the band stays vertical (not angled too far forward or backward) as you move downward.
- Both of your knees should remain inside the band as you squat.
- During the upward movement, keep the band in the overhead position and lift forcefully but in a controlled manner by pushing through the balls of your feet and extending your knees and hips. Keep your back flat, your arms overhead, your head and neck erect, and your eyes looking straight ahead.
- Repeat for the desired length of time or number of repetitions.

Medicine Ball Overhead Squat

- Select a medicine ball of an appropriate weight and hold it with a neutral grip, with your hands on either side of the ball.
- Keep your feet between hip- and shoulder-width apart, pointing forward or just slightly outward.
- Lift the medicine ball overhead and straighten your arms.
- Keep your back flat, flex your knees and hips in a controlled manner, and keep your bodyweight on the balls of your feet.
- Lift the medicine ball forcefully and with control by pushing through the balls of your feet and extending your knees and hips. Keep your back flat, your arms overhead, your head and neck erect, and your eyes looking straight ahead.
- Repeat for the desired length of time or number of repetitions.

Sandbag Overhead Squat

- Select a sandbag of an appropriate weight and hold the handles with a neutral grip.
- Keep your feet between hip- and shoulder-width apart, pointing forward or just slightly outward.
- Lift the sandbag overhead and straighten your arms.
- Maintain a flat back, flex your knees and hips in a controlled manner, and keep your bodyweight on the balls of your feet.
- Lift the sandbag forcefully and with control by pushing through the balls of your feet and extending your knees and hips. Keep your back flat, your arms overhead, your head and neck erect, and your eyes looking straight ahead.
- Repeat for the desired length of time or number of repetitions.

DUMBBELL BOX STEP-UP

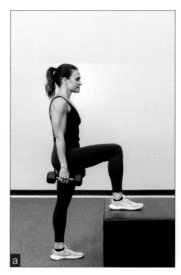
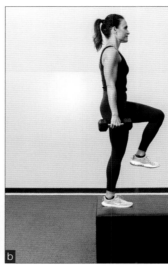

Fundamentals

- Capability to perform a squat with full range of motion, driving through the balls of the feet
- Sufficient core stability

Setup

- Choose a box or a bench with a stable surface that is knee height or lower, depending on your range of motion.
- Choose an appropriate set of dumbbells of equal weight and hold them at the sides of your body.
- Face the box, maintaining an upright posture, with your abs drawn in.
- Inhale prior to starting the movement.

Upward Movement

- Starting with your right leg, step up and place your right foot firmly on top of the box.
- Using your right leg, push through the ball of the foot to lift yourself onto the box.
- Maintain an erect body position and keep your hips square; your right leg should extend without going into hyperextension.
- Lift your left leg so your left foot reaches a height even with your right knee, but does not touch the box.

Downward Movement

- Return your left leg to the floor, keeping all of your weight on the right leg.
- Continue holding an upright posture as you return the left leg to the floor.
- Once your left foot is firmly placed on the floor behind the box, bring your right leg down so you are back in your starting position.
- Exhale at the completion of the movement.
- Complete the desired number of reps on your right leg and then switch to your left leg for the desired number of reps.

Variations in Fundamentals, Setup, and Movements

Medicine Ball Overhead Box Step-Up

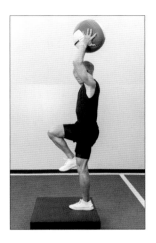

Fundamentals

- This exercise uses the same fundamentals as the box step-up, with the addition of the following: Enough strength and flexibility to hold a medicine ball overhead

Setup

- Select a medicine ball of an appropriate weight and hold it with a neutral grip, with your hands on either side of the ball.
- Position your feet between hip- and shoulder-width apart, pointing forward or just slightly outward.
- Lift the medicine ball overhead and straighten your arms.
- Maintain an erect torso, with your chest up, your shoulders back, your head and neck straight, and your eyes looking straight ahead.
- Before beginning the initial descent, inhale.

Movement

- Use the same movement cues as the box step-up in addition to the following: Continue holding the same upright body position with the medicine ball overhead as you return your left leg to the floor.

DUMBBELL FRONT LUNGE

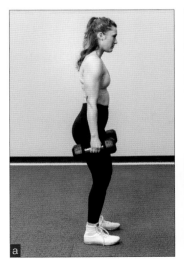 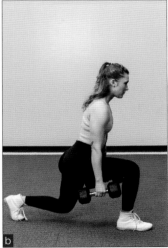

Fundamentals

- Capability to perform a lunge with full range of motion, driving through the balls of the feet
- Sufficient core stability

Setup

- Select two dumbbells of equal weight and hold them with a neutral grip.
- Position your feet between hip- and shoulder-width apart and point them forward.
- Maintain an erect torso, with your chest out and up, your shoulders back, your head and neck straight, and your eyes looking straight ahead.
- Before stepping forward, inhale.

Forward Movement

- Take an elongated step straight forward with one leg (lead leg), keeping your arms straight at your sides.
- Maintain an erect torso, with your shoulders aligned directly above your hips and your head held straight and facing forward as you step forward with the lead foot and it comes into contact with the floor on the ball of the foot, with the foot pointing straightforward.
- Your back leg remains in the setup position, but as your lead leg moves forward and your balance shifts to the ball of the foot, your back leg will begin to flex.
- You have reached the finish position of the forward movement when your back knee flexes 1 to 2 inches (2.5 to 5.0 centimeters) off the floor and when your lead leg is flexed to 90 degrees, with your lead knee aligned directly above or slightly in front of your ankle.
- At the completion of the forward movement, push back on your back leg.

Backward Movement

- Forcefully push off the floor with your lead foot by plantar flexing (extending the ankle) while also extending your lead knee and hip joints.
- As your lead foot returns to the starting position, your balance should shift to your back foot, resulting in your back foot regaining full contact with the floor.
- Your lead foot should return to its starting position: both feet should now be between hip- and shoulder-width apart and pointing forward. Avoid touching your lead foot to the floor until it has returned to the finish position. Once your lead foot has returned to the starting position, divide your bodyweight equally between both feet.
- Exhale at the completion of the backward movement.
- Repeat the exercise for a designated number of repetitions or length of time.

Variations in Fundamentals, Setup, and Movements

Kettlebell Overhead Lunge

Use the fundamentals, setup, and movement cues from the lunge exercise as well as the following:

Fundamentals

- Enough strength and flexibility to hold two kettlebells overhead

Setup

- Select two kettlebells of equal weight and grab them with a pronated grip (palms facing forward).
- Lift the kettlebells overhead and straighten your arms.

Forward Movement

- Take an elongated step straight forward with one leg (lead leg) while holding the kettlebells overhead.
- You have reached the finish position of the forward movement when your back knee is 1 to 2 inches (2.5 to 5.0 centimeters) off the floor, your lead leg is flexed to 90 degrees, and your lead knee is directly above or slightly in front of your ankle. The kettlebells should remain overhead through the entire movement.

Medicine Ball Overhead Lunge

Fundamentals

- Enough strength and flexibility to hold a medicine ball overhead

Setup

- Select a medicine ball of an appropriate weight and hold it with neutral grip overhead, keeping your arms straight.

Forward Movement

- Take an elongated step straight forward with one leg (lead leg) while holding the medicine ball overhead.
- You have reached the finish position of the forward movement you're your back knee is 1 to 2– inches (2.5 to 5.0 centimeters) off the floor, your lead leg is flexed to 90 degrees, and your lead knee is directly above or slightly in front of your ankle.

Sandbag Overhead Lunge

Fundamentals

- Enough strength and flexibility to hold sandbag overhead

Setup

- Select a sandbag of an appropriate weight and hold it with a pronated grip.
- Lift the sandbag overhead and straighten your arms.

Forward Movement

- Take an elongated step straight forward with one leg (lead leg) while holding sandbag overhead.
- You have reached the finish position of the forward movement when your back knee is 1 to 2 inches (2.5 to 5.0 centimeters) off the floor, your lead leg is flexed to 90 degrees, and your lead knee is directly above or slightly in front of your ankle.

DUMBBELL LATERAL LUNGE

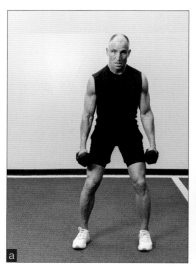
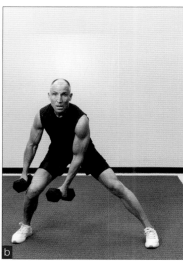

Fundamentals

- Capability to perform a lateral lunge with full range of motion
- Sufficient core stability

Setup

- Select two dumbbells of equal weight and hold them with a neutral grip.
- Position your feet hip-width apart and pointing forward, keeping your torso erect, your chest out and up, your shoulders back, your head and neck straight, and your eyes looking straight ahead.
- Before stepping laterally, inhale.

Lateral Movement

- Take an elongated step laterally (sideways) with one leg (lead leg), keeping the foot of your other leg flat on the floor and pointed straight forward.
- Keep your arms straight, with the dumbbells held at the sides, as your lead leg steps laterally and comes into contact with the floor.
- As your lead leg moves laterally, your balance should shift to the ball of your planted foot.
- Maintain an erect torso, with your shoulders aligned directly above the hips and the head erect and facing forward.
- You have reached the finish position when your lead leg is flexed to 90 degrees and your lead knee is directly above or slightly in front of your ankle. Your weight should be on the ball of your lead foot.

Return Movement

- Shift your balance back to your planted foot and forcefully push off the floor with the ball of your lead foot while extending your lead knee and hip joints.
- As your lead foot returns to the starting position, keep your balance on your planted foot until your lead foot regains full contact with the floor.
- Avoid touching your lead foot to the floor until it has returned to the finish position (unless balance is lost).
- Once your lead foot has returned to the starting position, divide your body-weight equally between both feet.
- Exhale at the completion of the return movement.
- Perform the desired length of time or number of repetitions for each leg.

Variations in Fundamentals, Setup, and Movements

Medicine Ball Overhead Lateral Lunge

Perform the overhead lateral lunge using the cues from the lateral lunge in addition to the following:

Fundamentals

- Enough strength and flexibility to hold a medicine ball overhead

Set Up

- Select a medicine ball of an appropriate weight and hold it with neutral grip overhead.
- Maintain an erect torso, with your chest up, your shoulders back, your head and neck straight, and your eyes looking straight ahead.

Lateral Movement

- As your lead leg moves laterally, your balance should shift to the ball of your planted foot. Keep the medicine ball directly overhead throughout the movement.

Return Movement

- Forcefully push off the floor with the ball of your lead foot while extending your lead knee and hip joints and holding the medicine ball overhead.

DUMBBELL BACKWARD LUNGE

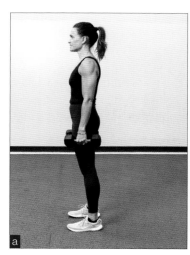 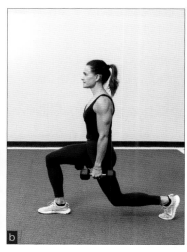

Fundamentals

- Capability to perform a backward lunge with full range of motion, driving through the balls of the feet
- Sufficient core stability

Setup

- Select two dumbbells of equal weight and hold them with a neutral grip.
- Position your feet between hip- and shoulder-width apart and point them forward.
- Maintain an erect torso, with your chest out and up, your shoulders back, your head and neck straight, and your eyes looking straight ahead.
- Before stepping backward, inhale.

Backward Movement

- Take an elongated step straight backward with one leg (back leg).
- Keep your arms straight, with the dumbbells held firmly at your sides, and your torso erect as the trail foot goes backward and meets the floor.
- Your front leg (lead leg) will remain in the starting position, and as your back leg moves backward and flexes, your balance should shift to the ball of your back foot.
- To maintain balance, ensure that your back leg moves directly backward from its original starting position.
- Keeping your torso erect, your shoulders aligned directly above your hips, and your head erect and facing forward, flex your lead knee to enable your back leg to bend toward the floor.
- You have reached the finish position when your back leg is 1 to 2 inches (2.5 to 5.0 centimeters) above the floor, your lead leg is flexed to 90 degrees, and your lead knee is aligned directly above or slightly in front of your ankle.
- At the completion of the backward movement, make a concentrated effort to "sit back" on your back leg, as if sitting on the front edge of a bench.

Forward Movement

- While maintaining an erect torso, shift your balance back to the lead foot and forcefully push off the floor with your back foot by plantar flexing while extending your lead knee and hip joints.
- Your back foot should then return to its starting position, with both feet between hip- and shoulder-width apart and pointing forward.
- Avoid touching your back foot to the floor until it is returned to the finish position (unless balance is lost).
- Exhale at the completion of the forward movement.
- Perform for the desired length of time or number of repetitions on each leg.

Variations in Fundamentals, Setup, and Movements

Medicine Ball Overhead Backward Lunge

Perform this exercise using the backward lunge cues in addition to the following:

Fundamentals

- Enough strength and flexibility to hold a medicine ball overhead

Setup

- Select a medicine ball of an appropriate weight and hold it with a neutral grip.
- Lift the medicine ball overhead and straighten your arms.
- Before beginning the backward movement, inhale.

Backward Movement

- Maintain an erect torso as the back foot moves backward and meets the floor.
- Keep your lead leg in the starting position as the back leg moves backward.
- Keeping your torso erect, with your shoulders aligned directly above your hips and your head erect and facing forward, flex your lead knee to enable your back leg to bend toward the floor, keeping the medicine ball overhead.
- You have reached the finish position when your back leg is 1 to 2 inches (2.5 to 5.0 centimeters) from the floor, your lead leg is flexed to 90 degrees, and your lead knee is directly above or slightly in front of your ankle.
- At the completion of the backward movement, make a concentrated effort to sit back on your back leg, as if sitting on the front edge of a bench.

Forward Movement

- Maintaining an erect torso and keeping medicine ball overhead, shift your balance back to the lead foot and forcefully push off the floor with the back foot by plantar flexing and extending your lead knee and hip joints.
- Repeat for the desired length of time or number of repetitions.

KETTLEBELL DEADLIFT

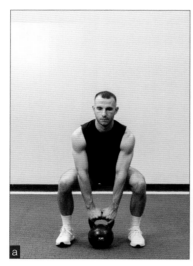 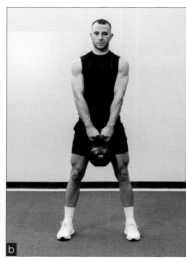

Fundamentals

- Capability to perform a squat with full range of motion
- Sufficient core stability

Setup

- Stand centered directly above one kettlebell on the floor, with your feet shoulder-width apart.
- Stabilize your core using correct body alignment.
- Keeping your weight on the balls of your feet, squat and grab the kettlebell with a two-handed pronated grip.
- Stand back up while keeping your arms straight.
- Maintain an erect torso, with your chest up, your shoulders back, your head and neck straight, and your eyes looking straight ahead.
- Before beginning the initial ascent, inhale.

Upward Movement

- Lift the kettlebell forcefully but in a controlled manner by pushing through the balls of your feet and extending your knees and hips. Keep your back flat, your head and neck erect, and your eyes looking straight ahead.
- Keep your knees aligned above to slightly in front of your ankles.
- Continue the upward movement by extending your lower-body joints at a consistent rate until you return to your original standing position.
- Exhale at the completion of the upward movement.

Downward Movement

- Keep your back flat, flex your knees and hips in a controlled manner, and keep your body-weight on the balls of your feet.
- Keep your knees above or slightly in front of your ankles throughout the downward movement.

- Continue the downward movement until the backs of your thighs are parallel to the floor, your heels begin to lift off the floor, and the kettlebell reaches the floor.
- When you reach the bottom position of the downward movement. avoid bouncing or increasing the rate of downward movement before beginning the upward movement.
- Repeat for the desired length of time or number of repetitions.

Variations in Setup and Upward Movement

Sandbag Deadlift

Setup

- Stand centered above the sandbag on the floor with your feet shoulder-width apart.
- Keeping your weight on the balls of your feet, squat and grab the sandbag with a two-handed neutral grip.

Upward Movement

- Lift the sandbag forcefully but in a controlled manner by pushing through the balls of your feet and extending your knees and hips. Keep your back flat, your arms at your sides, your head and neck erect, and your eyes looking straight ahead.
- Repeat for the desired length of time or number of repetitions.

KETTLEBELL STRAIGHT-LEG DEADLIFT

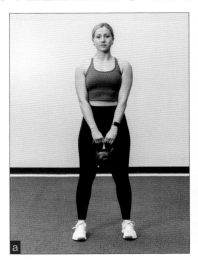
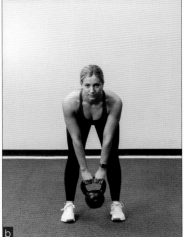

Fundamentals

- Sufficient core stability

Setup

- Hold a kettlebell with both hands using a pronated grip, resting it on the front of your thighs.
- Position your feet shoulder-width apart.
- Maintain an erect torso, with your chest up, your shoulders back, your head and neck straight, and your eyes looking straight ahead.
- Inhale prior to starting the downward movement.

Downward Movement

- Keeping your bodyweight on the balls of your feet, flex your knees slightly.
- Push your hips backward while simultaneously hinging at your hips to bend forward, allowing the kettlebell to slide down your thighs to the middle of your shins and keeping your torso parallel to the floor.

Upward Movement

- Push through the balls of your feet and return to the starting position, extending from your hips while maintaining a slight flex in your knees.
- Exhale at the completion of the upward movement.
- Repeat for the desired length of time or number of repetitions.

Variations in Setup and Movement

Use the following cues for each of these variations:

- Flex your knees slightly and push your hips backward while hinging at your hips to bend forward, allowing your hands to align with the middle of your shins and keeping your torso parallel to the floor.
- Before beginning the upward movement, inhale.
- For the upward movement, extend your hips and, hinging at your hips, come to an upright position with a slight flex in your knees.
- Exhale at the completion of the upward movement.

Resistance Band Straight-Leg Deadlift

- Stand in the middle of a large band, placing the balls of your feet securely on the band with your feet between hip- and shoulder-width apart and pointing forward or just slightly outward.
- Bring the band around the outsides of your feet.
- Grab both ends of the resistance band, one in each hand on the outsides of your legs, while keeping the band firmly and securely under your feet.
- Repeat for the desired length of time or number of repetitions.

Sandbag Straight-Leg Deadlift

- Hold a sandbag with both hands using a neutral grip.
- Position your feet shoulder-width apart.
- Hold the sandbag in front of your body, resting it on your thighs.
- Maintain an erect torso, with your chest up, your shoulders back, your head and neck straight, and your eyes looking straight ahead.
- Keeping your bodyweight on the balls of your feet, flex your knees slightly.
- For the downward movement, push your hips backward while hinging at your hips and bending forward, allowing the sandbag to slide down your thighs to the middle of your shins and keeping your torso parallel to the floor.
- Repeat for the desired length of time or number of repetitions.

DUMBBELL ONE-LEG STRAIGHT-LEG DEADLIFT

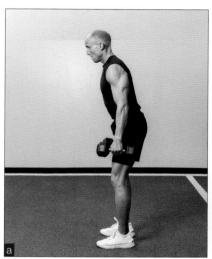 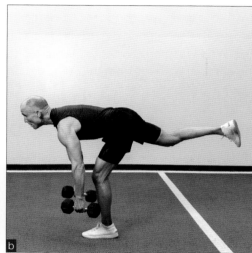

Fundamentals

- Capability to perform a straight leg deadlift with full range of motion, driving through the balls of the feet
- Ability to balance on one leg

Setup

- Select two dumbbells of equal weight and hold them with a neutral grip.
- Position your feet between hip- and shoulder-width apart and pointing forward.
- Your torso should remain erect, your chest out and up, your shoulders back, your head and neck straight, and your eyes looking straight ahead.
- Before initiating the exercise, inhale.

Downward Movement

- Flex your support leg at the knee before initiating the downward movement.
- Keeping your torso erect and your support knee slightly flexed. Hinge forward at the waist while lifting the non-support leg toward the rear, keeping it straight and in line with the torso, and lowering the dumbbells toward the floor in a slow and controlled manner.
- Keep your arms straight and hold the dumbbells along the support leg as you lower your torso toward the floor. The arm opposite your support leg should bring the dumbbell to the inside of your support leg, and the arm on the same side as your support leg should bring the dumbbell to the outside of your support leg.
- Continue flexing your hips and torso until the weights reach the midpoint of your shins or slightly below.
- Keep the weights close to the inside and outside of your support leg throughout the downward movement.

Upward Movement

- Slowly return your non-support leg back to the starting position while bringing the weights back up the inside and outside of your support leg.
- Keep your torso erect and your elbows extended.
- Once your non-support leg has returned to its starting position, stand erect.
- Exhale at the completion of the ascent.
- Repeat for the desired length of time or number of repetitions.

Variations in Setup and Downward Movement

Kettlebell One-Leg Straight-Leg Deadlift

Use the setup and movement cues for the dumbbell one-leg straight-leg deadlift as well as the following:

Setup

- Select two kettlebells of equal weight and hold them with a neutral grip.

Downward Movement

- Hinge forward at the waist while lifting your non-support leg to the rear, keeping it in line with your torso as you lower the kettlebells toward the floor in a slow and controlled manner.
- Keep your arms straight and hold the kettlebells on either side of your support leg as you lower your torso toward the floor. The arm opposite your support leg should bring the kettlebell to the inside of your support leg, and the arm on the same side as your support leg should bring the kettlebell to the outside of your support leg.
- Repeat for the desired length of time or number of repetitions.

FARMER'S WALK

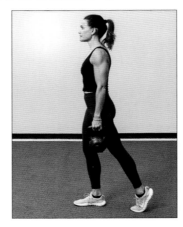

Fundamentals

- Capability to perform a deadlift
- Sufficient core stability
- Enough grip and upper- and lower-body strength to lift and carry two kettlebells

Setup

- Position two kettlebells of equal weight outside each foot.
- Stabilize your core using correct body alignment.
- Keeping your weight on the balls of your feet, squat and grab the kettlebells with a neutral grip (palms facing in) and keep the kettlebells outside each leg.
- Stand while keeping your arms straightened.
- Maintain an erect torso, with your chest up, your shoulders back, your head and neck straight, and your eyes looking straight ahead.
- Before beginning the movement forward, inhale.

Movement

- Walk 10 to 20 yards (9.1 to 18.3 meters) forward while holding a kettlebell in each hand.
- Turn around and walk back to the starting position before returning the kettlebells to the ground.

Variations in Fundamentals, Setup, and Movement

Sandbag Farmer's Walk

Fundamentals

- Enough grip and upper- and lower-body strength to lift and carry a sandbag

Setup

- Position two sandbags of equal weight outside each leg.
- Keeping your weight on the ball of your feet, squat and grab each sandbag with a neutral grip

Movement

- Walk 15 to 25 yards (13.7 to 22.9 meters) forward while holding the sandbags in each hand.
- Turn around and walk back to the starting position before returning the sandbags to the ground.
- Repeat the exercise for a designated number of repetitions or length of time.

DUMBBELL HIP THRUST

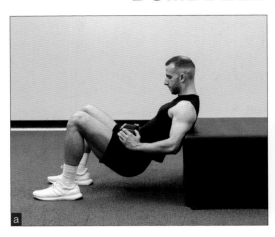 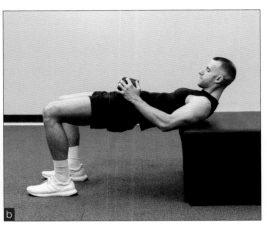

Fundamentals

- Capability to perform 10 bodyweight hip thrusts

Setup

- Bend the knees to 90 degrees and secure the upper back across an 18-inch (45.7-centimeter) plyometric box or bench.
- Place a dumbbell horizontally across your hips.
- Lower the buttocks until they are slightly off the floor.
- Before beginning the upward movement, inhale.

Upward Movement

- Lift your hips up until they are at the same height as your thighs and knees.
- Exhale at the completion of the upward movement.

Downward Movement

- While keeping your bodyweight on the balls of your feet, return your buttocks to the starting position, slightly off the floor.
- Repeat for the desired length of time or number of repetitions.

RESISTANCE BAND FORWARD WALK

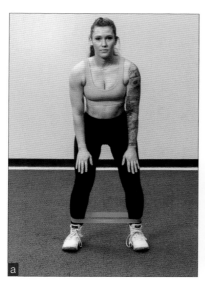 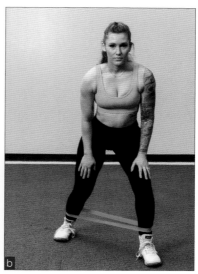

Fundamentals

- Capability to stand and maintain balance with the feet close together

Setup

- Place a mini band around your ankles.
- Stand with your feet hip-width apart and slightly flex your knees.

Movement

- With a slight flexion at your hips, take a wide step forward with one foot while keeping the band tight around your ankles.
- Then take a wide step forward with the other foot, so that it is level with the first foot. Maintain tension in the band.
- Move forward in this manner for 10 to 15 yards (9.1 to 13.7 meters) before turning around and repeating the steps to return to your starting position.

RESISTANCE BAND LATERAL WALK

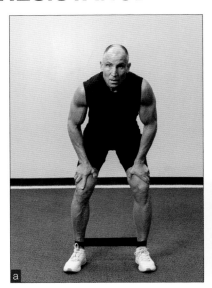 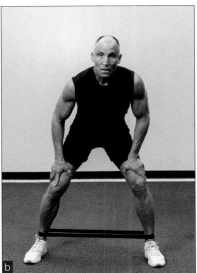

Fundamentals

- Capability to stand and maintain balance with your feet close together

Setup

- Place a mini band around both of your ankles.
- Stand with your feet hip-distance apart and slightly flex your knees.

Movement

- Utilizing your buttocks and outer thighs while slightly flexing at your hips, step sideways with one lead foot, so that the feet are shoulder-width apart.
- Then step in the same direction with the second foot, returning the feet to hip-width and keeping the band taut.
- Move sideways in this manner for 10 to 15 yards (9.1 to 13.7 meters) before returning to the starting location by using the opposite leg as the lead leg.

SUSPENSION ONE-LEG SQUAT

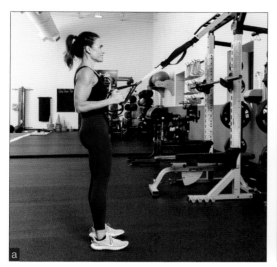 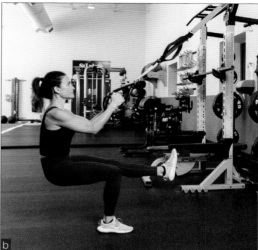

Fundamentals

- Capability to perform 20 suspension squats

Setup

- Adjust the suspension straps to a height where the angle of your knee forms a 90-degree angle with the floor when in bottom position, with your arms fully extended.
- Grasp the handles with a neutral or pronated grip.
- Step back to a point where your arms are fully extended at shoulder level.
- Position your feet hip-width apart, maintaining a neutral spine and a straight neck, and keeping your knees above your ankles.

Movement

- Keeping your bodyweight on the ball of the exercise foot, lift the opposite leg off the ground.
- Extend your hips back and flex at the exercise knee, maintaining a neutral spine and keeping the exercise knee aligned above or slightly in front of your ankle as you descend toward the floor.
- Continue the descent until your knee reaches a 90-degree angle.
- Reverse direction and return to the starting position.
- Repeat for the desired length of time or number of repetitions and do the same with the opposite leg.

SUSPENSION HIP BRIDGE

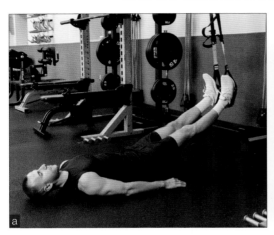 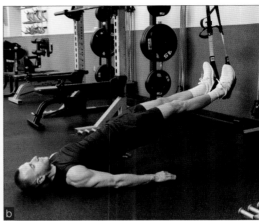

Fundamentals

- Capability to perform 10 bodyweight hip bridges

Setup

- Adjust the suspension straps to a height at which both of your heels can be placed in the foot straps and your body is in a supine incline position on the floor from your head to the backs of your upper thighs.
- Lie in a supine position and position your heels in the foot straps directly under the handles.

Movement

- Keeping your feet close together, lift your hips off the ground, maintaining a neutral spine and straight legs.
- Lower yourself back to the starting position.
- Repeat for the desired length of time or number of repetitions.

SUSPENSION BACKWARD LUNGE

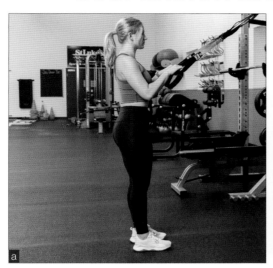 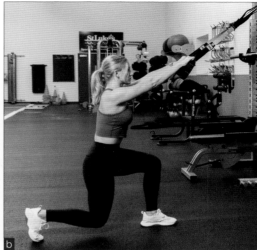

Fundamentals

- Capability to perform 10 bodyweight backward lunges with each leg

Setup

- Adjust the suspension straps to a height at which your front knee forms a 90-degree angle when in the bottom position, with your arms fully extended.
- Grasp the handles with a neutral or pronated grip.
- Step back to a point at which your arms are fully extended at shoulder level.
- Position your feet hip-width apart, maintaining a neutral spine and a straight neck, and keeping your knees above your ankles.

Movement

- Keeping your bodyweight on the balls of your feet, take a medium-to-large step back with your right foot and flex your right knee.
- Continue the descent until your knee reaches a 90-degree angle.
- Push off the ball of your left foot to return to a vertical position, and return your right leg to a position parallel to your left leg.
- Repeat the movement pattern, this time stepping back with your left foot.
- Repeat for the desired length of time or number of repetitions.

SUSPENSION LEG CURL

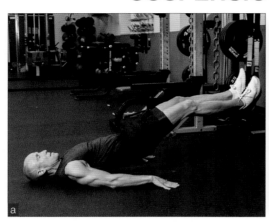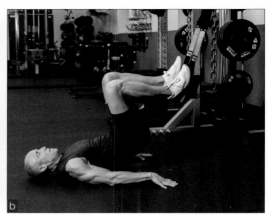

Fundamentals

- Capability to perform 10 bodyweight hip thrusts

Setup

- Lie in a supine position and place your heels in the foot straps directly under the handles.
- Adjust the suspension straps to a height at which both of your heels can be placed in the foot straps and your body is in an incline supine position on the floor from your head to the backs of your upper thighs.

Movement

- Keeping your feet close together, lift your hips off the ground, maintaining a neutral spine and straight leg position.
- While keeping your hips off the ground, pull the foot straps toward your buttocks by flexing at your knees.
- Extend your knees and lower back to return to the starting position.
- Repeat for the desired length of time or number of repetitions.

8

Upper-Body Exercises

A strong upper body enables you to perform daily tasks such as lifting, carrying, pushing, and pulling objects, maintaining control of them with your chest, upper back, shoulders, and arms. It also prevents injuries. Upper-body metabolic training enables you to increase your metabolism through improvements in lean body mass and increased caloric expenditure. Additionally, upper-body metabolic training increases cardiorespiratory fitness and bone health.

Upper-body metabolic training enables you to prevent injuries to the bones and connective tissues by developing practical strength that can be utilized in daily life when lifting, pushing, or pulling is required. An increase in upper-body strength enables you to walk and run faster by providing additional support to the lower body. Table 8.1 provides a listing of upper-body exercises.

Table 8.1 Upper-Body Exercises

Exercise name	Muscles used	Page number
Pull-up	Latissimus dorsi, trapezius, rhomboids, teres major, posterior deltoid, biceps brachii, brachialis, brachioradialis	110
Chin-up	Latissimus dorsi, trapezius, rhomboids, teres major, posterior deltoid, biceps brachii, brachialis, brachioradialis	111
Push-up (with medicine ball push-up, suspension elevated push-up, suspension push-up, and side push-up variations)	**Push-up, medicine ball push-up, and side-push up:** Pectoralis major, pectoralis minor, anterior deltoid, serratus anterior, triceps brachii; **Suspension elevated push-up and suspension push-up:** Pectoralis major, anterior deltoid, triceps, serratus anterior	112
Dip	Pectoralis major, pectoralis minor, anterior deltoid, serratus anterior, triceps brachii	114
Push-back	Pectoralis major, pectoralis minor, anterior deltoid, serratus anterior, triceps brachii	115
Y (with resistance band Y variation)	Rear deltoid, serratus anterior, triceps brachii	115
T (with resistance band T variation)	Rear deltoid, serratus anterior, triceps brachii	117
Triceps extension (with suspension triceps extension and sandbag overhead triceps extension variations)	Triceps brachii and core	118
Inverted biceps curl (with suspension biceps curl and sandbag biceps curl variations)	**Inverted biceps curl:** Biceps brachii and core; **suspension biceps curl and sandbag biceps curl:** Biceps brachii, brachialis, brachioradialis	120
Dumbbell bench press (with dumbbell alt-arm bench press variation)	**Dumbbell bench press:** Pectoralis major, pectoralis minor, anterior deltoid, serratus anterior, triceps brachii; **dumbbell alt-arm bench press:** Pectoralis major, pectoralis minor, anterior deltoid, serratus anterior, triceps brachii, core	122
Dumbbell incline press (with dumbbell alt-arm incline press variation)	**Dumbbell incline press:** Pectoralis major, pectoralis minor, deltoid, serratus anterior, triceps brachii; **dumbbell alt-arm incline press:** Pectoralis major, Pectoralis minor, deltoid, serratus anterior, triceps brachii, core	124
Fly (with suspension fly and suspension reverse fly variations)	**Fly:** Pectoralis major, pectoralis minor, deltoid, serratus anterior, triceps brachii; **Suspension fly:** Pectoralis major, anterior deltoid, triceps, serratus anterior; **Suspension reverse fly:** Trapezius, rhomboids, teres major, posterior deltoid	126
Pullover (with medicine ball pullover variation)	Latissimus dorsi, teres major, pectoralis major, pectoralis minor, posterior deltoid, serratus anterior, triceps brachii	128

Exercise name	Muscles used	Page number
Dumbbell one-arm row	Latissimus dorsi, trapezius, rhomboids, teres major, posterior deltoid, biceps brachii, brachialis, brachioradialis	129
Dumbbell renegade row	Latissimus dorsi, trapezius, rhomboids, teres major, posterior deltoid, biceps brachii, brachialis, brachioradialis, core	130
Dumbbell shoulder press (with resistance band shoulder press)	Anterior, medial and posterior deltoid; trapezius; serratus anterior; triceps brachii	131
Shoulder shrug	Trapezius, levator scapula, rhomboids	133
Dumbbell upright row (with resistance band upright row, suspension row, sandbag row, and sandbag upright row variations)	**Dumbbell upright row, resistance band upright row, and sandbag upright row:** Anterior, medial and posterior deltoid; trapezius, serratus anterior, brachialis, biceps brachii, brachioradialis; **suspension row, sandbag row:** latissimus dorsi, trapezius, rhomboids, teres major, posterior deltoid, biceps brachii, brachialis, brachioradialis	134
Dumbbell lateral raise (with resistance band lateral raise variation)	Anterior deltoid, trapezius, supraspinatus	137
Dumbbell front raise (with resistance band front raise variation)	Anterior deltoid, trapezius, supraspinatus, serratus anterior, rhomboids	138
Dumbbell bent-over raise	Infraspinatus, teres minor, trapezius, deltoids	140
Dumbbell supine triceps extension (with dumbbell one-arm triceps extension)	Triceps brachii	141
Dumbbell triceps kickback	Triceps brachii	143
Dumbbell alt-arm biceps curl	Biceps brachii, brachialis, brachioradialis	144
Dumbbell hammer curl (with resistance band hammer curl variation)	Biceps brachii, brachialis, brachioradialis	145
Dumbbell concentration curl	Biceps brachii, brachialis	146
Resistance band standing chest press (with resistance band standing row variation)	**Resistance band standing chest press:** Pectoralis major, Pectoralis minor, anterior deltoid, serratus anterior, triceps brachii; **resistance band standing row variation:** latissimus dorsi, trapezius, rhomboids, teres major, posterior deltoid, biceps brachii, brachialis, brachioradialis, core	147
Resistance band triceps pushdown	Triceps brachii	149
Medicine ball chest pass	Wrist supinator and pronator; pectoralis major; pectoralis minor; anterior, medial, and posterior deltoid; triceps brachii; quadriceps;	150
Decline push-up	Pectoralis major, anterior deltoid, triceps, serratus anterior	151

PULL-UP

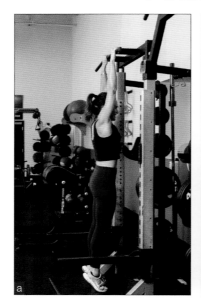 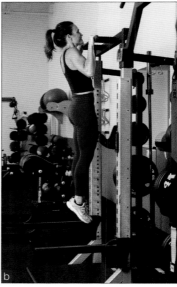

Fundamentals

- Basic upper-body (upper back, shoulders, and biceps) strength and endurance

Setup

- Step up onto a stable box.
- Extend arms and grasp the pull-up bar with a closed, pronated grip, with your hands slightly wider than shoulder-width apart.

Upward Movement

- Begin the upward movement by adducting your scapulae and upper arms.
- While pulling upward, your elbows should move down and back as your chest moves up and out.
- Pull upward until your chin passes the bar.
- Your torso should be leaning back slightly at the completion of the upward movement.
- Your lower body should remain fixed, with your knees straight throughout the upward movement.
- Avoid quickly leaning back farther or jerking your torso to pull yourself upward.

Downward Movement

- Return in a controlled manner to the starting position.
- Avoid extending your arms too rapidly during the downward movement.
- Repeat for the desired length of time or number of repetitions.

CHIN-UP

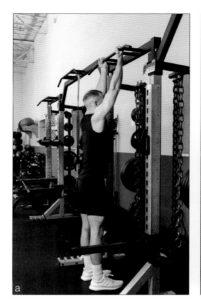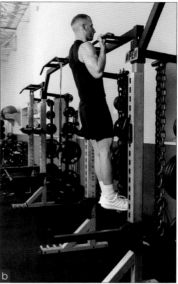

Fundamentals

- Basic upper-body strength and endurance

Setup

- Step up onto a stable box.
- Extend your arms and grasp the pull-up bar with a shoulder-width, closed, supinated grip.

Upward Movement

- Begin the upward movement by adducting your scapulae and flexing your elbows.
- While pulling yourself upward, your elbows should move down and along your sides, and your chest should move up and out.
- Continue pulling yourself upward until your chin reaches a level above the bar.
- Your torso should be leaning back slightly at the completion of the upward movement.
- Your lower body should remain fixed, with your knees straight throughout the upward movement.
- Avoid quickly leaning back farther or jerking your torso to help pull yourself upward.

Downward Movement

- Return in a controlled manner to the starting position.
- Avoid extending your arms too rapidly during the downward movement.
- Repeat for the desired length of time or number of repetitions.

PUSH-UP

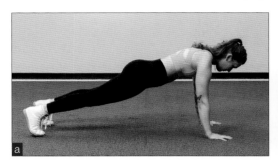 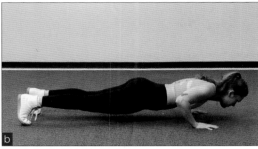

Fundamentals

- Basic upper-body strength and endurance (chest, shoulders, and triceps)

Setup

- Position your body in a plank position (your body should be in a straight line and balanced on your hands and toes, with your hands aligned directly under your shoulders and your feet hip-width apart).

Downward Movement

- Maintain a firm torso and lower your chest, hips, and trunk simultaneously toward the ground by bending your elbows until your upper arms become parallel to the ground.

Upward Movement

- Extend your elbows and press your body back up to the starting position, using your chest, shoulders, and triceps.
- Repeat for the desired length of time or number of repetitions.

Variations in Fundamentals, Setup, and Movements

Medicine Ball Push-Up

Fundamentals

- Ability to perform 15 standard push-ups with proper form

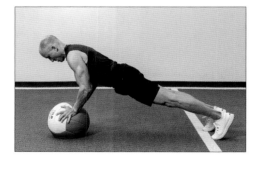

Setup and Movements

- Start in a plank position.
- Place both hands on a medicine ball aligned directly below your shoulders.
- Begin in the up position. Inhale before starting the downward movement.
- Keeping a firm torso, lower your body toward the medicine ball by bending your elbows until your chest touches the ball.
- Press back up until your arms are fully extended; maintain a firm torso.
- Repeat for the desired length of time or number of repetitions.

Suspension Elevated Push-Up

Fundamentals

- Ability to perform 10 bodyweight push-ups

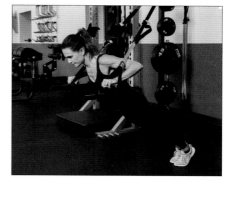

Setup and Movements

- Adjust the suspension straps to a height at which your body forms a 30- (more advanced) to 45-degree angle with floor when in the prone bottom position.
- Grasp the handles with a prone grip and position the straps underneath your arms.
- Position your body so that your body forms a slight angle with the floor.
- Lower your body in a controlled manner by flexing at your elbows, while maintaining a stable core and flat back, until your body forms a 30- to 45-degree angle with the floor. Reverse directions and return to the starting position by extending your arms.
- Repeat for the desired length of time or number of repetitions.

Suspension Push-Up

Fundamentals

- Ability to perform 20 bodyweight push-ups

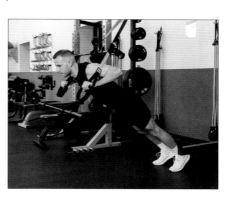

Setup and Movements

- Adjust the suspension straps to a height at which your body is parallel to the floor when in the prone bottom position.
- Grasp the handles with a prone grip and position the straps underneath your arms, as shown in the photo.
- Position your body in the prone position, with the arms straight and your body forming a slight angle with the floor (the stronger you are, the smaller the starting angle can be).
- Lower your body in a controlled manner by flexing at your elbows, maintaining a stable core and a flat back, until your body becomes parallel with the floor.
- Reverse directions and return to the starting position by extending your arms.
- Repeat for the desired length of time or number of repetitions.

Variation in Movement

Side Push-Up

Use the fundamentals and setup cues from the push-up exercise in addition to the following:

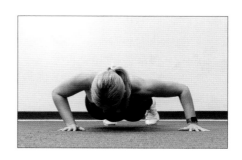

Downward Movement

- Maintain a firm torso and lower your chest, hips, and trunk simultaneously toward the ground by bending your elbows and leaning to one side until your upper arms become parallel to the ground.

Upward Movement

- Extend your elbows and press your body back up to the starting position, using the chest, shoulders, and triceps.
- Perform the exercise again, this time leaning to the opposite side.
- Repeat for the desired length of time or number of repetitions on each side.

DIP

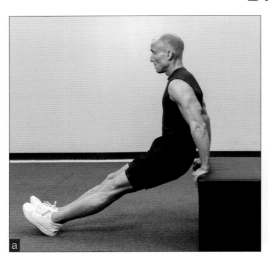 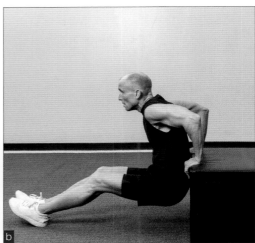

Fundamentals

- Basic upper-body strength and endurance (chest, shoulders, and triceps)

Setup

- Position yourself so that your hands are beside your body while you sit on the end of a chair, exercise step, or box.
- Position your feet so that your heels are on the floor.

Downward Movement

- Press your upper body slightly forward, so that you are no longer sitting on the chair, and lower your torso in a controlled manner by bending at your elbows until your upper arms are parallel with the floor.

Upward Movement

- Extend your elbows and use your chest, shoulders, and triceps to press your body back up to the starting position.
- Repeat for the desired length of time or number of repetitions.

PUSH-BACK

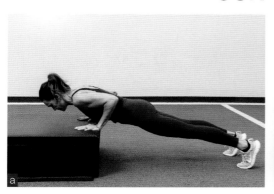 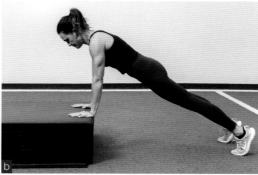

Fundamentals

- Basic upper-body strength and endurance (shoulders, upper back, and triceps)

Setup

- Position your body in a push-up position but with your hands on an exercise box, bench, or chair and aligned below your shoulders. Keep your hips up and your feet wider than hip-width.

Upward Movement

- Press your body up and back from the hands while keeping your hips higher than your shoulders.

Downward Movement

- Lower your upper body back to the initial starting position while maintaining hip elevation.
- Repeat for the desired length of time or number of repetitions.

Y

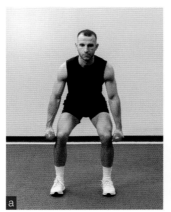 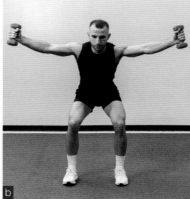

Fundamentals

- Basic upper-body strength and endurance (posterior shoulders and upper back), as well as basic glute strength

Setup

- From an erect position, flex at your hips, bringing your torso to approximately a 60-degree angle.
- Maintain a neutral spine and push your hips back.
- Begin with your arms straight and your hands directly below your shoulders.

Upward Movement

- Perform a Y movement pattern (moving the arms out at a 45-degree angle); keep your palms facing in.
- Continue the upward movement until your hands pass shoulder height.

Downward Movement

- Lower your arms back to the starting position in a controlled manner.
- Repeat for the desired length of time or number of repetitions.

Variations in Fundamentals, Setup, and Movements

Fundamentals

- Sufficient shoulder flexibility to perform a Y movement pattern
- Sufficient core stability

Resistance Band Y

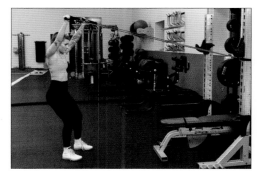

Setup and Movements

- Attach a resistance band to a sturdy anchor point, such as a stable rack, bench, or resistance machine, at chest level.
- Facing the anchor point, grab the resistance band at each end.
- Position your feet about hip-width apart staggered slightly.
- Bend slightly at your ankles, knees, and hips.
- Maintain an erect torso.
- Step away from the anchor point and extend your arms, keeping your palms facing down. Be sure to maintain tension in the band.
- Inhale prior to starting upward movement.
- Move your hands in an upward and outward arc until your arms are directly above your shoulders, forming a Y shape with your arms and body. Avoid leaning backward with your upper body.
- Exhale as you pull the handles up and out.

- Return your arms and hands to their starting position, extended in front of your chest, in a controlled manner.
- Inhale as you return your arms and hands to the starting position.
- Repeat for the desired length of time or number of repetitions.

T

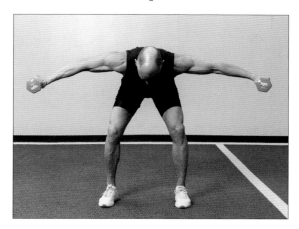

Fundamentals

- Basic upper-body strength and endurance (posterior shoulders and upper back), as well as glute strength

Setup

- From an erect position, flex at your hips, bringing your torso to approximately a 60-degree angle.
- Maintain a neutral spine and push your hips back.
- Begin with your arms straight and your hands directly below your shoulders.

Upward Movement

- Perform a T movement pattern by taking the arms horizontally away from the mid-line of the body, keeping your hands in a pronated position.
- Continue the upward movement until your hands pass shoulder height.

Downward Movement

- Return your arms to the starting position in a controlled manner.
- Repeat for the desired length of time or number of repetitions.

Variations in Fundamentals, Setup, and Movements

Fundamentals

- Sufficient shoulder flexibility and mobility to perform T movement pattern
- Sufficient core stability

Resistance Band T

Setup and Movements

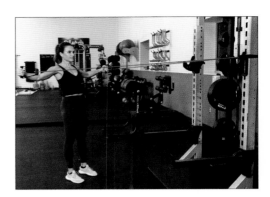

- Attach a resistance band to a sturdy anchor point, such as a stable rack, bench, or resistance machine, at chest level.
- Facing the anchor point, grab each end of the resistance band.
- Position your feet about hip-width apart in a staggered stance. Bend slightly at your ankles, knees, and hips.
- Maintain an erect torso.
- Step away from the anchor point and extend your arms, keeping your palms together. Be sure to maintain tension in the band.
- Inhale prior to starting upward movement.
- Pull your hands in a horizontal outward arc until your arms are pointing straight out from your shoulders, forming a T shape with your arms and body. Avoid leaning backward with your upper body.
- Exhale as you pull the handles outward.
- Return your hands and arms to their starting point, extended in front of your chest, in a controlled manner.
- Inhale as you return your hands and arms to the starting position.
- Repeat for the desired length of time or number of repetitions.

TRICEPS EXTENSION

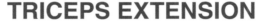
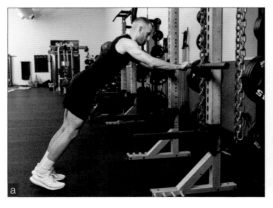
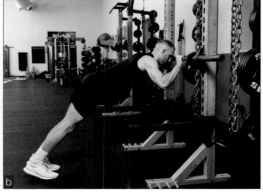

Fundamentals

- Basic upper-body strength and endurance (triceps brachii and core)

Setup

- Utilizing a Smith machine or power rack, adjust a barbell according to your strength level (the higher the barbell, the less resistance). Grab the barbell with an overhand shoulder-width grip.
- Maintain a neutral spine, keep your legs and arms straight, and shift your bodyweight to the balls of the feet while bracing your core.
- Begin with your arms straight.

Downward Movement

- Flex at your elbows and lower your body in a controlled manner until your forehead nearly reaches the barbell.

Upward Movement

- Push through your triceps and straighten your elbows until the starting position is reached.
- Repeat for the desired length of time or number of repetitions.

Variations in Fundamentals, Setup, and Movements

Suspension Triceps Extension

Fundamentals

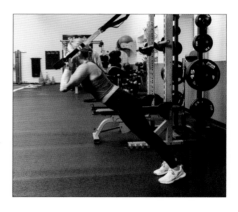

- Ability to perform 10 bodyweight triceps extensions on a Smith machine or a barbell mounted on a power rack from a prone, upright position.

Setup and Movements

- Adjust the suspension straps to a height at which your body forms a 30- (more advanced) to 45-degree angle with the floor when in the prone bottom position.
- Grasp the handles with a prone grip.
- Position your body in the prone top position so that your body forms a slight angle with the floor.
- Extend your arms away pushing your hands away from your body until the handles are at the height of your head.
- Lower your body in a controlled manner by flexing at your elbows and lowering your head toward the handles, maintaining a stable core and flat back and keeping the balls of your feet touching the ground, until your body forms a 30- to 45-degree angle with the floor, Keeping your upper arms firm and still, extend at your elbows and return to the upright prone starting position.
- Repeat for the desired length of time or number of repetitions.

Sandbag Overhead Triceps Extension

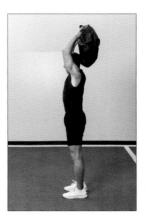

Fundamentals

- Shoulder and elbow flexibility and mobility needed to perform overhead triceps extension movement pattern
- Ability to lift and control resistance overhead
- Sufficient core stability

Setup and Movements

- Select a sandbag of appropriate weight.
- Grip the sandbag with a shoulder-width neutral grip.
- Position your feet shoulder-width apart.
- Hold the sandbag against your chest, with your elbows pointing down.
- Lift the sandbag above your head with both hands.
- Keeping your elbows and upper arms stationary, flex your elbows and lower the sandbag in a controlled manner behind your head to the back of your neck.
- Keep your head, shoulders, and upper back erect, and avoid arching your back.
- Lift the sandbag upward in a controlled manner by extending your elbows while keeping your upper arms stationary until your elbows are fully extended, with the sandbag directly above your head.
- Repeat for the desired length of time or number of repetitions.

INVERTED BICEPS CURL

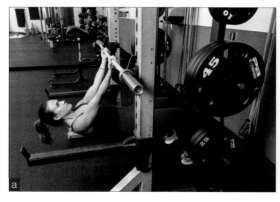 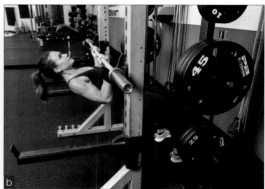

Fundamentals

- Basic upper-body strength and endurance (biceps brachii and core)

Setup

- Utilizing a Smith machine or power rack, adjust a barbell to suit your strength level (the higher the ball the less resistance). Position yourself under the barbell and grab the barbell with an underhand shoulder-width grip. Fully extend your arms.
- Maintain a neutral spine, keep your legs and torso in a straight line and knees bent at a 90-degree angle, and keep your bodyweight on the balls of your feet while bracing your core.

Upward Movement

- Pull through your biceps and flex your elbows, pulling your chest and head up to barbell height.

Downward Movement

- Extend at the elbows and lower your body in a controlled manner until your elbows are straight.
- Repeat for the desired length of time or number of repetitions.

Variations in Fundamentals, Setup, and Movements

Suspension Biceps Curl

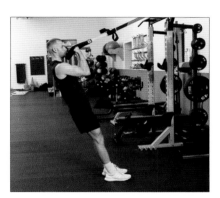

Fundamentals

- Ability to perform 10 bodyweight biceps curls on a Smith machine or a barbell on power rack from a prone upright position.

Setup and Movements

- Adjust the suspension straps to a height at which the body forms a 30- (more advanced) to 45-degree angle with the floor when in the supine bottom position.
- Grasp the handles with a supine grip.
- Position your body in the supine top position, so that it forms a slight supine angle with the floor, and so that your head is close to the handles.
- Lower your body in a controlled manner by extending at your elbows and lowering your body away from the handles, maintaining a stable core and flat back and keeping heels on the ground, until your body forms a 30- to 45-degree angle with the floor. Keeping your upper arms firm and still, flex at your elbows and return to the upright prone starting position.
- Repeat for the desired length of time or number of repetitions.

Sandbag Biceps Curl

Fundamentals

- Shoulder and elbow flexibility and mobility needed to perform biceps curl movement pattern
- Sufficient core stability

Setup and Movements

- Select a sandbag of appropriate weight.
- Grip the sandbag with a neutral shoulder-width grip.
- Position your feet shoulder-width apart.
- Hold the sandbag against your thighs with your elbows pointing down.
- Keep your elbows tight to the anterior portion of your torso and raise the sandbag in an upward arc by flexing your arms at your elbow.

- The movement should occur at your elbows, not at your shoulders.
- Avoid swinging the sandbag, arching your lower back, rising up on the toes, or shrugging your shoulders to lift the sandbag.
- Continue flexing your elbows until the sandbag reaches a point above chest level approximately 2 to 3 inches (5.0 to 7.6 centimeters) from your body.
- Avoid moving your elbows forward at the completion of the upward movement.
- Keep your elbows tight to the front portion of your torso and lower the sandbag in a controlled manner to the starting position.
- Maintain an erect upper body posture.
- Repeat for the desired length of time or number of repetitions.

DUMBBELL BENCH PRESS

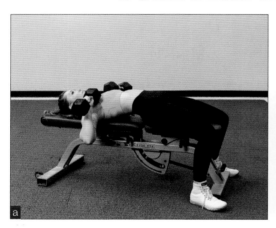 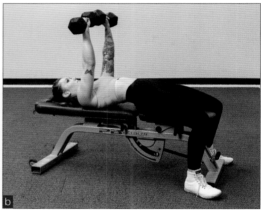

Fundamentals

- Ability to perform 10 push-ups with full range of motion using proper form
- Ability to lift and control resistance overhead
- Sufficient core stability

Setup

- Select two dumbbells of equal weight.
- Hold the dumbbells with a closed grip, so that the ends closest to your pinky fingers are against the fronts of your thighs (your hands should be facing in, and the handles should be parallel to each other)
- Sit down on the lower end of an adjustable bench and rest the dumbbells on the tops of the thighs.
- Lie back into the supine position, moving the dumbbells to the lateral aspect of your chest, near your armpit aligned at nipple level.
- Position your feet flat on the floor on either side of the bench, with your head, shoulders, and buttocks evenly and firmly on the bench.
- Rotate the dumbbells so that the thumb side of each dumbbell is against the lateral portion of your chest and both handles are in line with one another.
- Inhale prior to starting upward movement.

Upward Movement

- Press the dumbbells upward in a controlled manner.
- Avoid arching your lower back or lifting your buttocks off the bench.
- Do not allow the dumbbells to move out of control as you raise them.
- Press the dumbbells upward until your elbows are fully extended, but not locked.
- Bring the dumbbells at the completion of the movement, but do not bang them together.
- Exhale as you lift the dumbbells.

Downward Movement

- Lower and separate the dumbbells at the same rate as you bring them toward your mid-chest.
- The dumbbells should reach a point lateral to the chest, with both handles are in line with one another.
- Inhale as you lower the dumbbells.
- Repeat for the desired length of time or number of repetitions.

Variations in Movement

Dumbbell Alt-Arm Bench Press

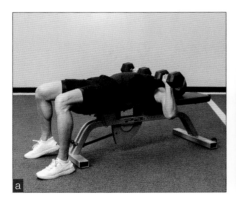 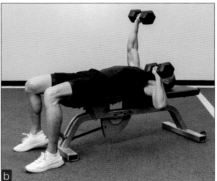

Using the fundamentals and setup cues for the bench press, perform this variation using the following movement cues:

Upward Movement

- Press one of the dumbbells upward in a controlled manner while keeping the other dumbbell in the starting position.
- Do not arch your lower back or lift your buttocks off the bench.
- Do not allow the dumbbell to move out of control as you raise it upward.
- Press the dumbbell upward until your elbow is fully extended, but not locked.
- Bring the dumbbell over the center of your chest at the completion of the movement.
- Exhale as you lift the dumbbell upward.

Downward Movement

- Lower the dumbbell in a controlled manner toward your mid-chest.
- The dumbbell should reach a point that is lateral to your chest, with the handle in line with the unused dumbbell on the other side.
- Inhale as you lower the dumbbell.
- Repeat the movement with the opposite arm for the desired length of time or number of repetitions.

DUMBBELL INCLINE PRESS

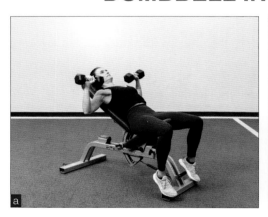 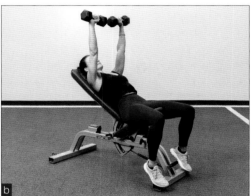

Fundamentals

- Capability to perform 10 push-ups with full range of motion using proper form
- Ability to lift and control resistance overhead
- Sufficient core stability

Setup

- Select two dumbbells of equal weight.
- Grasp the dumbbells with a closed, pronated grip. Align the dumbbells so that the ends closest to your pinky fingers are against the fronts of your thighs (your hands should be facing in, and the handles should be parallel to each other).
- Sit down on the lower end of an adjustable bench and rest the dumbbells on the tops of your thighs.
- Using your thighs to assist you, lift the dumbbells to your upper chest and recline at an angle of 30 to 45 degrees.
- Keep your head, shoulders, upper back, and buttocks in contact with the bench, and keep both feet securely on the floor.
- Inhale before starting the ascent.

Upward Movement

- Forcefully but evenly press the dumbbells up and slightly backward, exhaling as you do so.
- Continue pressing the dumbbells upward until your elbows are fully extended, but not forcefully locked.
- Bring the dumbbells together at the completion of the movement.

Downward Movement

- To maintain a stable position on the bench, lower both dumbbells at the same rate.
- The dumbbells should come to rest on the lateral portion of your upper chest, with both handles in line with one another.
- Inhale as you lower the dumbbells.
- Repeat for the desired length of time or number of repetitions.

Variations in Movement

Dumbbell Alt-Arm Incline Press

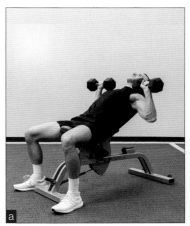 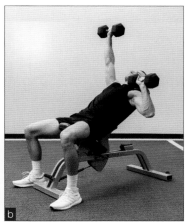

Using the fundamentals and setup cues for the incline press, perform this variation using the following movement cues:

Upward Movement

- Forcefully but evenly press one of the dumbbells up and slightly backward, keeping the other dumbbell stationary.
- Begin exhaling as you press the dumbbell upward.
- Continue pressing the dumbbell upward until your elbow is fully extended, but not fully locked.
- Bring the dumbbell above your chest at the completion of the movement.

Downward Movement

- Lower the dumbbell in a controlled manner until it comes to rest on the lateral portion of your upper chest, above your armpit.
- In the rest position, the handles of both dumbbells should be in line with one another.
- Inhale as you lower the dumbbell.
- Repeat the movement with the opposite arm for the desired length of time or number of repetitions.

FLY

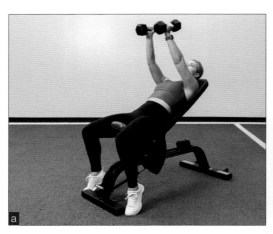 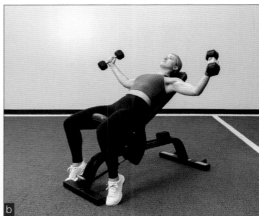

Fundamentals

- Capability to perform 10 push-ups with full range of motion using proper form
- Sufficient core stability

Setup

- Select two dumbbells of equal weight.
- Grip the dumbbells with a closed grip, with the ends closest to your pinky fingers against the fronts of your thighs (your hands should be facing in, and handles should be parallel to each other).
- Sit down on the lower end of the adjustable bench and rest the dumbbells on the tops of your thighs.
- Recline into the supine position and move the dumbbells to the lateral aspect of your chest, so that they are aligned at nipple level, near your armpits.
- Press the dumbbells up to an extended position (with your elbows slightly flexed directly above the chest).
- Position your feet flat on the floor and keep your head, shoulders, and buttocks evenly and firmly on the bench.
- Rotate the dumbbells to a neutral position (parallel to each other), rotating your elbows rotating out.
- Flex your elbows slightly before beginning the downward motion.

Downward Movement

- In a slow, controlled manner, lower the dumbbells in a wide arc.
- No movement should occur at the elbow joint—all movement should be at the shoulders.
- Inhale as you lower the dumbbells.
- As the downward motion continues, your elbows will go from pointing out to the side to pointing toward the floor.
- Continue the downward motion until the dumbbells are level with your chest and parallel to each other.

Upward Movement

- In a controlled manner, raise the dumbbells in an arc; simulate hugging a large pillar with your arms.
- Keep your elbows and wrists in a slightly flexed position throughout the upward motion.
- Exhale as the dumbbells are pressed upwards
- Continue moving the dumbbells in a wide arc until they are repositioned above your chest.
- Repeat for the desired length of time or number of repetitions.

Variations in Fundamentals, Setup, and Movements

Suspension Fly

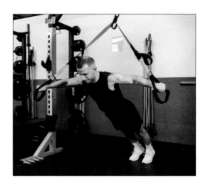

Fundamentals

- Ability to perform 10 suspension push-ups

Setup and Movements

- Adjust the suspension straps to a height at which your body forms a 45- (more advanced) to 60-degree angle with the floor when in the prone bottom position.
- Grasp the handles with a neutral grip and position the straps laterally to your upper shoulders.
- Position your body in the leaning downward slightly.
- Maintain a slight degree of elbow flexion.
- Lower your body in a controlled manner by moving your hands in an outward arc, maintaining a stable core and a flat back and keeping the balls of your feet touching the ground, until your body forms a 45- to 60-degree angle with the floor.
- Reverse directions and return to the starting position, with your arms extended.
- Repeat for the desired length of time or number of repetitions.

Suspension Reverse Fly

Fundamentals

- Ability to perform 20 suspension rows

Setup and Movements

- Adjust the suspension straps to a height at which your body forms a 45- (more advanced) to 60-degree angle with the floor when in the supine bottom position.
- Grasp the handles with a neutral grip and position your hands close together.
- Position your body in the supine position. Your body should form a slight angle with the floor. Maintain a slight degree of elbow flexion.
- Lower your body in a controlled manner by moving your hands in an outward arc. Maintain a stable core and a flat back, and keep your heels touching the ground until your body forms a 45- to 60-degree angle with the floor. Reverse directions and return to the starting position, with your arms extended.
- Repeat for the desired length of time or number of repetitions.

PULLOVER

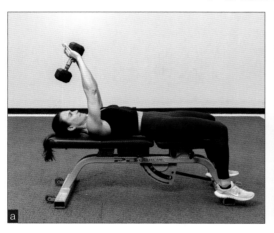
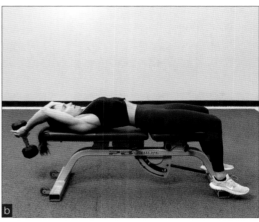

Fundamentals

- Capability to perform 10 push-ups with full range of motion using proper form
- Ability to lift and control resistance overhead
- Sufficient core stability

Setup

- Select a dumbbell of appropriate weight.
- Position your hands flat against the underside of the dumbbell. Your left index finger and thumb should be touching your right index finger and thumb.
- Sit down on the lower end of an adjustable bench and rest the dumbbell behind your head.
- Recline into a supine position so your head rests on the upper end of the bench.
- Your head, shoulders, and upper back, and buttocks should be firmly and evenly placed on the bench, and both feet should be securely planted on the floor on either side of the bench.
- Lift the dumbbell over your chest.
- Inhale before initiating the downward movement.

Downward Movement

- Flex your arm at the elbow and lower the dumbbell over your head in a controlled manner.
- Keep your elbows in a slightly flexed position while lowering the dumbbell over your head.
- Lower the dumbbell until your upper arms are approximately parallel to the floor.

Upward Movement

- Extend your arms at your shoulder joints in a slow, controlled manner until the dumbbell is above your chest.
- Your elbows should remain in a slightly flexed position.
- Exhale as you raise the dumbbell.
- Repeat for the desired length of time or number of repetitions.

Variations in Setup and Movement

Medicine Ball Pullover

Setup and Movements

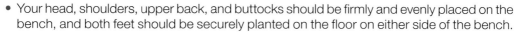

- Grip a medicine ball between your palms (one hand on either side of the medicine ball).
- Sit down on the lower end of an adjustable bench and rest the medicine ball behind your head.
- Recline into a supine position and rest your head on the upper end of the bench.
- Your head, shoulders, upper back, and buttocks should be firmly and evenly placed on the bench, and both feet should be securely planted on the floor on either side of the bench.
- Lift the medicine ball directly above your chest.
- Inhale before initiating the downward movement.
- Flex your arms at your elbows and lower the medicine ball over your head in a controlled manner.
- Keep your elbows in a slightly flexed position while lowering the medicine ball over your head.
- Lower the medicine ball until your upper arms are approximately parallel to the floor.
- Extend your arms at your elbows until the medicine ball is above your chest.
- Keep your elbows in a slightly flexed position.
- Exhale as you raise the medicine ball.
- Repeat for the desired length of time or number of repetitions.

DUMBBELL ONE-ARM ROW

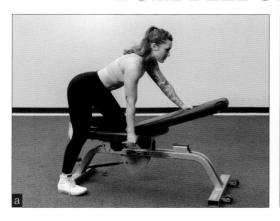

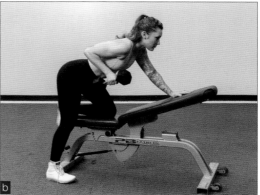

Fundamentals

- Sufficient core stability

Setup

- Select a dumbbell of appropriate weight and place it on the floor next to the upper left end of an adjustable bench.
- Set the bench incline to 30 degrees and stand at the upper end. Kneel on the bench with your right knee, keeping your left foot flat on the floor. Place your right hand at the upper end of the bench, and keep your bodyweight back toward the right heel, with a minimum amount of stress placed on the right hand.
- Position your slightly flexed left leg behind the back end of the bench but on the left side, with your toes pointing forward. Your upper extremity should remain parallel with the elevated bench.
- Reach down with your left hand and grasp the dumbbell with a closed, neutral grip (palm of the hand facing in). Hold the dumbbell (at a slightly upward angle) and fully extend your left elbow while keeping your shoulders parallel. Keep your back flat and your eyes focused straight ahead.
- Inhale just before raising the dumbbell.

Upward Movement

- Pull the dumbbell up toward your torso. Keep your wrist straight and your upper left arm and elbow next to the side of your body as you pull the dumbbell toward your rib cage, midway between your shoulder and your hip.
- Exhale as you lift the dumbbell.

Downward Movement

- Lower the dumbbell in a slow, controlled manner until your elbow is fully extended. Keep your shoulders parallel.
- Inhale as you return the dumbbell to the starting position.
- After completing the set with the left arm, place the dumbbell on the right side of the bench, stand on the right side, and repeat the procedure using your right arm for the desired length of time or number of repetitions.

DUMBBELL RENEGADE ROW

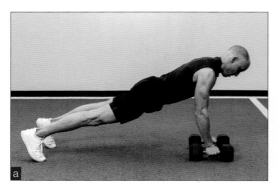
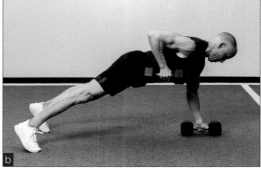

Fundamentals

- Capability to perform 20 push-ups with full range of motion using proper form
- Sufficient core stability

Setup

- Select a pair of dumbbells of appropriate weight and place them on the floor shoulder-width apart.
- Assume a plank position, with your hands shoulder-width apart, and hold a dumbbell in each hand.

Upward Movement

- Shifting your bodyweight to your left hand, pull the dumbbell in your right hand to the right side of your ribcage.
- Exhale as you lift the dumbbell.

Downward Movement

- Return to the starting position in a controlled manner and repeat the movement on your left side.
- Inhale as you lower the dumbbell.
- Repeat for the desired length of time or number of repetitions.

DUMBBELL SHOULDER PRESS

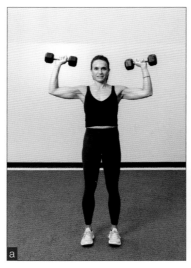 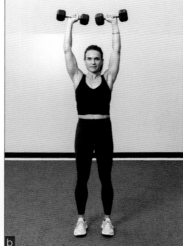

Fundamentals

- Capability to perform 10 push-ups with full range of motion using proper form
- Ability to lift and control resistance overhead
- Sufficient core stability

Setup

- Select two dumbbells of equal weight.
- Align the dumbbells so that the ends closest to your pinky fingers rest against the fronts of your thighs (your hands should be facing in, and the handles should be parallel to each other).

- Stand erect with your feet shoulder-width apart Lift the dumbbells in their starting position, at shoulder level.
- The dumbbells should be rotated so that the thumb sides are against the outsides of your shoulders and the handles are in line with one another.

Upward Movement

- Press the dumbbells upward and together in a controlled manner; do not arch your lower back.
- Your wrists should remain firm and straight, your forearms perpendicular to the floor, and your hands aligned with each other.
- Press the dumbbells upward until the elbows are fully extended, but not locked.
- At the completion of the movement, bring the dumbbells together over your head.
- Exhale as you lift the dumbbells.

Downward Movement

- Lower the dumbbells back to their starting position on the shoulders, making sure that the handles are in line with one another.
- Do not bounce the dumbbells off of your shoulders in the bottom position.
- Inhale as you lower the dumbbells.
- Repeat for the desired length of time or number of repetitions. This exercise may also be performed with kettlebells.

Variations in Setup and Movements

Resistance Band Shoulder Press

Setup and Movements

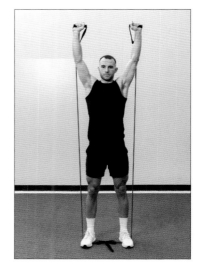

- Stand on the center of a resistance band, with your feet hip-width apart.
- Bend slightly at your ankles, knees, and hips.
- Maintain an erect torso.
- Bring the handles of the band above your shoulders so that your elbows are bent at a 90-degree angle.
- Press your arms straight up and bring your hands together overhead.
- Keep your shoulders down and avoid arching your back.
- Exhale as you lift your hands past the sticking point.
- Slowly lower your hands to the starting point.
- Inhale as you lower your hands.
- Repeat for the desired length of time or number of repetitions.

SHOULDER SHRUG

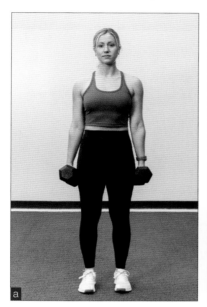 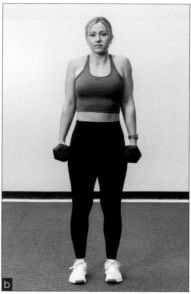

Fundamentals

- Capability to perform 10 push-ups with full range of motion using proper form
- Sufficient grip strength to hold heavier dumbbells at your sides
- Sufficient core stability

Setup

- Select two dumbbells of equal weight.
- Set your feet hip-width apart, pointing forward. Keep your torso erect, your chest out and up, your shoulders back, and your head and neck straight, with your eyes looking straight ahead.
- Hold the dumbbells at your sides with your palms facing in and your arms extended.
- Before initiating the upward movement, inhale.

Upward Movement

- Elevate your shoulders as much as possible while attempting to squeeze your shoulder blades together.
- Do not arch your lower back. Keep your elbows extended, but not locked, your wrists firm and straight, and your forearms and hands aligned with each other.
- Hold your shoulders at their highest point for one to two counts while simultaneously attempting to squeeze your shoulder blades together.
- Do not attempt to roll your shoulders forward or backward at the completion of the upward motion.
- Exhale as you lift the dumbbells past the sticking point.

Downward Movement

- Lower the shoulders to the starting position in a controlled manner.
- Avoid movements forward, backward, and side to side.
- Inhale as you lower your shoulders.
- Repeat for the desired length of time or number of repetitions.

DUMBBELL UPRIGHT ROW

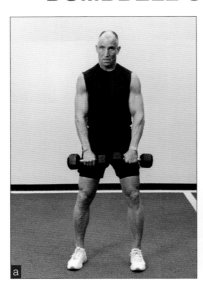 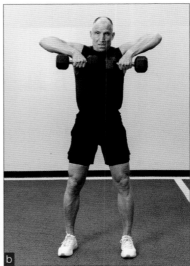

Fundamentals

- Capability to perform 10 push-ups with full range of motion using proper form
- Sufficient shoulder flexibility and mobility to perform upright-row movement pattern
- Sufficient core stability

Setup

- Select two dumbbells of equal weight.
- Position your feet hip-width apart and pointing forward. Keep your torso erect, your chest out and up, your shoulders back, and your head and neck straight, with your eyes looking straight ahead.
- Hold the dumbbells against the fronts of your thighs, with your elbows fully extended and the dumbbells aligned with each other.
- Before initiating the upward movement, inhale.

Upward Movement

- Begin the upward movement by lifting the dumbbells vertically along the front of your body, past the abdomen and chest, flexing your elbows and abducting your shoulders.
- The dumbbells should not swing away from your body or upward in an uncontrolled manner. Additionally, avoid rising up on your toes, extending your knees, and shrugging your shoulders to assist in the upward movement of the dumbbells.

- Continue pulling the dumbbells upward until your elbows are at shoulder height. Your wrists and the dumbbells should be elevated to a level between your sternum and your chin.
- Exhale at the completion of the upward movement.

Downward Movement

- Lower the dumbbells in a slow, controlled manner, keeping the dumbbells close to your body throughout the downward movement, until your elbows are fully extended, and the dumbbells are against the fronts of your thighs.
- Avoid bouncing the dumbbells against your thighs, rapidly extending your elbows, leaning forward with your torso, and shifting your bodyweight to the balls of your feet.
- Inhale as you lower the dumbbells during the downward movement.
- Repeat for the desired length of time or number of repetitions.

Variations in Fundamentals (Suspension Straps and Sandbag), Setup, and Movements

Resistance Band Upright Row

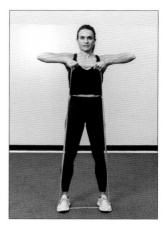

Setup and Movements

- Stand on the center of a resistance band, with your feet hip-width apart.
- Bend slightly at your ankles, knees, and hips.
- Maintain an erect torso.
- Hold the handles with your palms facing toward and resting on your thighs.
- Keeping your torso erect, lift the band, bringing your elbows up to shoulder level.
- Exhale as you lift your hands past the sticking point.
- Return to starting position.
- Inhale as you lower your hands.
- Repeat for the desired length of time or number of repetitions.

Suspension Row

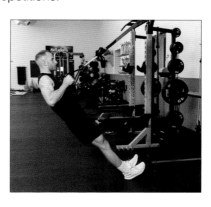

Fundamentals

- Ability to perform 10 bodyweight incline pull-ups on the Smith machine or on a barbell mounted on a power rack from an angled supine position

Setup and Movements

- Adjust the suspension straps to a height at which your body forms a 30- (more advanced) to 45-degree angle with the floor when in the supine bottom position.
- Grasp the handles with a supine grip.
- Position your body in the supine top position, with your body forming a slight supine angle.

- Lower your body in a controlled manner by extending at your elbows, maintaining a stable core and a flat back and keeping your heels touching the ground, until your body forms a 30- to 45-degree angle with the floor. Reverse directions and return to the starting position, with your arms extended.
- Repeat for the desired length of time or number of repetitions.

Sandbag Row

Fundamentals

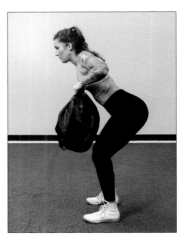

- Ability to perform straight-leg deadlift with proper form
- No history or presence of lower-back injuries
- Sufficient core stability

Setup and Movements

- Select a sandbag of appropriate weight.
- Adopt an athletic position, with your torso erect and with a slight bend in your ankles, knees, and hips.
- Lift and hold the sandbag with a neutral grip, with both hands across your mid-thighs.
- While tightening your core and with your knees and ankles slightly bent, push your hips back and flex at your waist.
- Keeping the sandbag close to your legs, extend your arms.
- Flex your elbows and pull the sandbag toward your abdomen.
- Repeat for the desired length of time or number of repetitions.

Sandbag Upright Row

Setup and Movements

- Select a sandbag of appropriate weight.
- Position your feet hip-width apart and pointing forward. Keep your torso erect, your chest out and up, your shoulders back, and your head and neck straight, with your eyes looking straight ahead.
- Hold the sandbag with a neutral grip against the fronts of your thighs, with your elbows fully extended.
- Begin the upward movement by flexing your elbows and abducting your shoulders to lift the sandbag vertically along the front of your body.
- Do not swing the sandbag away from the body or upward in an uncontrolled manner, and avoid rising up on your toes, extending your knees, or shrugging your shoulders to assist in the upward movement of the sandbag.
- Continue pulling the sandbag upward until your elbows are at shoulder height and your wrists and the sandbag are elevated to a level between the sternum and the chin.
- Lower the sandbag in a controlled manner, keeping it close to your body throughout the downward movement, until your elbows are fully extended, and the sandbag is against the fronts of your thighs.
- Avoid bouncing the sandbag against your thighs, rapidly extending your elbows, leaning forward with your torso, and shifting your bodyweight to the balls of your feet.
- Repeat for the desired length of time or number of repetitions.

DUMBBELL LATERAL RAISE

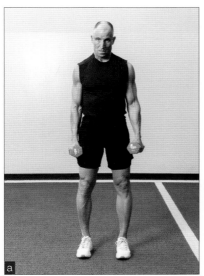 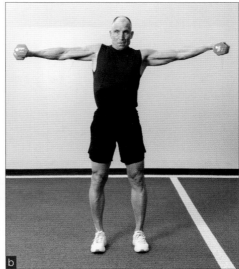

Fundamentals

- Sufficient shoulder flexibility and mobility to perform lateral-raise movement pattern
- Sufficient core stability

Setup

- Select two dumbbells of equal weight.
- Position your feet hip-width apart and pointing forward. Keep your torso erect, your chest out and up, your shoulders back, and head and neck straight, with your eyes looking straight ahead.
- Hold the dumbbells at your sides, with your palms facing in and your arms extended.
- Before initiating the upward movement, inhale.

Upward Movement

- Raise the dumbbells laterally (to the side) and upward in a controlled manner.
- Do not arch your lower back; keep your wrists firm and straight and your forearms and hands aligned with each other.
- Raise the dumbbells upward until they are even with your shoulders; keep your elbows extended, but not locked.
- Exhale as you lift the dumbbells past the sticking point

Downward Movement

- Lower the dumbbells in a controlled manner to their starting position, keeping your elbows extended, but not locked.
- Avoid movements forward, backward, and side to side.
- The dumbbells should not be bounced off the bottom position.
- Inhale as you lower the dumbbells.
- Repeat for the desired length of time or number of repetitions.

Variations in Setup and Movements

Resistance Band Lateral Raise

Setup and Movements

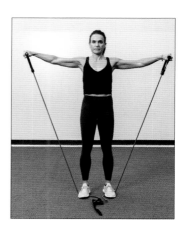

- Stand with both feet on the center of a resistance band, hip-width apart.
- Bend slightly at your ankles, knees, and hips.
- Maintain an erect torso.
- Hold the handles with your palms facing toward your outer thighs.
- Before initiating the upward movement, inhale.
- Keeping your torso erect, lift your hands in a lateral upward arc to shoulder level.
- Exhale as you lift your hands past the sticking point. Return to the starting position.
- Inhale as you lower your hands.
- Repeat for the desired length of time or number of repetitions.

DUMBBELL FRONT RAISE

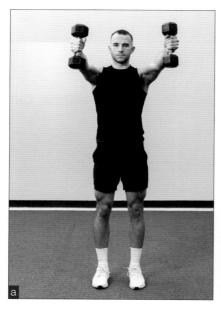
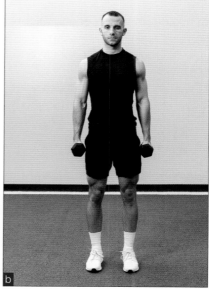

Fundamentals

- Sufficient shoulder flexibility and mobility to perform front-raise movement pattern
- Sufficient core stability

Setup

- Select two dumbbells of equal weight.
- Position your feet hip-width apart and pointing forward. Keep your torso erect, your chest out and up, your shoulders back, and your head and neck straight, with your eyes looking straight ahead.
- Hold the dumbbells at your sides with your palms facing in and your arms extended.
- Before initiating the upward movement, inhale.

Upward Movement

- Raise the dumbbells forward and upward in a controlled manner.
- Do not arch your lower back; keep your wrists firm and straight and your forearms and hands aligned with each other.
- Raise the dumbbells upward until they are at shoulder height; keep your elbows extended, but not locked.
- Exhale as you lift the dumbbells past the sticking point.

Downward Movement

- Lower the dumbbells in a controlled manner to their starting position, keeping your elbows extended, but not locked.
- Avoid movements forward, backward, and side to side.
- The dumbbells should not be bounced off the bottom position.
- Inhale as you lower the dumbbells.
- Repeat for the desired length of time or number of repetitions.

Variations in Setup and Movements

Resistance Band Front Raise

Setup and Movements

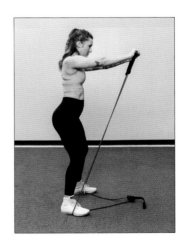

- Stand with both feet on the center of a resistance band, hip-width apart.
- Bend slightly at your ankles, knees, and hips.
- Maintain an erect torso.
- Hold the handles with your palms facing toward your thighs.
- Before initiating the upward movement, inhale.
- Keeping your torso erect, lift your hands in a forward and upward arc until they are level with your shoulders.
- Exhale as you lift your hands past the sticking point. Return to starting position.
- Inhale as you lower your hands.
- Repeat for the desired length of time or number of repetitions.

DUMBBELL BENT-OVER RAISE

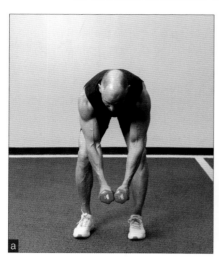 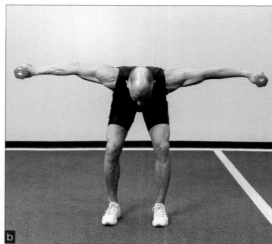

Fundamentals

- Sufficient shoulder flexibility and mobility to perform bent-over-raise movement pattern
- Sufficient core stability

Setup

- Select two dumbbells of equal weight, hold them with a closed grip, and rotate them to a neutral hand position (handles parallel to each other), with your elbows pointing out to the side.
- Position your feet shoulder-width apart and keep your knees slightly bent.
- Bend forward at your waist and keep your core firm.
- Extend your arms straight down from your shoulders, maintaining a slight flex in your elbows.

Upward Movement

- Keeping your wrists and elbows firm and straight and your forearms and hands aligned with each other, raise the dumbbells forward and upward together until they reach shoulder height.
- Do not arch your lower back.
- Exhale as you lift the dumbbells past the sticking point.

Downward Movement

- Lower the dumbbells in a controlled manner to their starting position, keeping your elbows extended, but not locked.
- Avoid movements forward, backward, and side to side.
- Inhale as you lower the dumbbells.
- Repeat for the desired length of time or number of repetitions.

DUMBBELL SUPINE TRICEPS EXTENSION

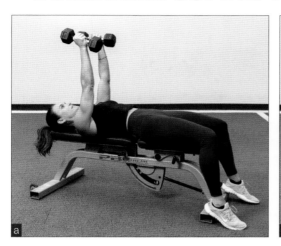
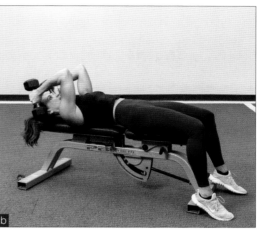

Fundamentals

- Sufficient shoulder and elbow flexibility and mobility to perform supine-triceps-extension movement pattern
- Ability to lift and control resistance overhead
- Sufficient core stability

Setup

- Select two dumbbells of equal weight and hold them with a closed grip.
- Sit down on the lower end of an adjustable bench and rest the dumbbells on the tops of your thighs. Align the dumbbells so that the ends closest to your pinky fingers are against the tops of your thighs (your hands should be facing in, and the handles should be parallel to each other).
- Recline into a supine position and rest your head on the other end of the bench.
- Your head, shoulders, upper back, and buttocks should be firmly and evenly placed on the bench, and both feet should be securely planted on the floor on either side of the bench.
- Lift the dumbbells up to a position above your shoulders where your arms are parallel to each other and perpendicular to the floor; this requires the dumbbells to be held parallel to each other, with your elbows extended.
- Your upper arms should be positioned so your elbows are directly above the shoulder.

Downward Movement

- Lower the dumbbells in a controlled manner toward the top of the forehead by bending your elbows; your upper arms should remain parallel to each other and perpendicular to the floor.
- Avoid arching your back during the downward motion.
- The dumbbells should come to either side of your head at their bottom position.
- Inhale during the downward motion.

Upward Movement

- Lift the dumbbells upward in a controlled manner by extending your elbows, keeping your elbows and upper arms stationary.
- Continue pressing the dumbbells upward until the elbows are fully extended, with the dumbbells directly above your shoulders.
- Exhale as you lift the dumbbells through the sticking point.
- Repeat for the desired length of time or number of repetitions.

Variations in Setup and Movements

Dumbbell One-Arm Triceps Extension

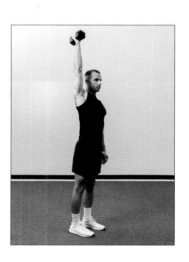

Setup

- Select a dumbbell of appropriate weight and hold it with a closed grip.
- Lift the dumbbell above your head with one hand, extending your elbow.
- Inhale prior to initiating the downward movement.

Downward Movement

- Keeping your elbow and upper arm stationary, flex your elbow and lower the dumbbell in a controlled manner behind your head to the back of your neck.
- Keep your head, shoulders, and upper back erect, and avoid arching your back.
- Inhale during the downward motion.

Upward Movement

- Lift the dumbbell upward in a controlled manner by extending your elbow, keeping your elbow and upper arm stationary, until your arm is fully extended, and the dumbbell is directly overhead.
- Exhale as you lift the dumbbell through the sticking point.
- Repeat for the desired length of time or number of repetitions.

DUMBBELL TRICEPS KICKBACK

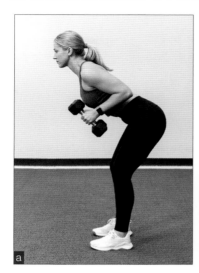 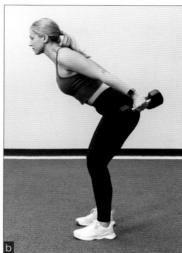

Fundamentals

- Sufficient shoulder and elbow flexibility and mobility to perform triceps-kickback movement pattern
- Sufficient core stability

Setup

- Select a dumbbell of appropriate weight and hold it with a closed grip.
- Stand with your legs staggered and your knees slightly flexed, bending forward at your waist but keeping your back straight.
- Lift your upper arm positioning your elbows against your sides with your palm facing in.
- Bend your elbow to approximately 60 degrees.
- Inhale prior to initiating the upward movement.

Upward Movement

- Keeping your elbow and upper arm stationary, extend your elbow and lift the dumbbell in a controlled manner until your elbow is straight, but not locked.
- Exhale during the ascent.

Downward Movement

- Lower the dumbbell in a controlled manner by flexing your elbow, keeping your elbow and upper arm stationary.
- Continue with the downward movement until your elbow returns to its starting position.
- Inhale through the downward movement.
- Repeat for the desired length of time or number of repetitions.

DUMBBELL ALT-ARM BICEPS CURL

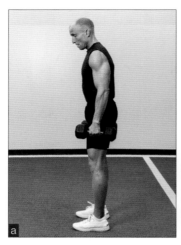
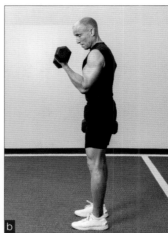

Fundamentals

- Sufficient shoulder and elbow flexibility and mobility to perform biceps-curl movement pattern
- Sufficient core stability

Setup

- Select two dumbbells of equal weight and hold them with a closed grip.
- Hold the dumbbells at your sides, with your elbows fully extended and your hands in a neutral position (palms facing in). Inhale just before lifting the first dumbbell.

Upward Movement

- Keeping your elbow tight against the front of your torso. raise one dumbbell in an upward arc by flexing your arm at the elbow and simultaneously supinating your hand (rotating the palm to a forward-facing position). The movement should occur at your elbow, not at your shoulders.
- Avoid swinging the dumbbell, arching your lower back, rising up on your toes, and shrugging your shoulders to lift the dumbbell.
- Continue flexing at your elbow until the dumbbell reaches a point above chest level, approximately 2 to 3 inches (5.0 to 7.6 centimeters) from your body.
- Avoid moving your elbow forward at the completion of the upward movement.
- Keep your opposite arm still and at your side during the upward movement.
- Exhale as the dumbbell passes the sticking point.

Downward Movement

- Keeping your elbow tight against the front of your torso, lower the dumbbell in a controlled manner, returning your hand to a neutral position as your elbow reaches full extension.
- Maintain an erect upper-body posture.
- Keep your opposite arm still and at your side until the repetition is completed, and then repeat the upward and downward movements with your opposite arm.
- Repeat for the desired length of time or number of repetitions.

DUMBBELL HAMMER CURL

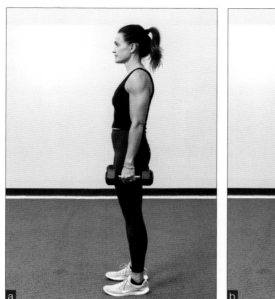 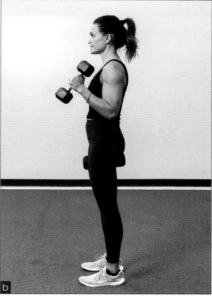

Fundamentals

- Sufficient shoulder and elbow flexibility and mobility to perform hammer-curl movement pattern
- Sufficient core stability

Setup

- Select two dumbbells of equal weight and hold them with a closed grip.
- Hold the dumbbells at your sides, with your elbows fully extended and your hands in a neutral position (palms facing in).
- Inhale just before lifting the first dumbbell.

Upward Movement

- Initiate the exercise by raising one dumbbell in a controlled upward arc, flexing your arm at the elbow.
- Keep your elbow tight against the front of your torso.
- The movement should occur at your elbow, not at your shoulder.
- Avoid swinging the dumbbell, arching your lower back, rising up on your toes, and shrugging your shoulders to lift the dumbbell.
- Continue flexing your elbow until the dumbbell reaches a point above chest level, approximately 2 to 3 inches (5.0 to 7.6 centimeters) from your body.
- Avoid moving your elbow forward at the completion of the upward movement.
- Exhale as the dumbbell passes the sticking point.
- Keep your opposite arm still at your side.

Downward Movement

- Lower the dumbbell in a controlled manner until your elbow is fully extended.
- Keep your elbow tight against the front of your torso as you lower the dumbbell. Inhale during the downward movement.
- Repeat for the desired length of time or number of repetitions.

Variations in Setup and Movements

Resistance Band Hammer Curl

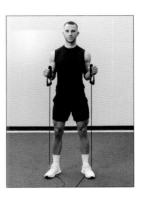

Setup and Movements

- Secure a long-looped resistance band under both feet, planting your feet shoulder-width apart.
- Bend slightly at your ankles, knees, and hips.
- Grab each side of the resistance band with your palms facing each other and elbows extended at your sides.
- Keeping your elbows and upper arms stationary, bend your elbows and pull the band in an upward arc motion until your hands are above chest level.
- Keep your head, shoulders, and upper back erect; avoid arching your back.
- Exhale during the upward motion.
- Lower your hands in a controlled manner by straightening your arms at your elbows, keeping your elbows and upper arms stationary, until your hands return to their starting point.
- Inhale during the downward movement.
- Repeat for the desired length of time or number of repetitions.

DUMBBELL CONCENTRATION CURL

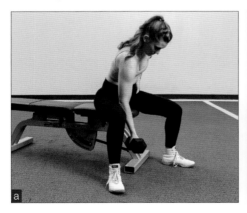
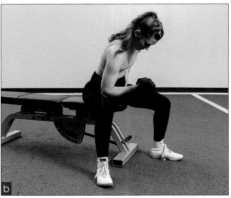

Fundamentals

- Sufficient shoulder and elbow flexibility and mobility to perform hammer-curl movement pattern
- Sufficient core stability

Setup

- Select a dumbbell and hold it with a closed grip.
- Sit on the end of a bench with your elbow resting on the inside of your thigh on the same side of your body.
- Allow the dumbbell to hang straight down, with your elbow fully extended and your hand supinated (palm facing forward).
- Inhale just before initiating the ascent.

Upward Movement

- Keeping your elbow tight against your inner thigh, lift the dumbbell in a controlled upward arc by flexing your arm at your elbow.
- The movement should occur at your elbow, not at your shoulder.
- Avoid swinging the dumbbell, arching your lower back, rising up on your toes, and shrugging your shoulders to lift the dumbbell.
- Continue flexing at your elbow until the dumbbell reaches a point above chest level, approximately 2 to 3 inches (5.0 to 7.6 centimeters) from your body.
- Avoid moving your elbow from your inner thigh.
- Exhale as the dumbbell passes the sticking point.

Downward Movement

- Keeping your elbow tight to your inner thigh, lower the dumbbell in a controlled manner, until your arm is fully extended.
- Inhale during the downward movement.
- Repeat for the desired length of time or number of repetitions and then switch arms.

RESISTANCE BAND
STANDING CHEST PRESS

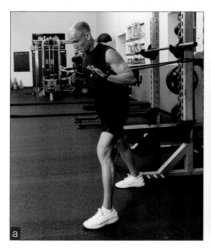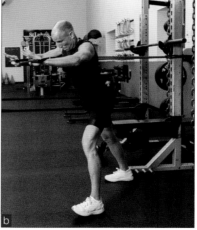

Fundamentals

- Functional shoulder strength and stability (ability to perform 15 push-ups)
- Sufficient core stability

Setup

- Attach a resistance band to a sturdy anchor point on stable rack, bench, or resistance machine at chest level.
- With your back to the anchor point, grab each end of the resistance band and place the ends under your armpits at chest level.
- Position your feet about hip-width apart and stagger one slightly in front of the other.
- Bend slightly at your ankles, knees, and hips.
- Maintain an erect torso with a slight forward lean for balance.
- Step away from the anchor point, putting tension into the band.
- Inhale prior to starting the upward movement.

Forward Movement

- Press hands forward and together in a controlled manner in front of your chest.
- Avoid leaning forward with your upper body.
- Exhale as you move the handles forward.

Backward Movement

- Return your hands in a controlled manner to their starting point, under your armpits at chest level.
- Inhale as the hands return to the starting position.
- Repeat for the desired length of time or number of repetitions.

Variations in Movements

Resistance Band Standing Row

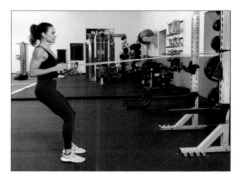

Backward Movement

- Pull your hands back in a controlled manner to your armpits.
- Avoid leaning backward with your upper body.
- Exhale as you pull the handles back.

Forward Movement

- Return your arms in a controlled manner to a fully extended position, keeping them at chest level.
- Inhale as you return your arms to the starting position.
- Repeat for the desired length of time or number of repetitions.

RESISTANCE BAND TRICEPS PUSHDOWN

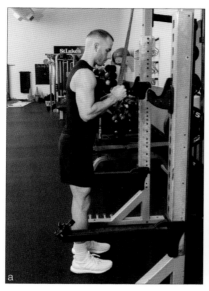 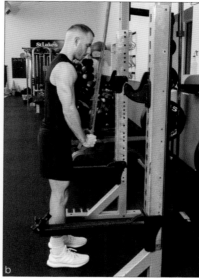

Fundamentals

- Sufficient shoulder and elbow flexibility and mobility to perform banded-triceps-pushdown movement pattern
- Sufficient core stability

Setup

- Secure a long-looped resistance band to an overhead power-rack support bar or secure door frame.
- Grab each side of the band with your palms facing each other; keep your elbows by your sides and your hands at chest level.

Downward Movement

- Keeping your elbows and upper arms stationary, extend your elbows and press downward, bringing your arms as close to full extension as possible.
- Keep your head, shoulders, and upper back erect; avoid arching your back.
- Exhale during the downward motion.

Upward Movement

- Lift your hands in a controlled manner, bending at your elbows while keeping your elbows and upper arms stationary, until your hands have returned to their starting point.
- Inhale during the upward movement.
- Repeat for the desired length of time or number of repetitions.

MEDICINE BALL CHEST PASS

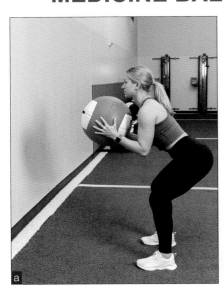 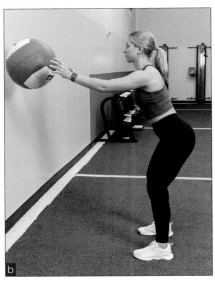

Fundamentals

- Ability to perform 15 push-ups

Setup

- Select a medicine ball of appropriate weight.
- Stand 3 to 6 feet from a solid wall.
- Position your feet between hip- and shoulder-width apart and point them forward or just slightly outward.
- Hold the medicine ball against your chest.
- Maintain an erect torso, with your chest up, your shoulders back, your head and neck straight, and your eyes looking straight ahead.
- Before beginning the initial movement, inhale.

Movement

Keeping your torso firm, pass the medicine ball against the wall for the desired length of time or number of repetitions.

DECLINE PUSH-UP

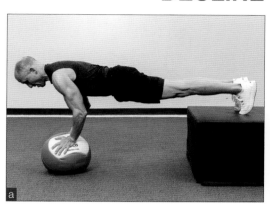 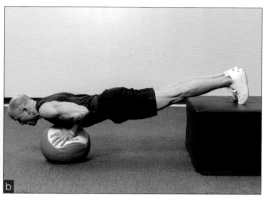

Fundamentals

- Ability to perform 15 push-ups

Setup

- Start in a plank position with your feet positioned on an elevated surface (bench, plyo-metric box, or physioball [for advanced exercisers]).
- Position your hands on either side of a medicine ball.

Movement

- While keeping your torso firm, lower your body toward the medicine ball by bending your elbows until your chest touches the ball.
- Press back up to the starting position, maintaining a firm torso.
- Repeat for the desired length of time or number of repetitions.

9

Core Exercises

Developing a strong and powerful lower and upper body for metabolic training is not as likely if you have a weak core. A strong core allows you to transfer energy to your upper and lower body, allowing for a more intense and effective workout. Additionally, the coordination and balance needed for rotational exercises and exercises in which positions are held for long periods of time make core strength essential to optimal fitness and sports performance.

Core exercises provide you with the strength and range of movement to carry out everyday functions and participate in a variety of activities, in addition to reducing the risk of injury. A high percentage of adults experience lower-back pain. Developing your core with metabolic training will help you limit unwanted stress and potential injury to your lower back. Training your core metabolically will enhance both anaerobic (exercise during which oxygen demands to muscles are being exceeded) and aerobic (exercise during which oxygen demands to muscles are being met) fitness by challenging posture and respiratory function.

In summary, core exercises form the foundation for a better metabolic workout and improved fitness and performance. Table 9.1 provides a listing of core exercises.

Table 9.1 Core Exercises

Exercise name	Muscles used	Page number
Abdominal crunch (with abdominal crunch: legs up variation)	Rectus abdominis, transversus abdominis, internal oblique, external oblique	155
Abdominal curl-up	Rectus abdominis, transversus abdominis, internal oblique, external oblique	156
Abdominal reach: legs up	Rectus abdominis, transversus abdominis, internal oblique, external oblique	157
Opposite-shoulder-to-knee crunch	Rectus abdominis, transversus abdominis, internal oblique, external oblique, serratus anterior, gluteus maximus	158
Front plank	Erector spinae; rectus abdominis; transversus abdominis; trapezius; rhomboids; anterior, medial, and posterior deltoid; pectoralis major and minor; serratus anterior; gluteus maximus; quadriceps; gastrocnemius	159
Side plank	Erector spinae; rectus abdominis; transversus abdominis; trapezius; rhomboids; anterior, medial, and posterior deltoid; pectoralis major and minor; serratus anterior; gluteus maximus; quadriceps; gastrocnemius	160
Birddog	Erector spinae; transverse abdominis; trapezius; rhomboids; anterior, medial, and posterior deltoid; pectorals; serratus anterior; gluteus maximus; quadriceps; hamstrings	161
Scissors	Iliopsoas, pectineus, sartorius, rectus femoris, tensor fasciae latae, internal and external obliques, rectus abdominis	162
Bicycle	Rectus abdominis, internal and external obliques, quadriceps, intercostals	162
Superman	Erector spinae, gluteus maximus, hamstrings	163
Medicine ball sit-up	Rectus abdominis, transverse abdominis, internal & external obliques	164
Medicine ball Russian twist	Internal and external obliques, rectus abdominis, transverse abdominis, erector spinae, supraspinatus, infraspinatus, teres minor, subscapularis, latissimus dorsi	164
Suspension hip and knee tuck	Iliopsoas, pectineus, sartorius, rectus femoris, internal and external obliques, rectus abdominis	165
Suspension pike	Iliopsoas; pectineus; sartorius; rectus femoris; internal and external obliques; rectus abdominis; anterior, medial, and posterior deltoid, biceps, triceps	166

ABDOMINAL CRUNCH

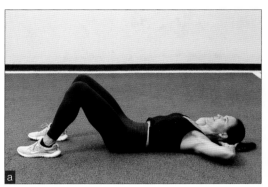
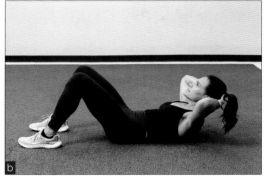

Fundamentals

- Basic core strength and endurance, trunk stability

Setup

- Lie supine (on your back) on the floor or on an exercise mat.
- Flex your hips and knees to a 90-degree angle, with your feet hip-width apart and flat on the floor.
- The focus of the exercise should be to move from your mid-thoracic region (middle back) and not your neck—your neck and head should remain stiff, as if a board were attached to the middle of your back.
- Place your hands behind your head (advanced, as pictured), with your hands supporting your lower back (beginner) or your hands supporting your lower back and your elbows lifted slightly, such that your arms do not lift your shoulders up and the load is shifted to your rectus abdominis (intermediate).

Upward Movement

- Pre-brace your core by contracting your muscles prior to initiating the upward movement.
- Keeping your head and neck rigid, lift them off the floor or mat no more than a few inches.
- Focus on moving from your mid-thoracic (mid-back) area.
- Avoid moving your neck (lifting or tucking your chin).

Downward Movement

- Keeping your core braced, return to the starting position in a controlled manner.
- Keep your head and neck rigid throughout the downward movement.

Variation in Setup

Abdominal Crunch: Legs Up

Using the same movements as the abdominal-crunch exercise, set up the abdominal crunch with legs up in the following way:

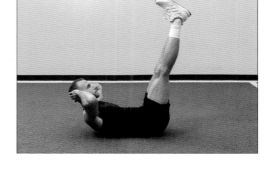

- Lie supine (on your back) on the floor or on an exercise mat. Flex your hips and lift your legs so that they form a 90-degree angle with your body and are perpendicular to the floor.
- Place your hands behind your head with your elbows lifted slightly, such that your arms do not lift your shoulders up and the load is shifted to your rectus abdominis.

ABDOMINAL CURL-UP

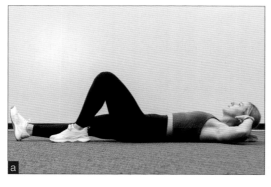

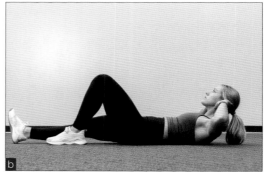

Fundamentals

- Basic core strength and endurance, trunk stability

Setup

- Lie supine (on your back) on the floor or on a mat.
- One leg should be bent, with the knee flexed to approximately a 90-degree angle, while the other leg remains straight on the floor or mat.
- The focus of the exercise should be to move from your mid-thoracic region (middle back) and not your neck, as is often done with abdominal crunches—your neck and head should remain stiff, as if a board were attached to the middle of your back.
- Place your hands on either side of your head (advanced, as pictured), supporting your lower back (beginner), or supporting your lower back with your elbows lifted slightly, such that your arms do not lift your shoulders up and the load is shifted to the rectus abdominis (intermediate).

Upward Movement

- Pre-brace your core by contracting your muscles prior to initiating the upward motion.
- Keeping your head and neck rigid, lift them off the floor or mat no more than a few inches, rotating them toward your bent opposite knee.
- Focus on moving from the mid-thoracic (mid-back) area.
- Avoid moving your neck (lifting or tucking your chin).

Downward Movement

- Keeping your core braced, return to the starting position in a controlled manner.
- Keep your head and neck rigid throughout the downward movement.

ABDOMINAL REACH: LEGS UP

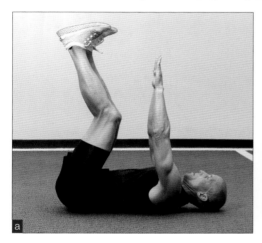 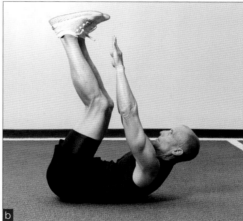

Fundamentals

- Basic core strength and endurance, trunk stability

Setup

- Lie supine (on your back) on the floor or on an exercise mat.
- Flex your hips and lift your legs so that they form a 90-degree angle with your body and are perpendicular to the floor.
- Straighten your arms directly above your shoulders, with your hands pointing toward your feet
- The focus of the exercise should be to move from your mid-thoracic region (middle back) and not your neck—your neck and head should remain stiff, as if a board were attached to the middle of your back.

Upward Movement

- Pre-brace your core by attempting to contract your muscles prior to initiating the upward movement.
- Keeping your head and neck rigid, lift them no more than a few inches off the floor or mat, simultaneously reaching toward your feet with your hands.
- Focus on moving from your mid-thoracic (mid-back) area.
- Avoid moving your neck (lifting or tucking your chin).

Downward Movement

- Keeping your core braced, return to the starting position in a controlled manner.
- Keep your head and neck rigid throughout the downward movement.

OPPOSITE-SHOULDER-TO-KNEE CRUNCH

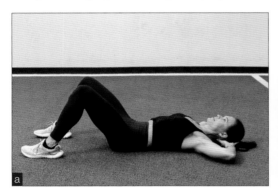 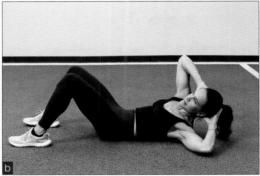

Fundamentals

- Basic core strength and endurance, trunk stability

Setup

- Lie supine (on your back) on the floor or on an exercise mat.
- Flex your hips and knees to form a 90-degree angle.
- The focus of the exercise should be to move from your mid-thoracic region (mid-back) and not your neck—your neck and head should remain stiff, as if a board were attached to the middle of your back.
- Place your hands behind your head with your elbows lifted slightly, so that your arms do not lift your shoulders up and the load is shifted to your rectus abdominis.

Upward Movement

- Pre-brace your core by contracting your muscles prior to initiating the upward movement.
- Keeping your head and neck rigid, lift one shoulder off the floor and rotate no more than a few inches to the opposite side.
- Focus on moving from your mid-thoracic (mid-back) and oblique area.
- Avoid moving your neck (lifting or tucking your chin).

Downward Movement

- Keeping your core braced, return to the starting position in a controlled manner.
- Keep your head and neck rigid throughout the downward movement.
- Repeat the movement on the opposite side.

FRONT PLANK

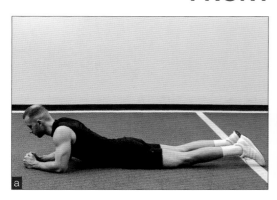 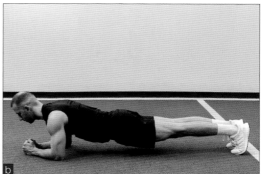

Fundamentals

- Basic core strength and endurance, trunk stability

Setup

- Lie prone (face down) on the floor or on an exercise mat.
- Support your bodyweight on both elbows, aligning them directly under your shoulders (shoulder-width apart), and on both knees.

Upward Movement

- Pre-brace your core by contracting your muscles prior to initiating the upward motion.
- Keep your head and neck rigid, looking toward a point in front of your hands.
- Focus on your core.
- Lift your knees off the floor or mat and straighten your torso, supporting your body on both elbows and both feet. Hold the position for the desired length of time

Downward Movement

- Keeping your core braced, return to the starting position in a controlled manner, lightly touching your knees to the floor or mat.
- Keep your head and neck rigid, focusing on a point in front of your hands, throughout the downward movement.

SIDE PLANK

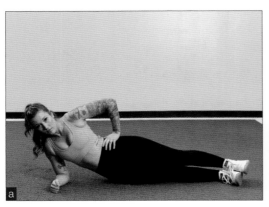 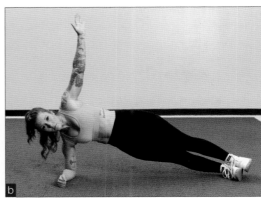

Fundamentals

- Basic core strength and endurance, trunk stability

Setup

- Lie on your side on the floor or on an exercise mat.
- Support your bodyweight with one elbow bent at 90 degrees and aligned directly under your shoulder. Your feet should be stacked on top of each other, with the foot on the same side as your elbow on the bottom.
- Place your opposite hand on your hip or reach it straight above your opposite shoulder.

Upward Movement

- Pre-brace your core by contracting your muscles prior to initiating the upward motion.
- Keep your head and neck rigid throughout the upward movement.
- Focus on moving from your core. Lift your torso from the floor or mat and straighten it, supporting your bodyweight on your elbow and your bottom foot. Hold the position for the desired length of time.

Downward Movement

- Keeping your core braced, return to the starting position in a controlled manner, lightly touching your bottom knee to the floor or mat.
- Keep your head and neck rigid, focusing on a point in front of your hands throughout the downward movement.

BIRDDOG

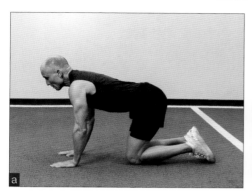
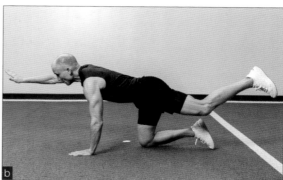

Fundamentals

- Basic core strength and endurance, trunk stability

Setup

- Begin on your hands and knees on the floor or on an exercise mat.
- Align your hands directly under your shoulders, and your knees directly under your hips.

Upward Movement: Right Arm and Left Leg

- In a controlled manner, lift your right arm forward and your left leg backward simultaneously, stopping when they become parallel with the floor.
- Keep your head and neck rigid throughout the upward movement.
- Focus on controlling the movement with your core.
- Avoid raising your right arm and left leg past horizontal.
- At the completion of the upward movement, hold your limbs parallel to the floor for about five seconds.

Downward Movement: Right Arm and Left Leg

- In a controlled manner, return your right arm and left leg to their starting positions.
- Keep your head and neck rigid throughout the downward movement. Upon completing the movement, repeat with your left arm and right leg.

SCISSORS

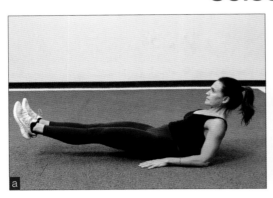 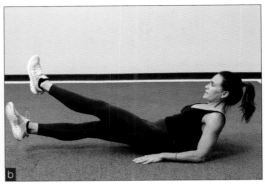

Fundamentals

- Basic core strength and endurance, trunk stability

Setup

- Lie supine on the floor or on a mat.
- Elevate your upper body by propping yourself up on your elbows.
- Extend your legs straight and elevate them 6 to 12 inches (15.2 to 30.5 centimeters) off the floor.

Movement

- Scissor your legs over and under each other.
- Engage your core and keep your lower back pressed onto the mat or floor throughout the movement.
- Move in a controlled manner.

BICYCLE

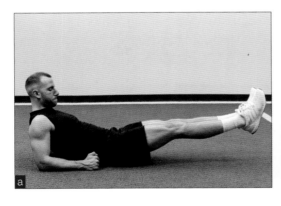 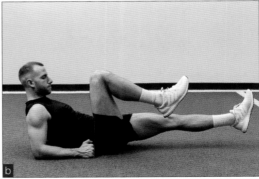

Fundamentals

- Basic core strength and endurance, trunk stability

Setup

- Lie supine on the floor or on a mat.
- Elevate your upper body by propping yourself up on both elbows.
- Extend your legs out straight and elevate them 6 to 12 inches (15.2 to 30.5 centimeters) off the floor.

Movement

- Rotate your legs forward and backward by extending one leg forward and away from your body's midline as the other leg flexes toward your body.
- Engage your core and keep your lower back pressed onto the mat or floor throughout the movement.
- Move in a controlled manner.

SUPERMAN

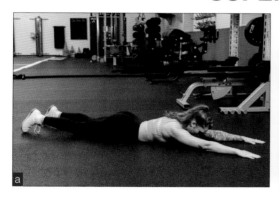 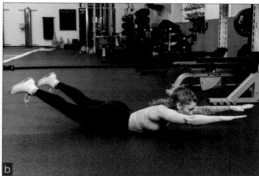

Fundamentals

- Basic core strength and endurance, trunk stability

Setup

- Lie prone on the floor or on a mat.
- Straighten your arms in front of you, keeping them shoulder-width apart.
- Straighten your legs behind you, keeping them hip-width apart.

Movement

- Lift your arms and legs simultaneously upward in a controlled manner, moving them as high as possible while keeping your torso on the mat or the floor.
- Engage your core and keep your torso pressed onto the mat or the floor throughout the movement.
- Move in a controlled manner.

MEDICINE BALL SIT-UP

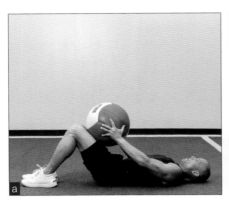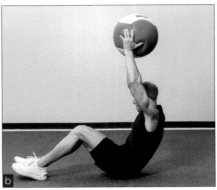

Fundamentals

- Capability to perform 10 sit-ups with full range of motion using proper form
- Sufficient shoulder and upper-body flexibility to hold a medicine ball overhead

Setup

- Select a medicine ball of appropriate weight.
- Lie supine with your knees bent and your feet flat on floor.
- Fully extend your arms, holding the medicine ball against your thighs.

Movement

- While lifting the medicine ball overhead with straight arms, perform a sit-up.
- The movement is finished when you are holding the medicine ball overhead and your torso is perpendicular to the ground.
- Return to the starting position and perform the desired number of repetitions.

MEDICINE BALL RUSSIAN TWIST

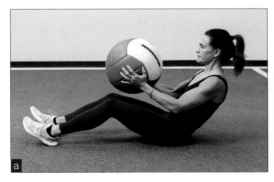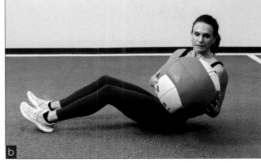

Fundamentals

- No history of back pain or injury
- Sufficient core stability

Setup

- Select a medicine ball of appropriate weight.
- Sit on the ground or on an exercise mat with your knees slightly bent and your heels in contact with the ground.
- Lean back and position your torso at approximately a 45-degree angle.

Movement

- Move the medicine ball from one side of your hips to the other by rotating your torso.
- Return to the starting position and perform the desired number of repetitions.

SUSPENSION HIP AND KNEE TUCK

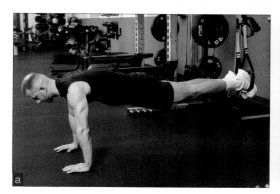 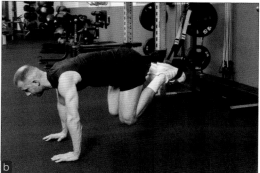

Fundamentals

- Ability to perform 10 bodyweight bird dogs with each arm consecutively

Setup

- Adjust the suspension straps to a height at which your body can be in the top position of a push-up, with your arms straight and your feet in the foot straps.
- Position your feet close together in the foot straps, and position your upper extremity in the top position of a push-up, keeping your spine neutral, your neck straight, and your knees above your ankles.
- Both your arms and your legs should be extended.

Movement

- Keeping your arms straight and your spine neutral, flex at your hips, bringing your knees toward your upper body.
- Reverse directions and return to the starting position.
- Repeat for the desired number of repetitions or length of time.

SUSPENSION PIKE

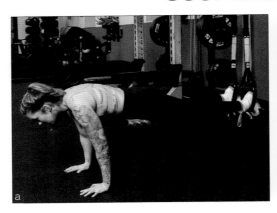 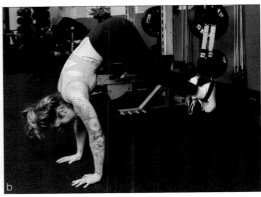

Fundamentals

- Ability to perform 20 suspension hip and knee tucks

Setup

- Adjust the suspension straps to a height at which your body can be in the top position of a push-up, with your arms straight and your feet in the foot straps.
- Position your feet close together in the foot straps, and position your upper extremity in the top position of a push-up, keeping your spine neutral, your neck straight, and your knees above your ankles.
- Both your arms and your legs should be extended.

Movement

- Keeping your arms and legs straight and your spine neutral, lift your hips until they are directly above your shoulders.
- Reverse directions and return to the starting position.
- Repeat for the desired number of repetitions or length of time.

10

Functional Training Exercises

Functional exercises in metabolic training mimic movements that may be a part of daily life, in contexts such as work, recreation (or sport), and everyday tasks. These exercises incorporate multiple groups of muscles working cohesively throughout the body.

In order to maximize the benefits of functional exercises, you should combine these movements with upper-body, lower-body, and core exercises. Select exercises that most closely resemble the movement patterns you are intending to improve or the fitness goals you are trying to reach. Functional exercises will help to improve your balance and coordination and will reduce the risk of injury. Functional exercises result in a higher caloric expenditure than upper-body, lower-body, and core exercises alone due to the recruitment of more muscle groups and the higher level of workout intensity.

Table 10.1 Functional Exercises

Exercise name	Muscles used	Page number
Heavy rope two-arm slams	Gluteus maximus; hamstrings; quadriceps; latissimus dorsi; abdominals; pectoralis major; pectoralis minor; anterior, medial, and posterior deltoid; trapezius; serratus anterior; biceps; and triceps	169
Heavy rope alt-arm slams	Gluteus maximus; hamstrings; quadriceps; latissimus dorsi; abdominals; pectoralis major; pectoralis minor; anterior, medial, and posterior deltoid; trapezius; serratus anterior; biceps; and triceps	170
Heavy rope scissors	Gluteus maximus; hamstrings; quadriceps; latissimus dorsi; abdominals; pectoralis major; pectoralis minor; anterior, medial, and posterior deltoid; trapezius; serratus anterior; biceps; and triceps	171
Heavy rope jumping jacks	Gluteus maximus; hamstrings; quadriceps; latissimus dorsi; abdominals; pectoralis major; pectoralis minor; anterior, medial, and posterior deltoid; trapezius; serratus anterior; biceps; and triceps	172
Heavy rope arm circles: clockwise	Gluteus maximus; hamstrings; quadriceps; latissimus dorsi; abdominals; pectoralis major; pectoralis minor; anterior, medial, and posterior deltoid; trapezius; serratus anterior; biceps; and triceps	173
Heavy rope two-hand shuffle slams (with heavy rope two-hand backpedal slams variation)	Gluteus maximus; hamstrings; quadriceps; latissimus dorsi; abdominals; pectoralis major, pectoralis minor; anterior, medial, and posterior deltoid; trapezius; serratus anterior; biceps; and triceps	174
Heavy rope kneeling two-arm slams (with heavy rope kneeling alt-arm slams variation)	Latissimus dorsi; abdominals; pectoralis major; pectoralis minor; anterior, medial, and posterior deltoid; trapezius; serratus anterior; biceps; and triceps	175
Heavy rope kneeling scissors	Latissimus dorsi; abdominals; pectoralis major; pectoralis minor; anterior, medial, and posterior deltoid; trapezius; serratus anterior; biceps; and triceps	176
Heavy rope two-arm unbalanced slams (with heavy rope alt-arm unbalanced slams variation)	Gluteus maximus; hamstrings; quadriceps; latissimus dorsi; abdominals; pectoralis major; pectoralis minor; anterior, medial, and posterior deltoid; trapezius; serratus anterior; biceps; and triceps	177
Heavy rope unbalanced scissors	Gluteus maximus; hamstrings; quadriceps; latissimus dorsi; abdominals; pectoralis major; pectoralis minor; anterior, medial, and posterior deltoid; trapezius; serratus anterior; biceps; and triceps	178

HEAVY ROPE TWO-ARM SLAMS

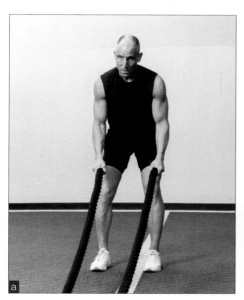 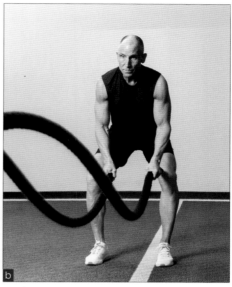

Fundamentals

- Sufficient lower-body strength and endurance to perform at least 10 consecutive body-weight squats
- Sufficient upper-body strength to lift a heavy rope overhead for at least 10 consecutive repetitions

Setup

- Anchor the rope to a stable rack, pillar, or wall mount.
- Grasp the rope below the endcaps with a firm, neutral grip (palms facing each other).
- Stabilize your body by bending your knees into a partial squat; keep your back flat and your head up.
- Keep your weight on the balls of your feet.

Movement

- Explosively extend your hips and lift your arms until the ropes and your arms are above a parallel position with the floor.
- Once the top position is reached, explosively squat back down and forcefully drive the ropes toward the ground.
- Repeat the movement for the desired length of time.

HEAVY ROPE ALT-ARM SLAMS

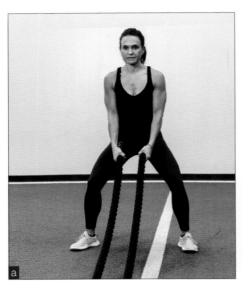 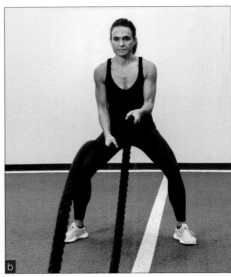

Fundamentals

- Sufficient lower-body strength and endurance to hold a partial squat 30 seconds
- Sufficient upper-body strength to lift a heavy rope to shoulder height for at least 10 consecutive repetitions with each arm

Setup

- Anchor the rope to a stable rack, pillar, or wall mount.
- Grasp the rope below the endcaps with a firm, neutral grip.
- Stabilize your body by bending your knees into a partial squat; keep your back flat and your head up.
- Keep your weight on the balls of your feet.

Movement

- While maintaining a partial squat, lift your arms and the rope up to a position where the arms are parallel to the floor.
- Still maintaining a partial squat, lift one arm up while explosively driving the other arm down; then reverse directions.
- Repeat the movement for the desired length of time.

HEAVY ROPE SCISSORS

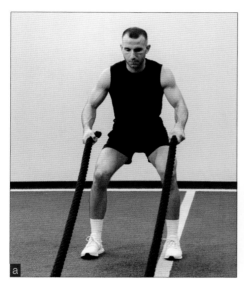 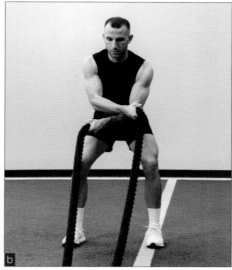

Fundamentals

- Sufficient lower-body strength and endurance to hold a partial squat for a desired time for 30 seconds
- Sufficient upper-body strength to lift a heavy rope to shoulder height for at least 10 consecutive repetitions with each arm

Setup

- Anchor the rope to a stable rack, pillar, or wall mount.
- Grasp the rope below the endcaps with a firm, neutral grip.
- Stabilize your body by bending your knees into a partial squat; keep your back flat and your head up.
- Keep your weight on the balls of your feet.

Movement

- While maintaining a partial squat, lift your arms and the rope up to a position where your arms are parallel to the floor.
- Still maintaining a partial squat, scissor your arms by explosively crossing your right arm over your left and then your left over your right.
- Repeat the movement for the desired length of time.

HEAVY ROPE JUMPING JACKS

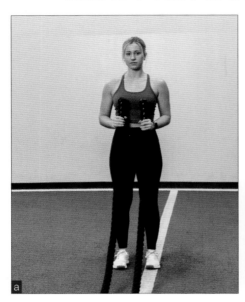 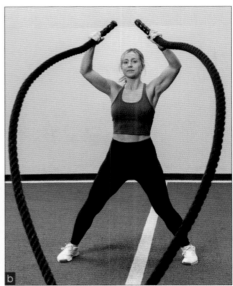

Fundamentals

- Ability to perform bodyweight jumping jacks consecutively for at least 30 seconds
- Sufficient upper-body strength to lift a heavy rope above shoulder height for at least 10 consecutive repetitions with each arm

Setup

- Anchor the rope to a stable rack, pillar, or wall mount.
- Grasp the rope below the endcaps with a firm, neutral, thumbs-up grip
- Stabilize your body by bending your knees into a partial squat; keep your back flat and your head up.
- Keep your weight on the balls of your feet.

Movement

- Perform a jumping jack, moving your feet laterally to shoulder-width position while explosively raising your hands and rope in an arc motion to a point above shoulder height.
- Return to the starting position.
- Repeat the movement for the desired length of time.

HEAVY ROPE ARM CIRCLES: CLOCKWISE

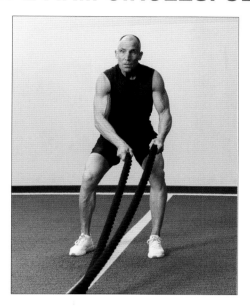

Fundamentals

- Sufficient lower-body strength and endurance to hold a partial squat for a desired time for 30 seconds
- Sufficient upper-body strength to lift a heavy rope to shoulder height for at least 10 consecutive repetitions with each arm

Setup

- Anchor the rope to a stable rack, pillar, or wall mount.
- Grasp the rope below the endcaps with a firm, neutral, thumbs-up grip.
- Stabilize your body by bending your knees into a partial squat; keep your back flat and your head up.
- Keep your weight on the balls of your feet.

Movement

- While maintaining a partial squat position, make large, explosive, clockwise rotations with your arms and the rope.
- Repeat the movement for the desired length of time.

Variation in Movement

Heavy Rope Arm Circles: Counterclockwise

- While maintaining a partial squat position, make large, explosive, counterclockwise rotations with your arms and the rope.
- Repeat the movement for the desired length of time.

HEAVY ROPE TWO-HAND SHUFFLE SLAMS

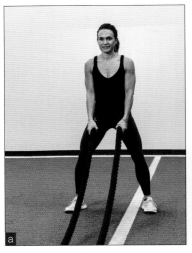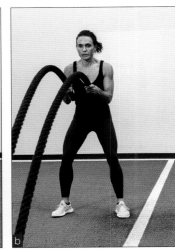

Fundamentals

- Ability to perform two-hand slams for 30 seconds
- Ability to perform a lateral shuffle while holding weighted dumbbells or kettlebells

Setup

- Anchor the rope to a stable rack, pillar, or wall mount.
- Grasp the rope below the endcaps with a firm, neutral grip.
- Stabilize your body by bending knees into a partial squat; keep your back flat and your head up.
- Keep your weight on the balls of your feet.

Movement

- Explosively extend your hips and lift your arms until the ropes and your arms are above a parallel position with the floor.
- Once you reach the top position, explosively squat back down and forcefully drive the ropes toward the ground.
- While explosively lifting and driving the ropes back to the floor, perform two shuffle steps to the right and back and then two shuffle steps to the left and back.
- Repeat the movement for the desired length of time.

Variations in Movement

Heavy Rope Two-Hand Backpedal Slams

- Explosively extend your hips and lift your arms until the ropes and your arms are above a parallel position with the floor.
- Once you reach the top position, explosively squat back down and forcefully drive the ropes toward the ground.

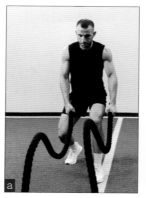 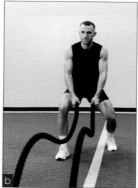

- While explosively lifting and driving the ropes back to the floor, perform two backpedal steps and then two forward steps to the starting position.
- Repeat the movement for the desired length of time.

HEAVY ROPE KNEELING TWO-ARM SLAMS

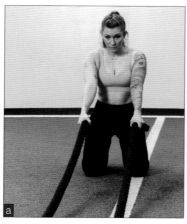 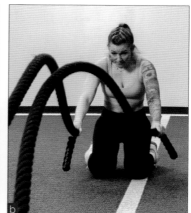

Fundamentals

- Sufficient upper-body and core strength to perform two-hand slams for at least 30 seconds while standing

Setup

- Anchor the rope to a stable rack, pillar, or wall mount.
- Grasp the rope below the endcaps with a firm, neutral grip.
- Stabilize your body by kneeling; keep your back flat and your head up.

Movement

- While maintaining a neutral spine, explosively lift your arms above a parallel position with the floor.
- Once you reach the top position, explosively drive the ropes toward the ground.
- Repeat the movement for the desired length time.

Variations in Fundamentals and Movement

Heavy Rope Kneeling Alt-Arm Slams

Fundamentals

- Sufficient upper-body and core strength to perform alternate-arm slams for at least 30 seconds while standing

Movement

- Maintaining a neutral spine, explosively lift your arms above a parallel position with the floor.
- Lift one arm up while explosively driving the other arm down; then reverse directions with each arm.
- Repeat the movement for the desired length of time.

HEAVY ROPE KNEELING SCISSORS

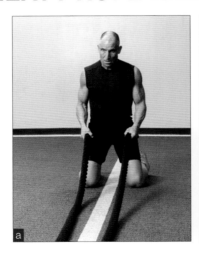 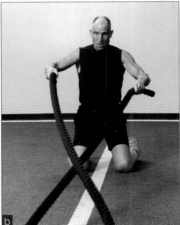

Fundamentals

- Sufficient upper-body and core strength to perform scissors for at least 30 seconds while standing

Setup

- Anchor the rope to a stable rack, pillar, or wall mount.
- Grasp the rope below the endcaps with a firm, neutral grip.
- Stabilize your body by kneeling; keep your back flat and your head up.

Movement

- Maintaining a neutral spine, explosively lift your arms above a parallel position with the floor.
- Scissor your arms by explosively crossing your right arm over your left and then your left over your right.
- Repeat the movement for the desired length of time.

HEAVY ROPE TWO-ARM UNBALANCED SLAMS

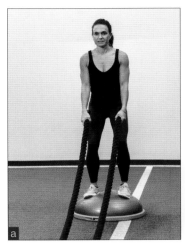 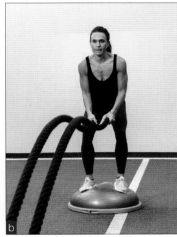

Fundamentals

- Sufficient upper-body, lower-body, and core strength to perform heavy rope two-hand slams for at least 30 seconds while standing

Setup

- Anchor the rope to a stable rack, pillar, or wall mount.
- Grasp the rope below the endcaps with a firm, neutral grip.
- Step onto an unbalanced mat or surface.
- Stabilize your body by bending knees into a partial squat; keep your back flat and your head up.
- Keep your weight on the balls of your feet.

Movement

- Explosively extend your hips and lift your arms until the ropes and your arms are above a parallel position with the floor.
- Once you reach the top position, explosively squat back down and forcefully drive the ropes toward the ground.
- Repeat the movement for the desired length of time.

Variations in Fundamentals and Movement

Heavy Rope Alt-Arm Unbalanced Slams

Fundamentals

- Sufficient upper-body, lower-body, and core strength to perform heavy rope alternate-arm slams for at least 30 seconds while standing

Movement

- Maintaining a partial squat, lift your arms and the rope to a position where your arms are parallel to the floor.
- Lift one arm up while explosively driving the other arm down; then reverse directions with each arm.
- Repeat the movement for the desired length of time.

HEAVY ROPE UNBALANCED SCISSORS

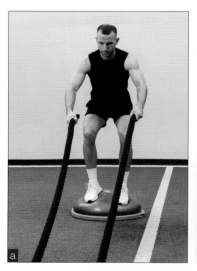 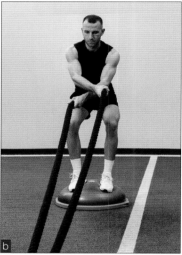

Fundamentals

- Sufficient upper-body, lower-body, and core strength to perform heavy rope scissors for at least 30 seconds while standing

Setup

- Anchor the rope to a stable rack, pillar, or wall mount.
- Grasp the rope below the endcaps with a firm, neutral grip.
- Step onto an unbalanced mat or surface.
- Stabilize your body by bending knees into a partial squat; keep your back flat and your head up.
- Keep your weight on the balls of your feet.

Movement

- Maintaining a partial squat, lift your arms and the rope to a position where your arms are parallel to the floor.
- Scissor your arms by explosively crossing your right arm over your left and then your left over your right.
- Repeat the movement for the desired length of time.

PART III

Metabolic-Training Programs

11

Programs for Endurance

Endurance is the ability to withstand hardship. In the context of physical activity, endurance is the ability to stave off fatigue and the ability to contract muscles repeatedly with little to no significant deprecation in ability or performance. Cardiorespiratory and muscular endurance can improve or maintain quality of life. Imagine being able to enjoy back-country hiking for several days, to complete your first half marathon or triathlon, or to stay physically active in your 60s, 70s, and beyond. Endurance activities such as running, biking, hiking, and swimming can improve cardiorespiratory capabilities, the ability to repeatedly contract muscles over longer periods of time, in addition to promoting a healthy body composition. However, endurance training does not improve strength and power capabilities. Metabolic-training methods can complement and improve traditional endurance activities with thoughtful programming. Exercise selection, exercise order, rest intervals, exercise intensity, and exercise duration have significant influence on training outcomes.

Cardiorespiratory and muscular endurance can be trained in a variety of ways, using a variety of methods. One of the advantages of metabolic training is that, with proper program design, it can improve both cardiorespiratory and muscular endurance over time. Example programs can be found in the second half of this chapter.

Benefits of Cardiorespiratory Endurance Training

Exercise physiologists have studied the effects of endurance training, observing general health and fitness improvements and determining optimal training methodologies. The American College of Sports Medicine recommends all healthy adults between the ages of 18 and 65 should participate in moderate-intensity aerobic activity for a minimum of 30 minutes five days per week or vigorous aerobic activity for a minimum of 20 minutes three days per week . The benefits of endurance training to the cardiorespiratory system include the following:

- Improved heat tolerance
- Improvement in lactate threshold
- Improvement in endurance performance

- Improvement in maximal exercise performance
- Improvement in recovery heart rate
- Increase in capillary density
- Increase in number and size of mitochondria in skeletal muscle
- Increase in exercise respiratory capacity
- Increase in maximal oxygen uptake
- Increase in cardiac output
- Decrease in exercise heart rate
- Decrease in resting heart rate
- Decrease in blood pressure in individuals with moderate to high blood pressure

Cardiorespiratory training methodologies typically used for endurance include the following:

- Metabolic training
- Running
- Biking
- Spinning
- Treadmill walking or running
- Elliptical
- Swimming
- Rowing
- Circuit weight training

Benefits of Muscular Endurance Training

Muscular endurance refers to the body's capacity to sustain repeated muscular actions, such as running for an extended period of time. Not surprisingly, muscular endurance is an important determinant of general health, fitness, and performance. Muscular endurance is improved through resistance training on a regular basis—three to five training sessions per week for at least eight weeks, for example—and it would stand to reason that metabolic training can improve muscular endurance when prioritized. Improvements in muscular endurance are realized through performing more repetitions of a selected exercise over time; for example, an individual capable of completing 30 push-ups without stopping could raise this number to 40 repetitions after several weeks of targeted and focused training.

Training for Muscular Endurance

Methods for training muscular endurance are nearly limitless. These methods are often but not exclusively used in metabolic training. There are several key considerations when training for muscular endurance. The first consideration is the inherent intensity and metabolic demand of the movement or exercise. Consider rapid bodyweight squats compared to biceps curls. The bodyweight squat is a multijoint movement, involving nearly all of the muscles of the lower body and requiring bodyweight to be displaced for a given number of repetitions. Biceps curls with dumbbells are performed with a fraction of the weight of a bodyweight squat and recruit the small muscles of the forearm. The metabolic demand of the bodyweight squats is significantly higher than the biceps curls. In other words, there is a direct positive correlation between the metabolic demand and the inherent intensity of the exercise. The following exercises are grouped according to the musculoskeletal strain they place on the body.

Muscular training methods for endurance include the following:

Higher metabolic demand

- Push-ups
- Pull-ups
- Squats and squat variations
- Lunges and lunge variations
- Bench press and bench variations
- Overhead press
- Cleans and clean variations
- Snatches and snatch variations

Lower metabolic demand

- Shoulder raises
- Biceps curls
- Triceps extensions
- Calf raises
- Abdominal crunches and variations
- Some torso-training exercises

Non-traditional, higher metabolic demand

- Battle ropes
- Sled pushes and pulls
- Kettlebell swings and variations
- Carrying exercises such as farmer's walks
- Multijoint medicine ball exercises
- Tire pulls, pushes, and flips
- Jumping jacks or star jumps
- Jumping rope
- Suspension trainer exercises: pushes, pulls, squats, and lunges

Guidelines and Goals of Endurance Training for Metabolic Conditioning

The following goals and guidelines will help you to create the safest and most effective training program for developing muscular endurance:

Exercise Technique

The goal is to use the best possible technique to perform each exercise. The best technique is also the safest technique.

Optimal exercise technique inherently varies from person to person. Variations exist for several reasons, including, but not limited to, individuality, experience, mastery of movement, and individual biomechanics. Keep in mind there is an acceptable range of variation in exercise technique. A qualified trainer can assist you if needed.

Exercise Order or Sequencing

The goal is to order or sequence exercises to manage fatigue.

Generally speaking, the exercises will be ordered changing from upper, lower, possibly mid-section, and back to upper and lower, respectively. However, keep in mind that sequencing the most demanding exercises back to back can result in excessive fatigue. So, it may be wise to incorporate less-fatiguing exercises intermittently throughout the workout.

Rating of Perceived Exertion

Rating of Perceived Exertion, or RPE, allows you to quantify the effort you feel you are exerting at a moment in time. There are several different scales that can be used, but the most common is 1-10, where 1 designates very light effort and 10 designates maximal effort.

When training for endurance, a reasonable RPE would be 6, 7, or 8 on a scale of 1-10. Depending on the individual and the goal of the training session, there may be easier or more difficult exercises. A bodyweight calf raise could be programmed directly after a 30-second treadmill sprint. The relatively light metabolic demand of the calf raise allows the body to recover from the more metabolically demanding treadmill sprint.

Fatigue Management

The goal is to modulate fatigue in such a way that the desired training effect is achieved.

Your workouts should be structured to minimize the accumulation of fatigue. This is accomplished by manipulating program variables such as exercise selection, exercise order, exercise intensity, and exercise duration. However, if you'd like to increase the metabolic demand at a particular time during the training session or for a specific area of the body, that can also be accomplished by way of program design.

Heart Rate

The goal is to manage your target heart rate to optimize endurance adaption.

Heart-rate response to exercise will vary from person to person. One person may have a higher heart rate at a given intensity compared to another person—thus, comparing heart rate from person to person has little to no value. To get the most out of training with heart rate, you should have a basic idea of your maximal or near-maximal HR, a high but sustainable HR, a lower, comfortable training HR, and your recovery HR.

Lactic-Acid Accumulation

The goal is to keep blood lactic acid below the level at which it cannot be cleared for the duration of the workout.

Resistance-training movements are generally anaerobic by nature, which means they produce lactic acid. Lactic acid will accumulate in the bloodstream during the course of a training session. Ideally, lactic-acid levels will be kept low enough to enable exercise to continue at a moderately high level.

Exercise Duration

The goal is to exercise to the point of reasonable fatigue but not exhaustion.

Endurance is best developed over time. Exercising to a reasonable level of fatigue means exercising enough to induce fatigue but not reaching a point at which you cannot recover within a day. Repeatedly exercising to exhaustion without adequate recovery will result in decreased performance.

Complement, not Compete

The goal of endurance-focused metabolic training is to improve your ability to tolerate prolonged physical exertion.

The optimal amount of metabolic endurance conditioning is determined by a number of factors, such as your adaptive capabilities and the degree to which endurance training stands to enhance your performance. Developing endurance should serve to complement and enhance your overall fitness, not compete against other performance goals.

Undulating Programming

The goal is to improve both metabolic and muscular endurance.

Perform two endurance-focused metabolic-conditioning sessions per week. One session should focus on metabolic endurance and the second should emphasize muscular endurance.

As stated above, endurance-focused metabolic training can emphasize metabolic demand or muscular demand. The loading parameters of the program will dictate where emphasis is placed. For instance, higher repetitions with shorter rest intervals will result in a greater metabolic demand than a muscular demand. Lower repetitions with longer rest intervals will yield a greater muscular demand than a metabolic demand. Keep in mind that multijoint, ground-based exercises are often more metabolically demanding than single-joint exercises. Tables 11.1 and 11.2 show two example workouts that target metabolic and muscular endurance.

Table 11.1 Sample Program Targeting Metabolic Endurance

Exercise	Sets	Repetitions, time, or distance	Rest interval
Jumping rope	4	1 min	30 sec
Push-ups	4	15 reps	30 sec
Step-ups	4	45 sec	30 sec
Weighted sled push	4	20 yd twice	30 sec
Bodyweight suspension trainer rows	4	15 reps	30 sec
Kettlebell swings	4	45 sec	30 sec
Planks	4	45 sec	30 sec

Table 11.2 Sample Program Targeting Muscular Strength

Exercise	Sets	Repetitions, time, or distance	Rest interval
Barbell back squat	4	6 reps	1 min
Barbell bench press	4	6 reps	1 min
Pull-ups	4	6 reps	1 min
Dumbbell backward lunge	4	10 reps: 5 each leg	1 min
Dumbbell curl to press	4	6 reps	1 min
Dumbbell row	4	6 reps	1 min
Cable chop	4	10 reps	1 min

The pods in the following exercise programs are a combination of three or more exercises performed with short rest periods between them for either a set number of repetitions or a prescribed amount of time.

Endurance Program 1A: Beginner

WARM-UP					
Exercise	Sets	Reps/time	Rest	Wt	Page #
March/walk	1	20 sec	10 sec	BW	N/A
Jumping jacks	1	20 sec	10 sec	BW	48
March/walk	1	20 sec	10 sec	BW	N/A
Single-leg squat (each leg)	1	20 sec	10 sec	BW	52
March/walk	1	20 sec	10 sec	BW	N/A
Mountain climbers	1	20 sec	10 sec	BW	49
March/walk	1	20 sec	10 sec	BW	N/A
Push-up	1	20 sec	10 sec	BW	112
March/walk	1	20 sec	10 sec	BW	N/A
Burpee	1	20 sec	10 sec	BW	50

LOWER BODY					
Exercise	Sets	Reps/time	Rest	Wt	Page #
Dumbbell box step-up	1	15 reps	15 sec	BW	86
Front lunge	1	15 reps	15 sec	BW	41
Lateral lunge	1	15 reps	15 sec	BW	42
Backward lunge	1	15 reps	15 sec	BW	43
Single-leg squat (each leg)	1	15 reps	15 sec	BW	52
Hip thrust	1	15 reps	15 sec	BW	100

CALISTHENICS					
Exercise	Sets	Reps/time	Rest	Wt	Page #
Jumping jacks	1	20 sec	10 sec	BW	48
Mountain climbers	1	20 sec	10 sec	BW	49
Groiner	1	20 sec	10 sec	BW	51
Single-leg squat (each leg)	1	20 sec	10 sec	BW	52
Front lunge	1	20 sec	10 sec	BW	41
Burpee	1	20 sec	10 sec	BW	50

UPPER BODY					
Exercise	Sets	Reps/time	Rest	Wt	Page #
Dumbbell bench press	1	15 reps	15 sec	10 lb, 15 lb, or 20 lb	122
Dumbbell one-arm row	1	15 reps	15 sec	10 lb, 15 lb, or 20 lb	129
Dumbbell shoulder press	1	15 reps	15 sec	8 lb, 10 lb, or 12 lb	131
Dumbbell bent-over raise	1	15 reps	15 sec	5 lb, or 8 lb	140
Dumbbell alt-arm biceps curl	1	15 reps	15 sec	10 lb, 12 lb, or 15 lb	144
Dumbbell supine triceps extension	1	15 reps	15 sec	10 lb, 12 lb, or 15 lb	141

CORE					
Exercise	Sets	Reps/time	Rest	Wt	Page #
Abdominal crunch	1	20 reps	15 sec	BW	155
Abdominal reach	1	20 reps	15 sec	BW	157
Front plank	1	30 sec	15 sec	BW	159
Side plank: right	1	30 sec	15 sec	BW	160
Side plank: left	1	30 sec	15 sec	BW	160
Birddog	1	30 sec	15 sec	BW	161

Wt = Weight; BW = Bodyweight

Endurance Program 1B: Intermediate

WARM-UP					
Exercise	Sets	Reps/time	Rest	Wt	Page #
Jog	1	30 sec	10 sec	BW	N/A
Jumping jacks	1	30 sec	10 sec	BW	48
Jog	1	30 sec	10 sec	BW	N/A
Single-leg squat (each leg)	1	30 sec	10 sec	BW	52
Jog	1	30 sec	10 sec	BW	N/A
Mountain climbers	1	30 sec	10 sec	BW	49
Jog	1	30 sec	10 sec	BW	N/A
Push-up	1	30 sec	10 sec	BW	112
Jog	1	30 sec	10 sec	BW	N/A
Burpee	1	30 sec	10 sec	BW	50
LOWER BODY					
Exercise	Sets	Reps/time	Rest	Wt	Page #
Dumbbell box step-up	1-2	15-20 reps	15 sec	8 lb, 10 lb, or 12 lb	86
Dumbbell front lunge	1-2	15-20 reps	15 sec	8 lb, 10 lb, or 12 lb	87
Dumbbell lateral lunge	1-2	15-20 reps	15 sec	8 lb, 10 lb, or 12 lb	90
Dumbbell backward lunge	1-2	15-20 reps	15 sec	8 lb, 10 lb, or 12 lb	92
Dumbbell squat	1-2	15-20 reps	15 sec	10 lb, 12 lb, or 15 lb	80
Dumbbell hip thrust	1-2	15-20 reps	15 sec	12 lb, 15 lb, or 20 lb	100
CALISTHENICS					
Exercise	Sets	Reps/time	Rest	Wt	Page #
Jumping jacks	1	30 sec	10 sec	BW	48
Mountain climbers	1	30 sec	10 sec	BW	49
Groiner	1	30 sec	10 sec	BW	51
Single-leg squat (each leg)	1	30 sec	10 sec	BW	52
Lunge	1	30 sec	10 sec	BW	41
Burpee	1	30 sec	10 sec	BW	50
UPPER BODY					
Exercise	Sets	Reps/time	Rest	Wt	Page #
Dumbbell bench press	1-2	15-20 reps	15 sec	10 lb, 15 lb, or 20 lb	122
Dumbbell one-arm row	1-2	15-20 reps	15 sec	10 lb, 15 lb, or 20 lb	129
Dumbbell shoulder press	1–2	15-20 reps	15 sec	8 lb, 10 lb, or 12 lb	131
Dumbbell bent-over raise	1-2	15-20 reps	15 sec	5 lb or 8 lb	140
Dumbbell alt-arm biceps curl	1-2	15-20 reps	15 sec	10 lb, 12 lb, or 15 lb	144
Dumbbell supine triceps extension	1-2	15-20 reps	15 sec	10 lb, 12 lb, or 15 lb	141
CORE					
Exercise	Sets	Reps/time	Rest	Wt	Page #
Abdominal crunch	1	30 reps	15 sec	BW	155
Abdominal reach	1	30 reps	15 sec	BW	157
Front plank	1	40 sec	15 sec	BW	159
Side plank: right	1	40 sec	15 sec	BW	160
Side plank: left	1	40 sec	15 sec	BW	160
Birddog	1	40 sec	15 sec	BW	161

Wt = Weight; BW = Bodyweight

Endurance Program 1C: Advanced

WARM-UP					
Exercise	Sets	Reps/time	Rest	Wt	Page #
Jog	1	40 sec	10 sec	BW	N/A
Jumping jacks	1	40 sec	10 sec	BW	48
Jog	1	40 sec	10 sec	BW	N/A
Single-leg squat (each leg)	1	40 sec	10 sec	BW	52
Jog	1	40 sec	10 sec	BW	N/A
Mountain climbers	1	40 sec	10 sec	BW	49
Jog	1	40 sec	10 sec	BW	N/A
Push-up	1	40 sec	10 sec	BW	112
Jog	1	40 sec	10 sec	BW	N/A
Burpee	1	40 sec	10 sec	BW	50
LOWER BODY					
Exercise	Sets	Reps/time	Rest	Wt	Page #
Dumbbell box step-up	2	15-20 reps	15 sec	12 lb, 15 lb, or 20 lb	86
Dumbbell front lunge	2	15-20 reps	15 sec	12 lb, 15 lb, or 20 lb	87
Dumbbell lateral lunge	2	15-20 reps	15 sec	12 lb, 15 lb, or 20 lb	90
Dumbbell backward lunge	2	15-20 reps	15 sec	12 lb, 15 lb, or 20 lb	92
Dumbbell squat	2	15-20 reps	15 sec	12 lb, 15 lb, or 20 lb	80
Dumbbell hip thrust	2	15-20 reps	15 sec	12 lb, 15 lb, or 20 lb	100
CALISTHENICS					
Exercise	Sets	Reps/time	Rest	Wt	Page #
Jumping jacks	1	40 sec	10 sec	BW	48
Mountain climbers	1	40 sec	10 sec	BW	49
Groiner	1	40 sec	10 sec	BW	51
Single-leg squat (each leg)	1	40 sec	10 sec	BW	52
Front lunge	1	40 sec	10 sec	BW	41
Burpee	1	40 sec	10 sec	BW	50
UPPER BODY					
Exercise	Sets	Reps/time	Rest	Wt	Page #
Dumbbell bench press	2	15-20 reps	15 sec	20 lb, 25 lb, or 30 lb	122
Dumbbell one-arm row	2	15-20 reps	15 sec	20 lb, 25 lb, or 30 lb	129
Dumbbell shoulder press	2	15-20 reps	15 sec	12 lb, 15 lb, or 20 lb	131
Dumbbell bent-over raise	2	15-20 reps	15 sec	8 lb, 10 lb, or 12 lb	140
Dumbbell alt-arm biceps curl	2	15-20 reps	15 sec	15 lb, 20 lb, or 25 lb	144
Dumbbell supine triceps extension	2	15-20 reps	15 sec	15 lb, 20 lb, or 25 lb	141
CORE					
Exercise	Sets	Reps/time	Rest	Wt	Page #
Abdominal crunch	1-2	40 reps	15 sec	BW	155
Abdominal reach	1	40 reps	15 sec	BW	157
Front plank	1	50 sec	15 sec	BW	159
Side plank: right	1	50 sec	15 sec	BW	160
Side plank: left	1	50 sec	15 sec	BW	160
Birddog	1	50 sec	15 sec	BW	161

Wt = Weight; BW = Bodyweight

Endurance Program 2A: Beginner

WARM-UP					
Exercise	Sets	Reps/time	Rest	Wt	Page #
March/walk	1	20 sec	10 sec	BW	N/A
Single-leg squat (each leg)	1	20 sec	10 sec	BW	52
March/walk	1	20 sec	10 sec	BW	N/A
Mountain climbers	1	20 sec	10 sec	BW	49
March/walk	1	20 sec	10 sec	BW	N/A
Jumping jacks	1	20 sec	10 sec	BW	48
March/walk	1	20 sec	10 sec	BW	N/A
Burpee	1	20 sec	10 sec	BW	50
March/walk	1	20 sec	10 sec	BW	N/A
Push-up	1	20 sec	10 sec	BW	112
LOWER BODY					
Exercise	Sets	Reps/time	Rest	Wt	Page #
Kettlebell deadlift	1	15 reps	15 sec	8 kg, 10 kg	94
Kettlebell goblet squat	1	15 reps	15 sec	8 kg, 10 kg	81
Resistance band forward walk	2	10 yd	15 sec	Light	101
Resistance band lateral walk: right	1	10 yd	15 sec	Light	102
Resistance band lateral walk: left	1	10 yd	15 sec	Light	102
Kettlebell straight-leg deadlift	1	15 reps	15 sec	8 kg, 10 kg	95
Dumbbell hip thrust	1	15 reps	15 sec	Light	100
CALISTHENICS					
Exercise	Sets	Reps/time	Rest	Wt	Page #
Mountain climbers	1	20 sec	10 sec	BW	49
Groiner	1	20 sec	10 sec	BW	51
Single-leg squat (each leg)	1	20 sec	10 sec	BW	52
Burpee	1	20 sec	10 sec	BW	50
Jumping jacks	1	20 sec	10 sec	BW	48
Front lunge	1	20 sec	10 sec	BW	41
UPPER BODY					
Exercise	Sets	Reps/time	Rest	Wt	Page #
Resistance band standing chest press	1	15 reps	15 sec	Light	147
Kettlebell one-arm row	1	15 reps	15 sec	6 kg, 8 kg, 10 kg	129
Kettlebell upright row	1	15 reps	15 sec	6 kg, 8 kg, 10 kg	134
Resistance band T	1	15 reps	15 sec	Light	117
Kettlebell alt-arm biceps curl	1	15 reps	15 sec	4 kg, 6 kg, 8 kg	144
Kettlebell overhead triceps extension	1	15 reps	15 sec	6 kg, 8 kg, 10 kg (22.0 lb	118
CORE					
Exercise	Sets	Reps/time	Rest	Wt	Page #
Abdominal crunch	1	20 reps	15 sec	BW	155
Abdominal reach	1	20 reps	15 sec	BW	157
Front plank	1	30 sec	15 sec	BW	159
Side plank: right	1	30 sec	15 sec	BW	160
Side plank: left	1	30 sec	15 sec	BW	160
Birddog	1	30 sec	15 sec	BW	161

Wt = Weight; BW = Bodyweight

Endurance Program 2B: Intermediate

WARM-UP					
Exercise	Sets	Reps/time	Rest	Wt	Page #
Jog	1	30 sec	10 sec	BW	N/A
Single-leg squat (each leg)	1	30 sec	10 sec	BW	52
Jog	1	30 sec	10 sec	BW	N/A
Mountain climbers	1	30 sec	10 sec	BW	49
Jog	1	30 sec	10 sec	BW	N/A
Jumping jacks	1	30 sec	10 sec	BW	48
Jog	1	30 sec	10 sec	BW	N/A
Burpee	1	30 sec	10 sec	BW	50
Jog	1	30 sec	10 sec	BW	N/A
Push-up	1	30 sec	10 sec	BW	112
LOWER BODY					
Exercise	Sets	Reps/time	Rest	Wt	Page #
Kettlebell deadlift	1-2	15 reps	15 sec	12 kg, 14 kg, 16 kg	94
Kettlebell goblet squat	1-2	15 reps	15 sec	12 kg, 14 kg, 16 kg	81
Resistance band forward walk	1-2	10 yd	15 sec	Light/moderate	101
Resistance band lateral walk: right	1-2	10 yd	15 sec	Light/moderate	102
Resistance band lateral walk: left	1-2	10 yd	15 sec	Light/moderate	102
Kettlebell straight-leg deadlift	1-2	15 reps	15 sec	12 kg, 14 kg, 16 kg	95
Dumbbell hip thrust	1-2	15 reps	15 sec	Light/moderate	100
CALISTHENICS					
Exercise	Sets	Reps/time	Rest	Wt	Page #
Mountain climbers	1	30 sec	10 sec	BW	49
Groiner	1	30 sec	10 sec	BW	51
Single-leg squat (each leg)	1	30 sec	10 sec	BW	52
Burpee	1	30 sec	10 sec	BW	50
Jumping jacks	1	30 sec	10 sec	BW	48
Front lunge	1	30 sec	10 sec	BW	41
UPPER BODY					
Exercise	Sets	Reps/time	Rest	Wt	Page #
Resistance band standing chest press	1-2	15 reps	15 sec	Moderate	147
Kettlebell one-arm row	1-2	15 reps	15 sec	12 kg, 14 kg, 16 kg	129
Kettlebell upright row	1-2	15 reps	15 sec	10 kg, 12 kg, 14 kg	134
Resistance band T	1-2	15 reps	15 sec	Moderate	118
Kettlebell alt-arm biceps curl	1-2	15 reps	15 sec	8 kg, 10 kg, 12 kg	144
Kettlebell overhead triceps extension	1-2	15 reps	15 sec	8 kg, 10 kg, 12 kg	120
CORE					
Exercise	Sets	Reps/time	Rest	Wt	Page #
Abdominal crunch	1	30 sec	15 sec	BW	155
Abdominal reach	1	30 sec	15 sec	BW	157
Front plank	1	40 sec	15 sec	BW	159
Side plank: right	1	40 sec	15 sec	BW	160
Side plank: left	1	40 sec	15 sec	BW	160
Birddog	1	40 sec	15 sec	BW	161

Wt = Weight; BW = Bodyweight

Endurance Program 2C: Advanced

WARM-UP					
Exercise	Sets	Reps/time	Rest	Wt	Page #
Jog	1	40 sec	10 sec	BW	N/A
Single-leg squat (each leg)	1	40 sec	10 sec	BW	52
Jog	1	40 sec	10 sec	BW	N/A
Mountain climbers	1	40 sec	10 sec	BW	49
Jog	1	40 sec	10 sec	BW	N/A
Jumping jacks	1	40 sec	10 sec	BW	48
Jog	1	40 sec	10 sec	BW	N/A
Burpee	1	40 sec	10 sec	BW	50
Jog	1	40 sec	10 sec	BW	N/A
Push-up	1	40 sec	10 sec	BW	112

LOWER BODY					
Exercise	Sets	Reps/time	Rest	Wt	Page #
Kettlebell deadlift	2	15 reps	15 sec	16 kg, 18 kg, 20 kg	94
Kettlebell goblet squat	2	15 reps	15 sec	14 kg, 16 kg, 18 kg	81
Resistance band forward walk	2	10 yd	15 sec	Moderate/heavy	101
Resistance band lateral walk: right	2	10 yd	15 sec	Moderate/heavy	102
Resistance band lateral walk: left	2	10 yd	15 sec	Moderate/heavy	102
Kettlebell straight-leg deadlift	2	15 reps	15 sec	14 kg, 16 kg, 18 kg	95
Dumbbell hip thrust	1-2	15 reps	15 sec	Moderate/heavy	100

CALISTHENICS					
Exercise	Sets	Reps/time	Rest	Wt	Page #
Mountain climbers	1	40 sec	10 sec	BW	49
Groiner	1	40 sec	10 sec	BW	51
Single-leg squat (each leg)	1	40 sec	10 sec	BW	52
Burpee	1	40 sec	10 sec	BW	50
Jumping jacks	1	40 sec	10 sec	BW	48
Front lunge	1	40 sec	10 sec	BW	41

UPPER BODY					
Exercise	Sets	Reps/time	Rest	Wt	Page #
Resistance band standing chest press	2	15 reps	15 sec	Moderate/Heavy	147
Kettlebell one-arm row	2	15 reps	15 sec	14 kg, 16 kg, 18 kg	129
Kettlebell upright row	2	15 reps	15 sec	12 kg, 14 kg, 16 kg	134
Resistance band T	2	15 reps	15 sec	Moderate/heavy	118
Kettlebell alt-arm biceps curl	2	15 reps	15 sec	10 kg, 12 kg, 14 kg	144
Kettlebell overhead triceps extension	2	15 reps	15 sec	10 kg, 12 kg, 14 kg	120

CORE					
Exercise	Sets	Reps/time	Rest	Wt	Page #
Abdominal crunch	1	40 reps	15 sec	BW	155
Abdominal reach	1	40 reps	15 sec	BW	157
Front plank	1	50 sec	15 sec	BW	159
Side plank: right	1	50 sec	15 sec	BW	160
Side plank: left	1	50 sec	15 sec	BW	160
Birddog	1	50 sec	15 sec	BW	161

Wt = Weight; BW = Bodyweight

Endurance Program 3A: Beginner

Note: Each exercise in a pod should be completed before moving to the next pod. A pod is a combination of three or more exercises performed with short rest periods between them for either a set number of repetitions or a prescribed amount of time.

WARM-UP					
Exercise	**Sets**	**Reps/time**	**Rest**	**Wt**	**Page #**
March/walk	1	20 sec	10 sec	BW	N/A
Single-leg squat (each leg)	1	20 sec	10 sec	BW	52
March/walk	1	20 sec	10 sec	BW	N/A
Mountain climbers	1	20 sec	10 sec	BW	49
March/walk	1	20 sec	10 sec	BW	N/A
Jumping jacks	1	20 sec	10 sec	BW	48
March/walk	1	20 sec	10 sec	BW	N/A
Burpee	1	20 sec	10 sec	BW	50
March/walk	1	20 sec	10 sec	BW	N/A
Push-up	1	20 sec	10 sec	BW	112

POD 1					
Exercise	**Sets**	**Reps/time**	**Rest**	**Wt**	**Page #**
Kettlebell two-hand swing	1	15 reps	15 sec	6 kg, 8 kg	62
Push-up	1	15 reps	15 sec	BW	112
Abdominal crunch	1	20 reps	15 sec	BW	155

POD 2					
Exercise	**Sets**	**Reps/time**	**Rest**	**Wt**	**Page #**
Dumbbell squat	1	15 reps	15 sec	10 lb, 12 lb, 15 lb	80
Dumbbell one-arm row	1	15 reps	15 sec	12 lb, 15 lb, 17.5 lb	129
Abdominal reach	1	20 reps	15 sec	BW	157

POD 3					
Exercise	**Sets**	**Reps/time**	**Rest**	**Wt**	**Page #**
Dumbbell front lunge	1	15 reps	15 sec	8 lb, 10 lb, 12 lb	87
Dumbbell shoulder press	1	15 reps	15 sec	8 lb, 10 lb, 12 lb	131
Scissors	1	30 sec	15 sec	BW	162

POD 4					
Exercise	**Sets**	**Reps/time**	**Rest**	**Wt**	**Page #**
Heavy rope two-arm slams	1	30 sec	15 sec	Rope	169
Heavy rope alt-arm slams	1	30 sec	15 sec	Rope	170
Heavy rope scissors	1	30 sec	15 sec	Rope	171

POD 5					
Exercise	**Sets**	**Reps/time**	**Rest**	**Wt**	**Page #**
Kettlebell goblet squat	1	15 reps	15 sec	6 kg, 8 kg, 10 kg	81
Dumbbell upright row	1	15 reps	15 sec	8 lb, 10 lb, 12 lb	134
Front plank	1	30 sec	15 sec	BW	159

POD 6					
Exercise	**Sets**	**Reps/time**	**Rest**	**Wt**	**Page #**
Mountain climbers	1	30 sec	10 sec	BW	49
Groiner	1	30 sec	10 sec	BW	51
Single-leg squat (each leg)	1	30 sec	10 sec	BW	52

(continued)

POD 7					
Exercise	**Sets**	**Reps/time**	**Rest**	**Wt**	**Page #**
Burpee	1	30 sec	10 sec	BW	50
Jumping jacks	1	30 sec	10 sec	BW	48
Front lunge	1	30 sec	10 sec	BW	41

POD 8					
Exercise	**Sets**	**Reps/time**	**Rest**	**Wt**	**Page #**
Dumbbell lateral lunge	1	15 reps	15 sec	8 lb, 10 lb, 12 lb	90
Dumbbell bench press	1	15 reps	15 sec	10 lb, 12 lb, 15 lb	122
Side plank: right	1	30 sec	15 sec	BW	160

POD 9					
Exercise	**Sets**	**Reps/time**	**Rest**	**Wt**	**Page #**
Dumbbell box step-up	1	15 reps	15 sec	8 lb, 10 lb, 12 lb	86
Dumbbell upright row	1	15 reps	15 sec	10 lb, 12 lb, 15 lb	134
Side plank: left	1	30 sec	15 sec	BW	160

POD 10					
Exercise	**Sets**	**Reps/time**	**Rest**	**Wt**	**Page #**
Dumbbell lateral box step-up	1	15 reps	15 sec	8 lb, 10 lb, 12 lb	86
Dumbbell front raise	1	15 reps	15 sec	5 lb, 8 lb, 10 lb	138
Superman	1	30 sec	15 sec	BW	163

POD 11					
Exercise	**Sets**	**Reps/time**	**Rest**	**Wt**	**Page #**
Dumbbell straight-leg deadlift	1	15 reps	15 sec	10 lb, 12 lb, 15 lb	95
Dumbbell bent-over raise	1	15 reps	15 sec	5 lb, 8 lb, 10 lb	140
Scissors	1	30 sec	15 sec	BW	162

POD 12					
Exercise	**Sets**	**Reps/time**	**Rest**	**Wt**	**Page #**
Weighted sled push	1	30 sec	15 sec	45 lb	74
Weighted sled pull and push	1	30 sec	15 sec	45 lb	75
Weighted sled push	1	30 sec	15 sec	45 lb	74

Wt = Weight; BW = Bodyweight

Endurance Program 3B: Intermediate

Note: Each exercise in a pod should be completed before moving to the next pod. A pod is a combination of three or more exercises performed with short rest periods between them for either a set number of repetitions or a prescribed amount of time.

WARM-UP					
Exercise	**Sets**	**Reps/time**	**Rest**	**Wt**	**Page #**
Jog in place / jump rope	1	40 sec	10 sec	BW	N/A
Single-leg squat (each leg)	1	40 sec	10 sec	BW	52
Jog in place / jump rope	1	40 sec	10 sec	BW	N/A
Mountain climbers	1	40 sec	10 sec	BW	49
Jog in place / jump rope	1	40 sec	10 sec	BW	N/A
Jumping jacks	1	40 sec	10 sec	BW	48
Jog in place / jump rope	1	40 sec	10 sec	BW	N/A
Burpee	1	40 sec	10 sec	BW	50
Jog in place / jump rope	1	40 sec	10 sec	BW	N/A
Push-up	1	40 sec	10 sec	BW	112

POD 1					
Exercise	Sets	Reps/time	Rest	Wt	Page #
Kettlebell two-hand swing	1-2	15 reps	15 sec	10 kg, 12 kg, 14 kg	62
Push-up	1-2	15 reps	15 sec	BW	112
Weighted abdominal crunch	1-2	30 reps	15 sec	10 lb	155
POD 2					
Exercise	Sets	Reps/time	Rest	Wt	Page #
Dumbbell squat	1-2	15 reps	15 sec	12 lb, 15 lb, 20 lb	80
Dumbbell one-arm row	1-2	15 reps	15 sec	15 lb, 20 lb, 25 lb	129
Weighted abdominal reach	1-2	30 reps	15 sec	10 lb	157
POD 3					
Exercise	Sets	Reps/time	Rest	Wt	Page #
Dumbbell front lunge	1-2	15 reps	15 sec	10 lb, 12 lb, 15 lb	87
Dumbbell shoulder press	1-2	15 reps	15 sec	10 lb, 12 lb, 15 lb	131
Scissors	1-2	40 sec	15 sec	BW	162
POD 4					
Exercise	Sets	Reps/time	Rest	Wt	Page #
Heavy rope two-arm slams	1	40 sec	15 sec	Rope	169
Heavy rope alt-arm slams	1	40 sec	15 sec	Rope	170
Heavy rope scissors	1	40 sec	15 sec	Rope	171
POD 5					
Exercise	Sets	Reps/time	Rest	Wt	Page #
Kettlebell goblet squat	1-2	15 reps	15 sec	8 , 10 kg, 12 kg	81
Dumbbell upright row	1-2	15 reps	15 sec	10 lb, 12 lb, 15 lb	134
Front plank	1-2	40 sec	15 sec	BW	159
POD 6					
Exercise	Sets	Reps/time	Rest	Wt	Page #
Mountain climbers	1	40 sec	10 sec	BW	49
Groiner	1	40 sec	10 sec	BW	51
Single-leg squat (each leg)	1	40 sec	10 sec	BW	52
POD 7					
Exercise	Sets	Reps/time	Rest	Wt	Page #
Burpee	1	40 sec	10 sec	BW	50
Jumping jacks	1	40 sec	10 sec	BW	48
Front lunge	1	40 sec	10 sec	BW	41
POD 8					
Exercise	Sets	Reps/time	Rest	Wt	Page #
Dumbbell lateral lunge	1-2	15 reps	15 sec	10 lb, 12 lb, 15 lb	90
Dumbbell bench press	1-2	15 reps	15 sec	15 lb, 20 lb, 25 lb	122
Side plank: right	1-2	40 sec	15 sec	BW	160
POD 9					
Exercise	Sets	Reps/time	Rest	Wt	Page #
Dumbbell box step-up	1-2	15 reps	15 sec	10 lb, 12 lb, 15 lb	86
Dumbbell upright row	1-2	15 reps	15 sec	15 lb, 20 lb, 25 lb	134
Side plank: left	1-2	40 sec	15 sec	BW	160

(continued)

Endurance Program 3B: Intermediate (continued)

POD 10					
Exercise	Sets	Reps/time	Rest	Wt	Page #
Dumbbell lateral box step-up	1-2	15 reps	15 sec	10 lb, 12 lb, 15 lb	86
Dumbbell front raise	1-2	15 reps	15 sec	8 lb, 10 lb, 12 lb	138
Superman	1-2	40 sec	15 sec	BW	163
POD 11					
Exercise	Sets	Reps/time	Rest	Wt	Page #
Dumbbell straight-leg deadlift	1-2	15 reps	15 sec	15 lb, 20 lb, 25 lb	95
Dumbbell bent-over raise	1-2	15 reps	15 sec	5 lb, 8 lb, 10 lb	140
Scissors	1-2	40 sec	15 sec	BW	162
POD 12					
Exercise	Sets	Reps/time	Rest	Wt	Page #
Weighted sled push	1	40 sec	15 sec	70 lb	74
Weighted sled pull and push	1	40 sec	15 sec	70 lb	75
Weighted sled push	1	40 sec	15 sec	70 lb	74

Wt = Weight; BW = Bodyweight

Endurance Program 3C: Advanced

Note: Each exercise in a pod should be completed before moving to the next pod. A pod is a combination of three or more exercises performed with short rest periods between them for either a set number of repetitions or a prescribed amount of time.

WARM-UP					
Exercise	Sets	Reps/time	Rest	Wt	Page #
Jog in place / jump rope	1	50 sec	10 sec	BW	N/A
Single-leg squat (each leg)	1	50 sec	10 sec	BW	52
Jog in place / jump rope	1	50 sec	10 sec	BW	N/A
Mountain climbers	1	50 sec	10 sec	BW	49
Jog in place / jump rope	1	50 sec	10 sec	BW	N/A
Jumping jacks	1	50 sec	10 sec	BW	48
Jog in place / jump rope	1	50 sec	10 sec	BW	N/A
Burpee	1	50 sec	10 sec	BW	50
Jog in place / jump rope	1	50 sec	10 sec	BW	N/A
Push-up	1	50 sec	10 sec	BW	112
POD 1					
Exercise	Sets	Reps/time	Rest	Wt	Page #
Kettlebell two-hand swing	1-2	15-20 reps	15 sec	10 kg, 12 kg, 14 kg	62
Push-up	1-2	15-20 reps	15 sec	BW	112
Weighted abdominal crunch	1-2	40 reps	15 sec	10 lb	155
POD 2					
Exercise	Sets	Reps/time	Rest	Wt	Page #
Dumbbell squat	1-2	15-20 reps	15 sec	12 lb, 15 lb, 20 lb	80
Dumbbell one-hand row	1-2	15-20 reps	15 sec	15 lb, 20 lb, 25 lb	129
Weighted abdominal reach	1-2	40 reps	15 sec	10 lb	157
POD 3					
Exercise	Sets	Reps/time	Rest	Wt	Page #
Dumbbell front lunge	1-2	15-20 reps	15 sec	10 lb, 12 lb, 15 lb	87
Dumbbell shoulder press	1-2	15-20 reps	15 sec	10 lb, 12 lb, 15 lb	131
Scissors	1-2	50 sec	15 sec	BW	162

POD 4					
Exercise	Sets	Reps/time	Rest	Wt	Page #
Heavy rope two-arm slams	1	40 sec	15 sec	Rope	169
Heavy rope alt-arm slams	1	40 sec	15 sec	Rope	170
Heavy rope scissors	1	40 sec	15 sec	Rope	171

POD 5					
Exercise	Sets	Reps/time	Rest	Wt	Page #
Kettlebell goblet squat	1-2	15-20 reps	15 sec	8 kg, 10 kg, 12 kg	81
Dumbbell upright row	1-2	15-20 reps	15 sec	10 lb, 12 lb, 15 lb	134
Front plank	1-2	50 sec	15 sec	BW	159

POD 6					
Exercise	Sets	Reps/time	Rest	Wt	Page #
Mountain climbers	1	50 sec	10 sec	BW	49
Groiner	1	50 sec	10 sec	BW	51
Single-leg squat (each leg)	1	50 sec	10 sec	BW	52

POD 7					
Exercise	Sets	Reps/time	Rest	Wt	Page #
Burpee	1	50 sec	10 sec	BW	50
Jumping jacks	1	50 sec	10 sec	BW	48
Front lunge	1	50 sec	10 sec	BW	41

POD 8					
Exercise	Sets	Reps/time	Rest	Wt	Page #
Dumbbell lateral lunge	1-2	15-20 reps	15 sec	10 lb, 12 lb, 15 lb	90
Dumbbell bench press	1-2	15-20 reps	15 sec	15 lb, 20 lb, 25 lb	122
Side plank: right	1-2	50 sec	15 sec	BW	160

POD 9					
Exercise	Sets	Reps/time	Rest	Wt	Page #
Dumbbell box step-up	1-2	15-20 reps	15 sec	10 lb, 12 lb, 15 lb	86
Dumbbell upright row	1-2	15-20 reps	15 sec	15 lb, 20 lb, 25 lb	134
Side plank: left	1-2	50 sec	15 sec	BW	160

POD 10					
Exercise	Sets	Reps/time	Rest	Wt	Page #
Dumbbell lateral box step-up	1-2	15-20 reps	15 sec	10 lb, 12 lb, 15 lb	86
Dumbbell front raise	1-2	15-20 reps	15 sec	8 lb, 10 lb, 12 lb	138
Superman	1-2	50 sec	15 sec	BW	163

POD 11					
Exercise	Sets	Reps/time	Rest	Wt	Page #
Dumbbell straight-leg deadlift	1-2	15-20 reps	15 sec	15 lb, 20 lb, 25 lb	95
Dumbbell bent-over raise	1-2	15-20 reps	15 sec	5 lb, 8 lb, 10 lb	140
Scissors	1-2	50 sec	15 sec	BW	162

POD 12					
Exercise	Sets	Reps/time	Rest	Wt	Page #
Weighted sled push	1	50 sec	15 sec	70 lb	74
Weighted sled pull and push	1	50 sec	15 sec	70 lb	75
Weighted sled push	1	50 sec	15 sec	70 lb	74

Wt = Weight; BW = Bodyweight

Endurance Program 4A: Beginner

Note: Each exercise in a pod should be completed before moving to the next pod. A pod is a combination of three or more exercises performed with short rest periods between them for either a set number of repetitions or a prescribed amount of time.

WARM-UP					
Exercise	Sets	Reps/time	Rest	Wt	Page #
March/walk	1	20 sec	10 sec	BW	N/A
Single-leg squat (each leg)	1	20 sec	10 sec	BW	52
March/walk	1	20 sec	10 sec	BW	N/A
Mountain climbers	1	20 sec	10 sec	BW	49
March/walk	1	20 sec	10 sec	BW	N/A
Jumping jacks	1	20 sec	10 sec	BW	48
March/walk	1	20 sec	10 sec	BW	N/A
Burpee	1	20 sec	10 sec	BW	50
March/walk	1	20 sec	10 sec	BW	N/A
Push-up	1	20 sec	10 sec	BW	112
POD 1					
Exercise	Sets	Reps/time	Rest	Wt	Page #
Dumbbell squat	1	15 reps	15 sec	10 lb, 12 lb, 15 lb	80
Kettlebell goblet squat	1	15 reps	15 sec	8 kg, 10 kg, 12 kg	81
Kettlebell straight-leg deadlift	1	15 reps	15 sec	10 kg, 12 kg, 14 kg	95
POD 2					
Exercise	Sets	Reps/time	Rest	Wt	Page #
Medicine ball slam	1	15 reps	15 sec	10 lb, 12 lb	66
Medicine ball alt-side slam	1	15 reps	15 sec	10 lb, 12 lb	67
Medicine ball overhead squat	1	15 reps	15 sec	10 lb, 12 lb	85
POD 3					
Exercise	Sets	Reps/time	Rest	Wt	Page #
Dumbbell front lunge	1	15 reps	15 sec	8 lb, 10 lb, 12 lb	87
Dumbbell lateral lunge	1	15 reps	15 sec	8 lb, 10 lb, 12 lb	90
Dumbbell backward lunge	1	15 reps	15 sec	8 lb, 10 lb, 12 lb	92
POD 4					
Exercise	Sets	Reps/time	Rest	Wt	Page #
Heavy rope two-arm slams	1	30 sec	15 sec	Rope	169
Heavy rope alt-arm slams	1	30 sec	15 sec	Rope	170
Heavy rope scissors	1	30 sec	15 sec	Rope	171
POD 5					
Exercise	Sets	Reps/time	Rest	Wt	Page #
Dumbbell box step-up: alt leg	1	15 reps	15 sec	8 lb, 10 lb, 12 lb	86
Resistance band lateral walk: right	1	15 reps	15 sec	8 lb, 10 lb, 12 lb	102
Resistance band lateral walk: left	1	15 reps	15 sec	8 lb, 10 lb, 12 lb	102
POD 6					
Exercise	Sets	Reps/time	Rest	Wt	Page #
Dumbbell bench press	1	15 reps	15 sec	12 lb, 15 lb, 20 lb	122
Dumbbell one-arm row	1	15 reps	15 sec	12 lb, 15 lb, 20 lb	129
Pullover	1	15 reps	15 sec	12 lb, 15 lb, 20 lb	128

POD 7					
Exercise	Sets	Reps/time	Rest	Wt	Page #
Dumbbell shoulder press	1	15 reps	15 sec	10 lb, 12 lb, 15 lb	131
Dumbbell upright row	1	15 reps	15 sec	10 lb, 12 lb, 15 lb	134
Dumbbell bent-over raise	1	15 reps	15 sec	8 lb, 10 lb, 12 lb	140
POD 8					
Exercise	Sets	Reps/time	Rest	Wt	Page #
Abdominal crunch	1	30 sec	15 sec	BW	155
Scissors	1	30 sec	15 sec	BW	162
Birddog	1	30 sec	15 sec	BW	161
POD 9					
Exercise	Sets	Reps/time	Rest	Wt	Page #
Weighted sled push	1	30 sec	15 sec	45 lb	74
Weighted sled pull and push	1	30 sec	15 sec	45 lb	75
Weighted sled drag	1	30 sec	15 sec	45 lb	76
POD 10					
Exercise	Sets	Reps/time	Rest	Wt	Page #
Front plank	1	30 sec	15 sec	BW	159
Side plank: right	1	30 sec	15 sec	BW	160
Side plank: left	1	30 sec	15 sec	BW	160

Wt = Weight; BW = Bodyweight

Endurance Program 4B: Intermediate

Note: Each exercise in a pod should be completed before moving to the next pod. A pod is a combination of three or more exercises performed with short rest periods between them for either a set number of repetitions or a prescribed amount of time.

WARM-UP					
Exercise	Sets	Reps/time	Rest	Wt	Page #
Jog in place / jump rope	1	40 sec	10 sec	BW	N/A
Single-leg squat (each leg)	1	40 sec	10 sec	BW	52
Jog in place / jump rope	1	40 sec	10 sec	BW	N/A
Mountain climbers	1	40 sec	10 sec	BW	49
Jog in place / jump rope	1	40 sec	10 sec	BW	N/A
Jumping jacks	1	40 sec	10 sec	BW	48
Jog in place / jump rope	1	40 sec	10 sec	BW	N/A
Burpee	1	40 sec	10 sec	BW	50
Jog in place / jump rope	1	40 sec	10 sec	BW	N/A
Push-up	1	40 sec	10 sec	BW	112
POD 1					
Exercise	Sets	Reps/time	Rest	Wt	Page #
Dumbbell squat	1-2	15 reps	15 sec	15 lb, 20 lb, 25 lb	80
Kettlebell deadlift	1-2	15 reps	15 sec	14 kg, 16 kg, 18 kg	94
Kettlebell one-leg straight-leg deadlift	1-2	15 reps	15 sec	8 kg, 10 kg, 12 kg	98

(continued)

Endurance Program 4B: Intermediate *(continued)*

POD 2					
Exercise	Sets	Reps/time	Rest	Wt	Page #
Medicine ball slam	1	15 reps	15 sec	12 lb, 14 lb	66
Medicine ball alt-side slam	1	15 reps	15 sec	12 lb, 14 lb	67
Medicine ball overhead squat	1	15 reps	15 sec	12 lb, 14 lb	85

POD 3					
Exercise	Sets	Reps/time	Rest	Wt	Page #
Dumbbell front lunge	1-2	15 reps	15 sec	10 lb, 12 lb, 15 lb	87
Dumbbell lateral lunge	1-2	15 reps	15 sec	10 lb, 12 lb, 15 lb	90
Dumbbell backward lunge	1-2	15 reps	15 sec	10 lb, 12 lb, 15 lb	92

POD 4					
Exercise	Sets	Reps/time	Rest	Wt	Page #
Heavy rope jumping jacks	1	40 sec	15 sec	Rope	172
Heavy rope arm circles: clockwise	1	40 sec	15 sec	Rope	173
Heavy rope arm circles: counterclockwise	1	40 sec	15 sec	Rope	173

POD 5					
Exercise	Sets	Reps/time	Rest	Wt	Page #
Dumbbell box step-up: alt leg	1-2	15 reps	15 sec	12 lb, 15 lb, 20 lb	86
Resistance band lateral walk: right	1-2	15 reps	15 sec	12 lb, 15 lb, 20 lb	102
Resistance band lateral walk: left	1-2	15 reps	15 sec	12 lb, 15 lb, 20 lb	102

POD 6					
Exercise	Sets	Reps/time	Rest	Wt	Page #
Dumbbell bench press	1-2	15 reps	15 sec	15 lb, 20 lb, 25 lb	122
Dumbbell one-arm row	1-2	15 reps	15 sec	15 lb, 20 lb, 25 lb	129
Pullover	1-2	15 reps	15 sec	20 lb, 25 lb	128

POD 7					
Exercise	Sets	Reps/time	Rest	Wt	Page #
Dumbbell shoulder press	1-2	15 reps	15 sec	12 lb, 15 lb, 20 lb	131
Dumbbell upright row	1-2	15 reps	15 sec	12 lb, 15 lb, 20 lb	134
Dumbbell bent-over raise	1-2	15 reps	15 sec	8 lb, 10 lb, 12 lb	140

POD 8					
Exercise	Sets	Reps/time	Rest	Wt	Page #
Weighted abdominal crunch	1-2	40 reps	15 sec	10 lb	155
Scissors	1-2	40 sec	15 sec	BW	162
Birddog	1-2	40 sec	15 sec	BW	161

POD 9					
Exercise	Sets	Reps/time	Rest	Wt	Page #
Weighted sled push	1	40 sec	15 sec	70 lb	74
Weighted sled pull and push	1	40 sec	15 sec	70 lb	75
Weighted sled drag	1	40 sec	15 sec	70 lb	76

POD 10					
Exercise	Sets	Reps/time	Rest	Wt	Page #
Front plank	1-2	40 sec	15 sec	BW	159
Side plank: right	1-2	40 sec	15 sec	BW	160
Side plank: left	1-2	40 sec	15 sec	BW	160

Wt = Weight; BW = Bodyweight

Endurance Program 4C: Advanced

Note: Each exercise in a pod should be completed before moving to the next pod. A pod is a combination of three or more exercises performed with short rest periods between them for either a set number of repetitions or a prescribed amount of time.

WARM-UP					
Exercise	Sets	Reps/time	Rest	Wt	Page #
Jog in place / jump rope	1	50 sec	10 sec	BW	N/A
Single-leg squat (each leg)	1	50 sec	10 sec	BW	52
Jog in place / jump rope	1	50 sec	10 sec	BW	N/A
Mountain climbers	1	50 sec	10 sec	BW	49
Jog in place / jump rope	1	50 sec	10 sec	BW	N/A
Jumping jacks	1	50 sec	10 sec	BW	48
Jog in place / jump rope	1	50 sec	10 sec	BW	N/A
Burpee	1	50 sec	10 sec	BW	50
Jog in place / jump rope	1	50 sec	10 sec	BW	N/A
Push-up	1	50 sec	10 sec	BW	112
POD 1					
Exercise	Sets	Reps/time	Rest	Wt	Page #
Dumbbell squat	1-2	15-20 reps	15 sec	20 lb, 25 lb, 30 lb	80
Kettlebell deadlift	1-2	15-20 reps	15 sec	16 kg, 18 kg, 20 kg	94
Kettlebell one-leg straight-leg deadlift	1-2	15-20 reps	15 sec	10 kg, 12 kg, 14 kg	98
POD 2					
Exercise	Sets	Reps/time	Rest	Wt	Page #
Medicine ball slam	1	20 reps	15 sec	14 lb, 16 lb	66
Medicine ball alt-side slam	1	20 reps	15 sec	14 lb, 16 lb	67
Medicine ball overhead squat	1	20 reps	15 sec	14 lb, 16 lb	85
POD 3					
Exercise	Sets	Reps/time	Rest	Wt	Page #
Dumbbell front lunge	1-2	15-20 reps	15 sec	15 lb, 20 lb, 25 lb	87
Dumbbell lateral lunge	1-2	15-20 reps	15 sec	15 lb, 20 lb, 25 lb	90
Dumbbell backward lunge	1-2	15-20 reps	15 sec	15 lb, 20 lb, 25 lb	92
POD 4					
Exercise	Sets	Reps/time	Rest	Wt	Page #
Heavy rope jumping jacks	1	50 sec	15 sec	Rope	172
Heavy rope arm circles: clockwise	1	50 sec	15 sec	Rope	173
Heavy rope arm circles: counterclockwise	1	50 sec	15 sec	Rope	173
POD 5					
Exercise	Sets	Reps/time	Rest	Wt	Page #
Dumbbell box step-up: alt leg	1-2	15-20 reps	15 sec	15 lb, 20 lb, 25 lb	86
Resistance band lateral walk: right	1-2	15-20 reps	15 sec	15 lb, 20 lb, 25 lb	102
Resistance band lateral walk: left	1-2	15-20 reps	15 sec	15 lb, 20 lb, 25 lb	102
POD 6					
Exercise	Sets	Reps/time	Rest	Wt	Page #
Dumbbell bench press	1-2	15-20 reps	15 sec	20 lb, 25 lb, 30 lb	122
Dumbbell one-arm row	1-2	15-20 reps	15 sec	20 lb, 25 lb, 30 lb	129
Pullover	1-2	15-20 reps	15 sec	25 lb, 30 lb	128

(continued)

Endurance Program 4C: Advanced *(continued)*

POD 7					
Exercise	Sets	Reps/time	Rest	Wt	Page #
Dumbbell shoulder press	1-2	15-20 reps	15 sec	15 lb, 20 lb, 25 lb	131
Dumbbell upright row	1-2	15-20 reps	15 sec	15 lb, 20 lb, 25 lb	134
Dumbbell bent-over raise	1-2	15-20 reps	15 sec	10 lb, 12 lb, 15 lb	140
POD 8					
Exercise	Sets	Reps/time	Rest	Wt	Page #
Weighted abdominal crunch	1-2	50 sec	15 sec	10 lb	155
Scissors	1-2	50 sec	15 sec	BW	162
Birddog	1-2	50 sec	15 sec	BW	161
POD 9					
Exercise	Sets	Reps/time	Rest	Wt	Page #
Weighted sled push	1	50 sec	15 sec	90 lb	74
Weighted sled pull and push	1	50 sec	15 sec	90 lb	75
Weighted sled drag	1	50 sec	15 sec	90 lb	76
POD 10					
Exercise	Sets	Reps/time	Rest	Wt	Page #
Front plank	1-2	50 sec	15 sec	BW	159
Side plank: right	1-2	50 sec	15 sec	BW	160
Side plank: left	1-2	50 sec	15 sec	BW	160

Wt = Weight; BW = Bodyweight

12

Programs for Fat Loss

Losing fat is a common goal among people who exercise for general health and fitness. Many competitive athletes are also interested in controlling their lean mass to fat ratio in their bodies, also known as the body-fat percentage. Exercising regularly, optimizing fat utilization during exercise, and gaining or retaining lean muscle, in addition to dietary strategies, can help you achieve the results you want.

Fat Loss and Metabolic Training

Fat loss in the context of metabolic conditioning refers to the loss of adipose, or fat tissue. We want to point out a distinction between fat loss and weight loss. Weight loss is the reduction in overall bodyweight, which includes the loss of water and muscle, in addition to fat. Ideally, you want to lose body fat and retain muscle, thus improving your overall body composition. The metabolic-training strategies and programs in this chapter will help you to do just this.

Methods for Measuring Fat Loss

A few methods of measuring fat loss are worth mentioning here. Weighing yourself on a scale will measure any losses in bodyweight, but will not specifically measure fat loss. Losing weight can directly benefit athletic performance as well as general health and fitness, but, as mentioned earlier, losing weight is not necessarily the same as losing fat. Fat loss can be measured in several different ways.

Bioelectrical Impedance Analysis

The most commonly used method of measuring body fat is bioelectrical impedance analysis. Bioelectrical impedance analysis measures how fast an electrical current travels through the body. Electrical current travels more slowly through fat, so the more fat, the slower the current. A specific formula is used to determine your body composition using this method. Many commercially available scales have the capability to conduct bioelectrical impedance analysis. As opposed to traditional scales, these scales measure both bodyweight and body composition. Some scales can even be paired with an app that records date, weight, body composition, and several additional metrics, allowing you to track your progress. There are also readily available handheld bioelectrical devices. To ensure accuracy, make sure you are well hydrated when measuring body composition using bioelectrical impedance.

Skin-Fold Calipers

Skin-fold calipers can also be used to assess body composition by measuring the amount of skin and sub-cutaneous fat lying just above the body's muscle. Measurements are taken at several different locations on the body, and the results are entered into specific formula to determine body composition. To get the most accurate measurement, the calipers need to be calibrated and the person performing the test needs to know how to take the measurement properly. Where to measure on the body, how to position the caliper relative to the pinch, and how hard to pinch will all determine the accuracy of the measurement. Skin folds can also be measured over time to track trends. Cross-referencing skin-fold measurements, body composition, and bodyweight can help you gauge your progress over time.

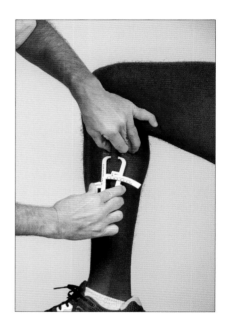

Dual-Energy X-Ray Absorptiometry

The most accurate method for measuring body fat is the DEXA scan. Dual-Energy X-Ray Absorptiometry, or DEXA, is a medical imaging test that uses low-level X-rays to measure bone density, body composition, and body fat. Medical experts consider DEXA scans to be the most useful, the easiest, and the most inexpensive test for diagnosing certain diseases associated with bone density. The test is quick and painless.

The results of a DEXA scan can help medical professionals in identifying health issues, such as loss of muscle after a surgery, hormonal imbalances, heart disease, and diabetes. If you are looking to maximize your training program's effectiveness, you may want to contact your doctor to learn more about the DEXA scan.

Fat Utilization Factors

Fat utilization, also known as fat oxidation, supplies working muscles with energy during exercise. The fat used for exercise can come from several different sources, including adipose tissue, fat within the muscle itself, cholesterol, and dietary fat. There are several factors that have been shown to affect fat utilization. These factors include exercise intensity, exercise duration, training status, nutrition, and sex.

- *Exercise intensity.* Maximal fat oxidation has been reported to occur at an exercise intensity between 45 and 75 percent of $\dot{V}O_2$max. Sixty-five percent of

$\dot{V}O_2$max is conventionally thought of as the intensity at which maximal fat oxidation occurs. Unless you have been clinically measured, you most likely don't know the intensity at which you maximize fat oxidation. A rule of thumb is to work at an intensity at which you could sustain a conversation but probably would not want to. Continuous exercise at an intensity above maximal fat oxidation causes your body to use carbohydrates as its main energy source; at these higher intensities, fat oxidation is not optimized.

• *Exercise duration.* The duration of an exercise session has been shown to influence fat oxidation. Prolonged exercise sessions trigger changes in the source of the fat being used to sustain the exercise. There are other factors that influence the source of energy being used as well, such as your current nutritional state.

• *Training status.* Training status is another factor that influences fat utilization. Endurance-trained individuals can use fat as a fuel source more effectively than people who are sedentary . Trained individuals can also burn fat at a higher relative intensity than their sedentary counterparts can. Practically speaking, establishing a consistent pattern of exercise over time will enable you to burn fat more effectively.

• *Nutrition.* Carbohydrate, protein, and fat consumption and schedule have been shown to affect your body's ability to respond and adapt to exercise. High-fat diets have been shown to have some performance benefits, though their practical application is limited. Manipulating your diet beyond conventional healthy recommendations is not advisable. When it comes to losing fat, you will achieve the best results by calibrating your exercise and diet to establish a healthy caloric deficit over time.

• *Sex.* Studies have shown that premenopausal women have a significantly greater ability to oxidize fat during exercise than men. This is due to the role of estrogen, the female sex hormone, in regulating fat oxidation.

High-Intensity Intermittent Exercise

HIIE consists of brief, near-all-out efforts lasting from six seconds to four minutes followed by low-intensity rest. The duration of the training session is relatively brief, often lasting no more than 20 to 30 minutes. HIIE seems to be an effective method for losing fat, improving cardiorespiratory function, improving anaerobic and aerobic fitness, reducing bodyweight, improving blood chemistry, possibly suppressing appetite, and promoting overall health. HIIE could be particularly appealing given the short training-session duration and, in addition to being an effective approach in and of itself, should be considered a viable option to supplement your overall fitness program. Metabolic training can be designed to elicit the same HIIE response, using programs like those presented in the remainder of this chapter.

The pods in the following exercise programs are a combination of three or more exercises performed with short rest periods between them for either a set number of repetitions or a prescribed amount of time.

Fat Loss Program 1A: Beginner

WARM-UP					
Exercise	Sets	Reps/time	Rest	Wt	Page #
March/walk	1	20 sec	10 sec	BW	N/A
Single-leg squat (each leg)	1	20 sec	10 sec	BW	52
March/walk	1	20 sec	10 sec	BW	N/A
Jumping jacks	1	20 sec	10 sec	BW	48
March/walk	1	20 sec	10 sec	BW	N/A
Push-up	1	20 sec	10 sec	BW	112
March/walk	1	20 sec	10 sec	BW	N/A
Mountain climbers	1	20 sec	10 sec	BW	49
March/walk	1	20 sec	10 sec	BW	N/A
Burpee	1	20 sec	10 sec	BW	50
LOWER BODY					
Exercise	Sets	Reps/time	Rest	Wt	Page #
Dumbbell split squat	1	15 reps	15 sec	8 lb, 10 lb, 12 lb	82
March/walk	1	30 sec	15 sec	BW	N/A
Dumbbell box step-up	1	15 reps	15 sec	8 lb, 10 lb, 12 lb	86
Jumping jacks	1	30 sec	15 sec	BW	48
Dumbbell squat	1	15 reps	15 sec	10 lb, 12 lb, 15 lb	80
March/walk	1	30 sec	15 sec	BW	N/A
Kettlebell goblet squat	1	15 reps	15 sec	6 kg, 8 kg, 10 kg	81
Mountain climbers	1	30 sec	15 sec	BW	49
Bodyweight/dumbbell front lunge	1	15 reps	15 sec	8 lb, 10 lb, 12 lb	87
March/walk	1	30 sec	15 sec	BW	N/A
Kettlebell deadlift	1	15 reps	15 sec	10 kg, 12 kg, 14 kg	94
Single-leg squat (each leg)	1	30 sec	15 sec	BW	52
Kettlebell straight-leg deadlift	1	15 reps	15 sec	8 kg, 10 kg, 12 kg	95
March/walk	1	30 sec	15 sec	BW	N/A
UPPER BODY					
Exercise	Sets	Reps/time	Rest	Wt	Page #
Resistance band standing chest press	1	15 reps	15 sec	Light/moderate	147
March/walk	1	30 sec	15 sec	BW	N/A
Resistance band upright row	1	15 reps	15 sec	Light/moderate	135
Jumping jacks	1	30 sec	15 sec	BW	48
Resistance band upright row	1	15 reps	15 sec	Light/moderate	135
March/walk	1	30 sec	15 sec	BW	N/A
Resistance band T	1	15 reps	15 sec	Light	118
Single-leg squat (each leg)	1	30 sec	15 sec	BW	52
Kettlebell alt-arm biceps curl	1	15 reps	15 sec	Light/moderate	144
March/walk	1	30 sec	15 sec	BW	N/A
Kettlebell overhead triceps extension	1	15 reps	15 sec	6 kg, 8 kg, 10 kg	120
Mountain climbers	1	30 sec	15 sec	BW	49

CORE					
Exercise	Sets	Reps/time	Rest	Wt	Page #
Abdominal curl-up	1	20 reps	15 sec	BW	156
Bicycle	1	30 sec	15 sec	BW	162
Front plank	1	30 sec	15 sec	BW	159
Side plank: right	1	30 sec	15 sec	BW	160
Side plank: left	1	30 sec	15 sec	BW	160
Superman	1	30 sec	15 sec	BW	163

Wt = Weight; BW = Bodyweight

Fat Loss Program 1B: Intermediate

WARM-UP					
Exercise	Sets	Reps/time	Rest	Wt	Page #
Jog in place/jump rope	1	30 sec	10 sec	BW	N/A
Single-leg squat (each leg)	1	30 sec	10 sec	BW	52
Jog in place/jump rope	1	30 sec	10 sec	BW	N/A
Jumping jacks	1	30 sec	10 sec	BW	48
Jog in place/jump rope	1	30 sec	10 sec	BW	N/A
Push-up	1	30 sec	10 sec	BW	112
Jog in place/jump rope	1	30 sec	10 sec	BW	N/A
Mountain climbers	1	30 sec	10 sec	BW	49
Jog in place/jump rope	1	30 sec	10 sec	BW	N/A
Burpee	1	30 sec	10 sec	BW	50
LOWER BODY					
Exercise	Sets	Reps/time	Rest	Wt	Page #
Dumbbell split squat	1-2	20 reps	15 sec	12 lb, 15 lb, 20 lb	82
Jog in place/jump rope	1	40 sec	15 sec	BW	N/A
Dumbbell box step-up	1-2	20 reps	15 sec	10 lb, 12 lb, 15 lb	86
Jumping jacks	1	40 sec	15 sec	BW	48
Dumbbell squat	1-2	20 reps	15 sec	15 lb, 20 lb, 25 lb	80
Jog in place/jump rope	1	40 sec	15 sec	BW	N/A
Kettlebell goblet squat	1-2	20 reps	15 sec	12 kg, 14 kg, 16 kg	81
Mountain climbers	1	40 sec	15 sec	BW	49
Dumbbell front lunge	1-2	20 reps	15 sec	10 lb, 12 lb, 15 lb	87
Jog in place/jump rope	1	40 sec	15 sec	BW	N/A
Kettlebell deadlift	1-2	20 reps	15 sec	14 kg, 16 kg, 18 kg	94
Single-leg squat (each leg)	1	40 sec	15 sec	BW	52
Kettlebell straight-leg deadlift	1-2	20 reps	15 sec	12 kg, 14 kg, 16 kg	95
Jog in place/jump rope	1	40 sec	15 sec	BW	N/A

(continued)

Fat Loss Program 1B: Intermediate *(continued)*

UPPER BODY					
Exercise	Sets	Reps/time	Rest	Wt	Page #
Resistance band standing chest press	1-2	20 reps	15 sec	Moderate/heavy	147
Jog in place/jump rope	1	40 sec	15 sec	BW	N/A
Resistance band upright row	1-2	20 reps	15 sec	Moderate/heavy	135
Jumping jacks	1	40 sec	15 sec	BW	48
Resistance band upright row	1-2	20 reps	15 sec	Moderate/heavy	135
Jog in place/jump rope	1	40 sec	15 sec	BW	N/A
Resistance band T	1-2	20 reps	15 sec	Light/moderate	118
Single-leg squat (each leg)	1	40 sec	15 sec	BW	52
Kettlebell alt-arm biceps curl	1-2	20 reps	15 sec	8 kg, 10 kg, 12 kg	144
Jog in place/jump rope	1	40 sec	15 sec	BW	N/A
Kettlebell overhead triceps extension	1-2	20 reps	15 sec	10 kg, 12 kg, 14 kg	120
Mountain climbers	1	40 sec	15 sec	BW	49
CORE					
Exercise	Sets	Reps/time	Rest	Wt	Page #
Front plank	1	40 sec	15 sec	BW	159
Side plank: right	1	40 sec	15 sec	BW	160
Side plank: left	1	40 sec	15 sec	BW	160
Birddog	1	40 sec	15 sec	BW	161
Weighted abdominal crunch	1	30 reps	15 sec	5-10 lb	155
Weighted abdominal reach	1	30 reps	15 sec	5-10 lb	157
Opposite-shoulder-to-knee crunch	1	30 reps	15 sec	BW	158
Scissors	1	40 sec	15 sec	BW	162
Bicycle	1	40 sec	15 sec	BW	162

Wt = Weight; BW = Bodyweight

Fat Loss Program 1C: Advanced

WARM-UP					
Exercise	Sets	Reps/time	Rest	Wt	Page #
Jog in place/jump rope	1	40 sec	10 sec	BW	N/A
Single-leg squat (each leg)	1	40 sec	10 sec	BW	52
Jog in place/jump rope	1	40 sec	10 sec	BW	N/A
Jumping jacks	1	40 sec	10 sec	BW	48
Jog in place/jump rope	1	40 sec	10 sec	BW	N/A
Push-up	1	40 sec	10 sec	BW	112
Jog in place/jump rope	1	40 sec	10 sec	BW	N/A
Mountain climbers	1	40 sec	10 sec	BW	49
Jog in place/jump rope	1	40 sec	10 sec	BW	N/A
Burpee	1	40 sec	10 sec	BW	50

LOWER BODY					
Exercise	Sets	Reps/time	Rest	Wt	Page #
Dumbbell split squat	1-2	20 reps	15 sec	15 lb, 20 lb, 25 lb	82
Jog in place/jump rope	1	50 sec	15 sec	BW	N/A
Dumbbell box step-up	1-2	20 reps	15 sec	12 lb, 15 lb, 20 lb	86
Jumping jacks	1	50 sec	15 sec	BW	48
Dumbbell squat	1-2	20 reps	15 sec	20 lb, 25 lb, 30 lb	80
Jog in place/jump rope	1	50 sec	15 sec	BW	N/A
Kettlebell goblet squat	1-2	20 reps	15 sec	16 kg, 18 kg 20 kg	81
Mountain climbers	1	50 sec	15 sec	BW	49
Dumbbell front lunge	1-2	20 reps	15 sec	15 lb, 20 lb, 25 lb	87
Jog in place/jump rope	1	50 sec	15 sec	BW	N/A
Kettlebell deadlift	1-2	20 reps	15 sec	16 kg, 18 kg 20 kg	94
Single-leg squat (each leg)	1	50 sec	15 sec	BW	52
Kettlebell straight-leg deadlift	1-2	20 reps	15 sec	14 kg, 16 kg, 18 kg	95
Jog in place/jump rope	1	50 sec	15 sec	BW	N/A
UPPER BODY					
Exercise	Sets	Reps/time	Rest	Wt	Page #
Resistance band standing chest press	1-2	20 reps	15 sec	Heavy	147
Jog in place/jump rope	1	50 sec	15 sec	BW	N/A
Resistance band upright row	1-2	20 reps	15 sec	Heavy	135
Jumping jacks	1	50 sec	15 sec	BW	48
Resistance band upright row	1-2	20 reps	15 sec	Heavy	135
Jog in place/jump rope	1	50 sec	15 sec	BW	N/A
Resistance band T	1-2	20 reps	15 sec	Moderate	118
Single-leg squat (each leg)	1	50 sec	15 sec	BW	52
Kettlebell alt-arm biceps curl	1-2	20 reps	15 sec	12 kg, 14 kg, 16 kg	144
Jog in place/jump rope	1	50 sec	15 sec	BW	N/A
Kettlebell overhead triceps extension	1-2	20 reps	15 sec	14 kg, 16 kg, 18 kg	120
Mountain climbers	1	50 sec	15 sec	BW	49
CORE					
Exercise	Sets	Reps/time	Rest	Wt	Page #
Front plank	1	50 sec	15 sec	BW	159
Side plank: right	1	50 sec	15 sec	BW	160
Side plank: left	1	50 sec	15 sec	BW	160
Birddog	1	50 sec	15 sec	BW	161
Weighted abdominal crunch	1	40 reps	15 sec	5-10 lb	155
Weighted abdominal reach	1	40 reps	15 sec	5-10 lb	157
Opposite-shoulder-to-knee crunch	1	40 reps	15 sec	BW	158
Scissors	1	50 sec	15 sec	BW	162
Bicycle	1	50 sec	15 sec	BW	162

Wt = Weight; BW = Bodyweight

Fat Loss Program 2A: Beginner

WARM-UP					
Exercise	Sets	Reps/time	Rest	Wt	Page #
March/walk in place	1	20 sec	10 sec	BW	N/A
Mountain climbers	1	20 sec	10 sec	BW	49
March/walk in place	1	20 sec	10 sec	BW	N/A
Burpee	1	20 sec	10 sec	BW	50
March/walk in place	1	20 sec	10 sec	BW	N/A
Single-leg squat (each leg)	1	20 sec	10 sec	BW	52
March/walk in place	1	20 sec	10 sec	BW	N/A
Jumping jacks	1	20 sec	10 sec	BW	48
March/walk in place	1	20 sec	10 sec	BW	N/A
Push-up	1	20 sec	10 sec	BW	112
LOWER BODY					
Exercise	Sets	Reps/time	Rest	Wt	Page #
Resistance band overhead squat	1	15 reps	15 sec	Light/moderate	84
March/walk in place	1	30 sec	15 sec	BW	N/A
Kettlebell overhead squat	1	15 reps	15 sec	6 kg, 8 kg, 10 kg	83
Burpee	1	30 sec	15 sec	BW	50
Dumbbell lateral lunge	1	15 reps	15 sec	8 lb, 10 lb, 12 lb	90
March/walk in place	1	30 sec	15 sec	BW	N/A
Dumbbell backward lunge	1	15 reps	15 sec	8 lb, 10 lb, 12 lb	92
Jumping jacks	1	30 sec	15 sec	BW	48
Kettlebell deadlift	1	15 reps	15 sec	10 kg, 12 kg, 14 kg	94
March/walk in place	1	30 sec	15 sec	BW	N/A
Kettlebell overhead lunge	1	15 reps	15 sec	6 kg, 8 kg, 10 kg	88
Mountain climbers	1	30 sec	15 sec	BW	49
Kettlebell one-leg straight-leg deadlift	1	15 reps	15 sec	6 kg, 8 kg, 10 kg	97
March/walk in place	1	30 sec	15 sec	BW	N/A
UPPER BODY					
Exercise	Sets	Reps/time	Rest	Wt	Page #
Kettlebell pullover	1	15 reps	15 sec	8 kg, 10 kg, 12 kg	128
March/walk in place	1	30 sec	15 sec	BW	N/A
Kettlebell one-arm row	1	15 reps	15 sec	8 kg, 10 kg, 12 kg	129
Jumping jacks	1	30 sec	15 sec	BW	48
Kettlebell shoulder press	1	15 reps	15 sec	4 kg, 6 kg, 8 kg	131
March/walk in place	1	30 sec	15 sec	BW	N/A
Resistance band Y	1	15 reps	15 sec	Light	116
Single-leg squat (each leg)	1	30 sec	15 sec	BW	52
Kettlebell alt-arm biceps curl	1	15 reps	15 sec	4 kg, 6 kg, 8 kg	144
March/walk in place	1	30 sec	15 sec	BW	N/A
Kettlebell overhead triceps extension	2	15 reps	15 sec	6 kg, 8 kg, 10 kg	120
Mountain climbers	1	30 sec	15 sec	BW	49

CORE					
Exercise	Sets	Reps/time	Rest	Wt	Page #
Opposite-shoulder-to-knee crunch	1	20 reps	15 sec	BW	158
Scissors	1	30 sec	15 sec	BW	162
Bicycle	1	30 sec	15 sec	BW	162
Front plank	1	30 sec	15 sec	BW	159
Side plank: right	1	30 sec	15 sec	BW	160
Side plank: left	1	30 sec	15 sec	BW	160
Birddog	1	30 sec	15 sec	BW	161
Abdominal crunch	1	20 reps	15 sec	BW	155
Abdominal reach	1	20 reps	15 sec	BW	157
Opposite-shoulder-to-knee crunch	1	30 reps	15 sec	BW	158
Scissors	1	30 sec	15 sec	BW	162
Bicycle	1	30 sec	15 sec	BW	162

Wt = Weight; BW = Bodyweight

Fat Loss Program 2B: Intermediate

WARM-UP					
Exercise	Sets	Reps/time	Rest	Wt	Page #
Jog in place/jump rope	1	30 sec	10 sec	BW	N/A
Mountain climbers	1	30 sec	10 sec	BW	49
Jog in place/jump rope	1	30 sec	10 sec	BW	N/A
Burpee	1	30 sec	10 sec	BW	50
Jog in place/jump rope	1	30 sec	10 sec	BW	N/A
Single-leg squat (each leg)	1	30 sec	10 sec	BW	52
Jog in place/jump rope	1	30 sec	10 sec	BW	N/A
Jumping jacks	1	30 sec	10 sec	BW	48
Jog in place/jump rope	1	30 sec	10 sec	BW	N/A
Push-up	1	30 sec	10 sec	BW	112
LOWER BODY					
Exercise	Sets	Reps/time	Rest	Wt	Page #
Resistance band overhead squat	1-2	20 reps	15 sec	Moderate/heavy	84
Jog in place/jump rope	1	40 sec	15 sec	BW	N/A
Kettlebell overhead squat	1-2	20 reps	15 sec	8 kg, 10 kg, 12 kg	83
Burpee	1	40 sec	15 sec	BW	50
Dumbbell lateral lunge	1-2	20 reps	15 sec	12 lb, 15 lb, 20 lb	90
Jog in place/jump rope	1	40 sec	15 sec	BW	N/A
Dumbbell backward lunge	1-2	20 reps	15 sec	12 lb, 15 lb, 20 lb	92
Jumping jacks	1	40 sec	15 sec	BW	48
Kettlebell deadlift	1-2	20 reps	15 sec	14 kg, 16 kg, 18 kg	94
Jog in place/jump rope	1	40 sec	15 sec	BW	N/A

(continued)

Fat Loss Program 2B: Intermediate *(continued)*

LOWER BODY *(CONTINUED)*					
Exercise	Sets	Reps/time	Rest	Wt	Page #
Kettlebell overhead lunge	1-2	20 reps	15 sec	8 kg, 10 kg, 12 kg	88
Mountain climbers	1	40 sec	15 sec	BW	49
Kettlebell one-leg straight-leg deadlift	1-2	20 reps	15 sec	8 kg, 10 kg, 12 kg	98
Jog in place/jump rope	1	40 sec	15 sec	BW	N/A
UPPER BODY					
Exercise	Sets	Reps/time	Rest	Wt	Page #
Kettlebell pullover	1-2	20 reps	15 sec	10 kg, 12 kg, 14 kg	128
Jog in place/jump rope	1	40 sec	15 sec	BW	N/A
Kettlebell one-arm row	1-2	20 reps	15 sec	10 kg, 12 kg, 14 kg	129
Jumping jacks	1	40 sec	15 sec	BW	48
Kettlebell shoulder press	1-2	20 reps	15 sec	6 kg, 8 kg, 10 kg	131
Jog in place/jump rope	1	40 sec	15 sec	BW	N/A
Resistance band Y	1-2	20 reps	15 sec	Light/moderate	116
Single-leg squat (each leg)	1	40 sec	15 sec	BW	52
Kettlebell alt-arm biceps curl	1-2	20 reps	15 sec	6 kg, 8 kg, 10 kg	144
Jog in place/jump rope	1	40 sec	15 sec	BW	N/A
Kettlebell overhead triceps extension	1-2	20 reps	15 sec	8 kg, 10 kg, 12 kg	120
Mountain climbers	1	40 sec	15 sec	BW	49
CORE					
Exercise	Sets	Reps/time	Rest	Wt	Page #
Opposite-shoulder-to-knee crunch	1	30 reps	15 sec	BW	158
Scissors	1	40 sec	15 sec	BW	162
Bicycle	1	40 sec	15 sec	BW	162
Front plank	1	40 sec	15 sec	BW	159
Side plank: right	1	40 sec	15 sec	BW	160
Side plank: left	1	40 sec	15 sec	BW	160
Birddog	1	40 sec	15 sec	BW	161
Weighted abdominal crunch	1	30 reps	15 sec	5-10 lb	155
Weighted abdominal reach	1	30 reps	15 sec	5-10 lb	157
Opposite-shoulder-to-knee crunch	1	30 reps	15 sec	BW	158
Scissors	1	40 sec	15 sec	BW	162
Bicycle	1	40 sec	15 sec	BW	162

Wt = Weight; BW = Bodyweight

Fat Loss Program 2C: Advanced

WARM-UP					
Exercise	Sets	Reps/time	Rest	Wt	Page #
Jog in place/jump rope	1	40 sec	10 sec	BW	N/A
Mountain climbers	1	40 sec	10 sec	BW	49
Jog in place/jump rope	1	40 sec	10 sec	BW	N/A
Burpee	1	40 sec	10 sec	BW	50
Jog in place/jump rope	1	40 sec	10 sec	BW	N/A
Single-leg squat (each leg)	1	40 sec	10 sec	BW	52
Jog in place/jump rope	1	40 sec	10 sec	BW	N/A
Jumping jacks	1	40 sec	10 sec	BW	48
Jog in place/jump rope	1	40 sec	10 sec	BW	N/A
Push-up	1	40 sec	10 sec	BW	112
LOWER BODY					
Exercise	Sets	Reps/time	Rest	Wt	Page #
Resistance band overhead squat	1-2	20 reps	15 sec	Heavy	84
Jog in place/jump rope	1	50 sec	15 sec	BW	N/A
Kettlebell overhead squat	1-2	20 reps	15 sec	10 kg, 12 kg, 14 kg	83
Burpee	1	50 sec	15 sec	BW	50
Dumbbell lateral lunge	1-2	20 reps	15 sec	15 lb, 20 lb, 25 lb	90
Jog in place/jump rope	1	50 sec	15 sec	BW	N/A
Dumbbell backward lunge	1-2	20 reps	15 sec	15 lb, 20 lb, 25 lb	92
Jumping jacks	1	50 sec	15 sec	BW	48
Kettlebell deadlift	1-2	20 reps	15 sec	16 kg, 18 kg 20 kg	94
Jog in place/jump rope	1	50 sec	15 sec	BW	N/A
Kettlebell overhead lunge	1-2	20 reps	15 sec	10 kg, 12 kg, 14 kg	88
Mountain climbers	1	50 sec	15 sec	BW	49
Kettlebell one-leg straight-leg deadlift	1-2	20 reps	15 sec	10 kg, 12 kg, 14 kg	98
Jog in place/jump rope	1	50 sec	15 sec	BW	N/A
UPPER BODY					
Exercise	Sets	Reps/time	Rest	Wt	Page #
Kettlebell push-up	1-2	50 sec	15 sec	BW	112
Jog in place/jump rope	1	50 sec	15 sec	BW	N/A
Kettlebell renegade row	1-2	20 reps	15 sec	10 kg, 12 kg, 14 kg	130
Jumping jacks	1	50 sec	15 sec	BW	48
Kettlebell shoulder press	1-2	20 reps	15 sec	8 kg, 10 kg, 12 kg	131
Jog in place/jump rope	1	50 sec	15 sec	BW	N/A
Resistance band Y	1-2	20 reps	15 sec	Moderate	116
Single-leg squat (each leg)	1	50 sec	15 sec	BW	52
Kettlebell alt-arm biceps curl	1-2	20 reps	15 sec	8 kg, 10 kg, 12 kg	144
Jog in place/jump rope	1	50 sec	15 sec	BW	N/A
Kettlebell overhead triceps extension	1-2	20 reps	15 sec	10 kg, 12 kg, 14 kg	120
Mountain climbers	1	50 sec	15 sec	BW	49

(continued)

Fat Loss Program 2C: Advanced *(continued)*

CORE					
Exercise	Sets	Reps/time	Rest	Wt	Page #
Opposite-shoulder-to-knee crunch	1	40 reps	15 sec	BW	158
Scissors	1	50 sec	15 sec	BW	162
Bicycle	1	50 sec	15 sec	BW	162
Front plank	1	50 sec	15 sec	BW	159
Side plank: right	1	50 sec	15 sec	BW	160
Side plank: left	1	50 sec	15 sec	BW	160
Birddog	1	50 sec	15 sec	BW	161
Weighted abdominal crunch	1	40 reps	15 sec	5-10 lb	155
Weighted abdominal reach	1	40 reps	15 sec	5-10 lb	157
Opposite-shoulder-to-knee crunch	1	40 reps	15 sec	BW	158
Scissors	1	50 sec	15 sec	BW	162
Bicycle	1	50 sec	15 sec	BW	162

Wt = Weight; BW = Bodyweight

Fat Loss Program 3A: Beginner

Note: Each exercise in a pod should be completed before moving to the next pod. A pod is a combination of three or more exercises performed with short rest periods between them for either a set number of repetitions or a prescribed amount of time.

WARM-UP					
Exercise	Sets	Reps/time	Rest	Wt	Page #
Jumping jacks	1	20 sec	10 sec	BW	48
Walk/march in place	1	20 sec	10 sec	BW	N/A
Burpee	1	20 sec	10 sec	BW	50
Walk/march in place	1	20 sec	10 sec	BW	N/A
Push-up	1	20 sec	10 sec	BW	112
Walk/march in place	1	20 sec	10 sec	BW	N/A
Single-leg squat (each leg)	1	20 sec	10 sec	BW	52
Walk/march in place	1	20 sec	10 sec	BW	N/A
Mountain climbers	1	20 sec	10 sec	BW	49
Walk/march in place	1	20 sec	10 sec	BW	N/A
POD 1					
Exercise	Sets	Reps/time	Rest	Wt	Page #
Dumbbell squat	1	15 reps	15 sec	10 lb, 12 lb, 15 lb	80
Jumping jacks	1	30 sec	15 sec	BW	48
Dumbbell goblet squat	1	15 reps	15 sec	10 lb, 12 lb, 15 lb	81

POD 2					
Exercise	Sets	Reps/time	Rest	Wt	Page #
Dumbbell front lunge	1	15 reps	15 sec	10 lb, 12 lb, 15 lb	87
Single-leg squat (each leg)	1	30 sec	15 sec	BW	52
Dumbbell backward lunge	1	15 reps	15 sec	10 lb, 12 lb, 15 lb	92
POD 3					
Exercise	Sets	Reps/time	Rest	Wt	Page #
Medicine ball overhead lateral lunge: right	1	15 reps	15 sec	10 lb, 12 lb, 15 lb	91
Burpee	1	30 sec	15 sec	BW	50
Medicine ball overhead lateral lunge: left	1	15 reps	15 sec	10 lb, 12 lb, 15 lb	91
POD 4					
Exercise	Sets	Reps/time	Rest	Wt	Page #
Heavy rope two-arm slams	1	30 sec	15 sec	Rope	169
Mountain climbers	1	30 sec	15 sec	Rope	49
Heavy rope scissors	1	30 sec	15 sec	Rope	171
POD 5					
Exercise	Sets	Reps/time	Rest	Wt	Page #
Dumbbell bench press	1	15 reps	15 sec	12 lb, 15 lb, 20 lb	122
Push-up	1	30 sec	15 sec	BW	112
Dumbbell incline press	1	15 reps	15 sec	10 lb, 12 lb, 15 lb	124
POD 6					
Exercise	Sets	Reps/time	Rest	Wt	Page #
Dumbbell one-arm row: right	1	15 reps	15 sec	12 lb, 15 lb, 20 lb	129
Jumping jacks	1	30 sec	15 sec	BW	48
Dumbbell one-arm row: left	1	15 reps	15 sec	12 lb, 15 lb, 20 lb	129
POD 7					
Exercise	Sets	Reps/time	Rest	Wt	Page #
Dumbbell shoulder press	1	15 reps	15 sec	10 lb, 12 lb, 15 lb	131
Dumbbell biceps curl	1	15 reps	15 sec	10 lb, 12 lb, 15 lb	144
Dumbbell triceps kickback	1	15 reps	15 sec	8 lb, 10 lb, 12 lb	143
POD 8					
Exercise	Sets	Reps/time	Rest	Wt	Page #
Weighted sled push	1	30 sec	15 sec	45 lb	74
Groiner	1	30 sec	15 sec	BW	51
Weighted sled drag	1	30 sec	15 sec	45 lb	76
POD 9					
Exercise	Sets	Reps/time	Rest	Wt	Page #
Abdominal crunch	1	30 sec	15 sec	BW	155
Scissors	1	30 sec	15 sec	BW	162
Superman	1	30 sec	15 sec	BW	163

(continued)

Fat Loss Program 3A: Beginner (continued)

POD 10					
Exercise	Sets	Reps/time	Rest	Wt	Page #
Front plank	1	30 sec	15 sec	BW	159
Side plank: right	1	30 sec	15 sec	BW	160
Side plank: left	1	30 sec	15 sec	BW	160

Wt = Weight; BW = Bodyweight

Fat Loss Program 3B: Intermediate

Note: Each exercise in a pod should be completed before moving to the next pod. A pod is a combination of three or more exercises performed with short rest periods between them for either a set number of repetitions or a prescribed amount of time.

WARM-UP					
Exercise	Sets	Reps/time	Rest	Wt	Page #
Jumping jacks	1	30 sec	10 sec	BW	48
Jog in place/jumping jacks	1	30 sec	10 sec	BW	N/A
Burpee	1	30 sec	10 sec	BW	50
Jog in place/jumping jacks	1	30 sec	10 sec	BW	N/A
Push-up	1	30 sec	10 sec	BW	112
Jog in place/jumping jacks	1	30 sec	10 sec	BW	N/A
Single-leg squat (each leg)	1	30 sec	10 sec	BW	52
Jog in place/jumping jacks	1	30 sec	10 sec	BW	N/A
Mountain climbers	1	30 sec	10 sec	BW	49
Jog in place/jumping jacks	1	30 sec	10 sec	BW	N/A
POD 1					
Exercise	Sets	Reps/time	Rest	Wt	Page #
Dumbbell squat	1-2	15-20 reps	15 sec	15 lb, 20 lb, 25 lb	80
Jumping jacks	1	40 sec	15 sec	BW	48
Dumbbell goblet squat	1-2	15-20 reps	15 sec	15 lb, 20 lb, 25 lb	81
POD 2					
Exercise	Sets	Reps/time	Rest	Wt	Page #
Dumbbell front lunge	1-2	15-20 reps	15 sec	12 lb, 15 lb, 20 lb	87
Single-leg squat (each leg)	1	40 sec	15 sec	BW	52
Dumbbell backward lunge	1-2	15-20 reps	15 sec	12 lb, 15 lb, 20 lb	92
POD 3					
Exercise	Sets	Reps/time	Rest	Wt	Page #
Medicine ball overhead lateral lunge: right	1-2	15-20 reps	15 sec	12 lb, 15 lb, 20 lb	91
Burpee	1	40 sec	15 sec	BW	50
Medicine ball overhead lateral lunge: left	1-2	15-20 reps	15 sec	12 lb, 15 lb, 20 lb	91

POD 4					
Exercise	Sets	Reps/time	Rest	Wt	Page #
Heavy rope two-arm slams	1	40 sec	15 sec	Rope	169
Mountain climbers	1	40 sec	15 sec	BW	49
Heavy rope scissors	1	40 sec	15 sec	Rope	171

POD 5					
Exercise	Sets	Reps/time	Rest	Wt	Page #
Dumbbell bench press	1-2	15-20 reps	15 sec	15 lb, 20 lb, 25 lb	122
Push-up	1	40 sec	15 sec	BW	112
Dumbbell incline press	1-2	15-20 reps	15 sec	12 lb, 15 lb, 20 lb	124

POD 6					
Exercise	Sets	Reps/time	Rest	Wt	Page #
Dumbbell one-arm row: right	1-2	15-20 reps	15 sec	15 lb, 20 lb, 25 lb	129
Jumping jacks	1	40 sec	15 sec	BW	48
Dumbbell one-arm row: left	1-2	15-20 reps	15 sec	15 lb, 20 lb, 25 lb	129

POD 7					
Exercise	Sets	Reps/time	Rest	Wt	Page #
Dumbbell shoulder press	1-2	15-20 reps	15 sec	12 lb, 15 lb, 20 lb	131
Dumbbell biceps curl	1-2	15-20 reps	15 sec	12 lb, 15 lb, 20 lb	144
Dumbbell triceps kickback	1-2	15-20 reps	15 sec	10 lb, 12 lb, 15 lb	143

POD 8					
Exercise	Sets	Reps/time	Rest	Wt	Page #
Weighted sled push	1	40 sec	15 sec	70 lb	74
Groiner	1	40 sec	15 sec	BW	51
Weighted sled drag	1	40 sec	15 sec	70 lb	76

POD 9					
Exercise	Sets	Reps/time	Rest	Wt	Page #
Abdominal crunch	1	40 sec	15 sec	BW	155
Scissors	1	40 sec	15 sec	BW	162
Superman	1	40 sec	15 sec	BW	163

POD 10					
Exercise	Sets	Reps/time	Rest	Wt	Page #
Front plank	1	40 sec	15 sec	BW	159
Side plank: right	1	40 sec	15 sec	BW	160
Side plank: left	1	40 sec	15 sec	BW	160

Wt = Weight; BW = Bodyweight

Fat Loss Program 3C: Advanced

Note: Each exercise in a pod should be completed before moving to the next pod. A pod is a combination of three or more exercises performed with short rest periods between them for either a set number of repetitions or a prescribed amount of time.

WARM-UP					
Exercise	Sets	Reps/time	Rest	Wt	Page #
Jumping jacks	1	40 sec	10 sec	BW	48
Jog in place/jumping jacks	1	40 sec	10 sec	BW	N/A
Burpee	1	40 sec	10 sec	BW	50
Jog in place/jumping jacks	1	40 sec	10 sec	BW	N/A
Push-up	1	40 sec	10 sec	BW	112
Jog in place/jumping jacks	1	40 sec	10 sec	BW	N/A
Single-leg squat (each leg)	1	40 sec	10 sec	BW	52
Jog in place/jumping jacks	1	40 sec	10 sec	BW	N/A
Mountain climbers	1	40 sec	10 sec	BW	49
Jog in place/jumping jacks	1	40 sec	10 sec	BW	N/A
POD 1					
Exercise	Sets	Reps/time	Rest	Wt	Page #
Dumbbell squat	2	20 reps	15 sec	20 lb, 25 lb, 30 lb	80
Jumping jacks	1	50 sec	15 sec	BW	48
Dumbbell goblet squat	2	20 reps	15 sec	20 lb, 25 lb, 30 lb	81
POD 2					
Exercise	Sets	Reps/time	Rest	Wt	Page #
Dumbbell front lunge	2	20 reps	15 sec	15 lb, 20 lb, 25 lb	87
Single-leg squat (each leg)	1	50 sec	15 sec	BW	52
Dumbbell backward lunge	2	20 reps	15 sec	15 lb, 20 lb, 25 lb	92
POD 3					
Exercise	Sets	Reps/time	Rest	Wt	Page #
Medicine ball overhead lateral lunge: right	2	20 reps	15 sec	15 lb, 20 lb, 25 lb	91
Burpee	1	50 sec	15 sec	BW	50
Medicine ball overhead lateral lunge: left	2	20 reps	15 sec	15 lb, 20 lb, 25 lb	91
POD 4					
Exercise	Sets	Reps/time	Rest	Wt	Page #
Heavy rope two-arm slams	1	50 sec	15 sec	Rope	169
Mountain climbers	1	50 sec	15 sec	BW	49
Heavy rope scissors	1	50 sec	15 sec	Rope	171
POD 5					
Exercise	Sets	Reps/time	Rest	Wt	Page #
Dumbbell bench press	2	20 reps	15 sec	20 lb, 25 lb, 30 lb	122
Push-up	1	50 sec	15 sec	BW	112
Dumbbell incline press	2	20 reps	15 sec	15 lb, 20 lb, 25 lb	124

POD 6					
Exercise	Sets	Reps/time	Rest	Wt	Page #
Dumbbell one-arm row: right	2	20 reps	15 sec	20 lb, 25 lb, 30 lb	129
Jumping jacks	1	50 sec	15 sec	BW	48
Dumbbell one-arm row: left	2	20 reps	15 sec	20 lb, 25 lb, 30 lb	129
POD 7					
Exercise	Sets	Reps/time	Rest	Wt	Page #
Dumbbell shoulder press	2	20 reps	15 sec	15 lb, 20 lb, 25 lb	131
Dumbbell biceps curl	2	20 reps	15 sec	15 lb, 20 lb, 25 lb	144
Dumbbell triceps kickback	2	20 reps	15 sec	12 lb, 15 lb, 20 lb	143
POD 8					
Exercise	Sets	Reps/time	Rest	Wt	Page #
Weighted sled push	1	50 sec	15 sec	90 lb	74
Groiner	1	50 sec	15 sec	BW	51
Weighted sled drag	1	50 sec	15 sec	90 lb	76
POD 9					
Exercise	Sets	Reps/time	Rest	Wt	Page #
Abdominal crunch	1	50 sec	15 sec	BW	155
Scissors	1	50 sec	15 sec	BW	162
Superman	1	50 sec	15 sec	BW	163
POD 10					
Exercise	Sets	Reps/time	Rest	Wt	Page #
Front plank	1	50 sec	15 sec	BW	159
Side plank: right	1	50 sec	15 sec	BW	160
Side plank: left	1	50 sec	15 sec	BW	160

Wt = Weight; BW = Bodyweight

Fat Loss Program 4A: Beginner

Note: Each exercise in a pod should be completed before moving to the next pod. A pod is a combination of three or more exercises performed with short rest periods between them for either a set number of repetitions or a prescribed amount of time.

WARM-UP					
Exercise	Sets	Reps/time	Rest	Wt	Page #
March/walk	1	20 sec	10 sec	BW	N/A
Single-leg squat (each leg)	1	20 sec	10 sec	BW	52
March/walk	1	20 sec	10 sec	BW	N/A
Mountain climbers	1	20 sec	10 sec	BW	49
March/walk	1	20 sec	10 sec	BW	N/A
Jumping jacks	1	20 sec	10 sec	BW	48
March/walk	1	20 sec	10 sec	BW	N/A
Burpee	1	20 sec	10 sec	BW	50
March/walk	1	20 sec	10 sec	BW	N/A
Push-up	1	20 sec	10 sec	BW	112

(continued)

Fat Loss Program 4A: Beginner *(continued)*

POD 1					
Exercise	Sets	Reps/time	Rest	Wt	Page #
Kettlebell goblet squat	1	15 reps	15 sec	8 kg, 10 kg, 12 kg	81
Single-leg squat (each leg)	1	30 sec	15 sec	BW	52
Kettlebell straight-leg deadlift	1	15 reps	15 sec	10 kg, 12 kg, 14 kg	95
POD 2					
Exercise	Sets	Reps/time	Rest	Wt	Page #
Dumbbell bench press	1	15 reps	15 sec	12 lb, 15 lb, 20 lb	122
Burpee	1	30 sec	15 sec	BW	50
Kettlebell one-arm row	1	15 reps	15 sec	8 kg, 10 kg, 12 kg	129
POD 3					
Exercise	Sets	Reps/time	Rest	Wt	Page #
Medicine ball overhead squat	1	15 reps	15 sec	10 lb	85
Mountain climbers	1	30 sec	15 sec	BW	49
Medicine ball overhead lunge	1	15 reps	15 sec	10 lb	89
POD 4					
Exercise	Sets	Reps/time	Rest	Wt	Page #
Heavy rope arm circles: clockwise	1	30 sec	15 sec	Rope	173
Heavy rope two-hand shuffle slams	1	30 sec	15 sec	Rope	174
Heavy rope arm circles: counterclockwise	1	30 sec	15 sec	Rope	173
POD 5					
Exercise	Sets	Reps/time	Rest	Wt	Page #
Kettlebell shoulder press	1	15 reps	15 sec	6 kg, 8 kg, 10 kg	131
Push-up	1	30 sec	15 sec	BW	112
Dumbbell bent-over raise	1	15 reps	15 sec	5 lb, 8 lb, 10 lb	140
POD 6					
Exercise	Sets	Reps/time	Rest	Wt	Page #
Medicine ball burpee	1	30 sec	15 sec	10 lb	70
Medicine ball Russian twist	1	30 sec	15 sec	10 lb	164
Medicine ball squat and jump	1	30 sec	15 sec	10 lb	71
POD 7					
Exercise	Sets	Reps/time	Rest	Wt	Page #
Resistance band shoulder press	1	15 reps	15 sec	Light	132
Dumbbell hammer curl	1	15 reps	15 sec	10 lb, 12 lb, 15 lb	145
Dumbbell supine triceps extension	1	15 reps	15 sec	8 lb, 10 lb, 12 lb	141
POD 8					
Exercise	Sets	Reps/time	Rest	Wt	Page #
Weighted sled pull and push	1	30 sec	15 sec	45 lb	75
Groiner	1	30 sec	15 sec	BW	51
Kettlebell farmer's walk	1	30 sec	15 sec	8 kg, 10 kg, 12 kg	98

POD 9					
Exercise	Sets	Reps/time	Rest	Wt	Page #
Medicine ball sit-up	1	30 sec	15 sec	10 lb	164
Medicine ball Russian twist	1	30 sec	15 sec	10 lb	164
Medicine ball chop	1	30 sec	15 sec	10 lb	72
POD 10					
Exercise	Sets	Reps/time	Rest	Wt	Page #
Bicycle	1	30 sec	15 sec	BW	162
Scissors	1	30 sec	15 sec	BW	162
Superman	1	30 sec	15 sec	BW	163

Wt = Weight; BW = Bodyweight

Fat Loss Program 4B: Intermediate

Note: Each exercise in a pod should be completed before moving to the next pod. A pod is a combination of three or more exercises performed with short rest periods between them for either a set number of repetitions or a prescribed amount of time.

WARM-UP					
Exercise	Sets	Reps/time	Rest	Wt	Page #
Jog in place/jump rope	1	30 sec	10 sec	BW	N/A
Single-leg squat (each leg)	1	30 sec	10 sec	BW	52
Jog in place/jump rope	1	30 sec	10 sec	BW	N/A
Mountain climbers	1	30 sec	10 sec	BW	49
Jog in place/jump rope	1	30 sec	10 sec	BW	N/A
Jumping jacks	1	30 sec	10 sec	BW	48
Jog in place/jump rope	1	30 sec	10 sec	BW	N/A
Burpee	1	30 sec	10 sec	BW	50
Jog in place/jump rope	1	30 sec	10 sec	BW	N/A
Push-up	1	30 sec	10 sec	BW	112
POD 1					
Exercise	Sets	Reps/time	Rest	Wt	Page #
Kettlebell goblet squat	1-2	15-20 reps	15 sec	12 kg, 14 kg, 16 kg	81
Single-leg squat (each leg)	1-2	40 sec	15 sec	BW	52
Kettlebell straight-leg deadlift	1-2	15-20 reps	15 sec	12 kg, 14 kg, 16 kg	95
POD 2					
Exercise	Sets	Reps/time	Rest	Wt	Page #
Dumbbell bench press	1-2	15-20 reps	15 sec	15 lb, 20 lb, 25 lb	122
Burpee	1	40 sec	15 sec	BW	50
Kettlebell one-arm row	1-2	15-20 reps	15 sec	12 kg, 14 kg, 16 kg	129

(continued)

Fat Loss Program 4B: Intermediate *(continued)*

POD 3					
Exercise	Sets	Reps/time	Rest	Wt	Page #
Medicine ball overhead squat	1-2	15-20 reps	15 sec	12 lb, 14 lb	85
Mountain climbers	1	40 sec	15 sec	BW	49
Medicine ball overhead lunge	1-2	15-20 reps	15 sec	12 lb, 14 lb	89

POD 4					
Exercise	Sets	Reps/time	Rest	Wt	Page #
Heavy rope arm circles: clockwise	1	40 sec	15 sec	Rope	173
Heavy rope two-hand shuffle slams	1	40 sec	15 sec	Rope	174
Heavy rope arm circles: counterclockwise	1	40 sec	15 sec	Rope	173

POD 5					
Exercise	Sets	Reps/time	Rest	Wt	Page #
Kettlebell shoulder press	1-2	15-20 reps	15 sec	8 kg, 10 kg, 12 kg	131
Push-up	1-2	30 sec	15 sec	BW	112
Dumbbell bent-over raise	1-2	15-20 reps	15 sec	8 lb, 10 lb, 12 lb	140

POD 6					
Exercise	Sets	Reps/time	Rest	Wt	Page #
Medicine ball burpee	1	40 sec	15 sec	12 lb, 14 lb	70
Medicine ball Russian twist	1	40 sec	15 sec	12 lb, 14 lb	164
Medicine ball squat and jump	1	40 sec	15 sec	12 lb, 14 lb	71

POD 7					
Exercise	Sets	Reps/time	Rest	Wt	Page #
Resistance band shoulder press	1-2	15-20 reps	15 sec	Moderate	132
Dumbbell hammer curl	1-2	15-20 reps	15 sec	12 lb, 15 lb, 20 lb	145
Dumbbell supine triceps extension	1-2	15-20 reps	15 sec	8 lb, 10 lb, 12 lb	141

POD 8					
Exercise	Sets	Reps/time	Rest	Wt	Page #
Weighted sled pull and push	1	40 sec	15 sec	70 lb	75
Groiner	1	40 sec	15 sec	BW	51
Kettlebell farmer's walk	1	40 sec	15 sec	12 kg, 14 kg, 16 kg	98

POD 9					
Exercise	Sets	Reps/time	Rest	Wt	Page #
Medicine ball sit-up	1	40 sec	15 sec	12 lb, 14 lb	164
Medicine ball Russian twist	1	40 sec	15 sec	12 lb, 14 lb	164
Medicine ball chop	1	40 sec	15 sec	12 lb, 14 lb	72

POD 10					
Exercise	Sets	Reps/time	Rest	Wt	Page #
Bicycle	1	40 sec	15 sec	BW	162
Scissors	1	40 sec	15 sec	BW	162
Superman	1	40 sec	15 sec	BW	163

Wt = Weight; BW = Bodyweight

Fat Loss Program 4C: Advanced

WARM-UP					
Exercise	Sets	Reps/time	Rest	Wt	Page #
Jog in place/jump rope	1	40 sec	10 sec	BW	N/A
Single-leg squat (each leg)	1	40 sec	10 sec	BW	52
Jog in place/jump rope	1	40 sec	10 sec	BW	N/A
Mountain climbers	1	40 sec	10 sec	BW	49
Jog in place/jump rope	1	40 sec	10 sec	BW	N/A
Jumping jacks	1	40 sec	10 sec	BW	48
Jog in place/jump rope	1	40 sec	10 sec	BW	N/A
Burpee	1	40 sec	10 sec	BW	50
Jog in place/jump rope	1	40 sec	10 sec	BW	N/A
Push-up	1	40 sec	10 sec	BW	112
POD 1					
Exercise	Sets	Reps/time	Rest	Wt	Page #
Kettlebell goblet squat	1-2	20 reps	15 sec	14 kg, 16 kg, 18 kg	81
Single-leg squat (each leg)	1-2	50 sec	15 sec	BW	52
Kettlebell straight-leg deadlift	1-2	20 reps	15 sec	14 kg, 16 kg, 18 kg	95
POD 2					
Exercise	Sets	Reps/time	Rest	Wt	Page #
Dumbbell bench press	1-2	20 reps	15 sec	20 lb, 25 lb, 30 lb	122
Burpee	1-2	50 sec	15 sec	BW	50
Kettlebell one-arm row	1-2	20 reps	15 sec	14 kg, 16 kg, 18 kg	129
POD 3					
Exercise	Sets	Reps/time	Rest	Wt	Page #
Medicine ball overhead squat	1-2	20 reps	15 sec	14 lb, 16 lb	85
Mountain climbers	1	50 sec	15 sec	BW	49
Medicine ball overhead lunge	1-2	20 reps	15 sec	14 lb, 16 lb	89
POD 4					
Exercise	Sets	Reps/time	Rest	Wt	Page #
Heavy rope arm circles: clockwise	1	50 sec	15 sec	Rope	173
Heavy rope two-hand shuffle slams	1	50 sec	15 sec	BW	174
Heavy rope arm circles: counterclockwise	1	50 sec	15 sec	Rope	173
POD 5					
Exercise	Sets	Reps/time	Rest	Wt	Page #
Kettlebell shoulder press	1-2	20 reps	15 sec	10 kg, 12 kg, 14 kg	131
Push-up	1	50 sec	15 sec	BW	112
Dumbbell bent-over raise	1-2	20 reps	15 sec	10 lb, 12 lb, 15 lb	140

(continued)

Fat Loss Program 4C: Advanced *(continued)*

POD 6					
Exercise	**Sets**	**Reps/time**	**Rest**	**Wt**	**Page #**
Medicine ball burpee	1-2	50 sec	15 sec	14 lb, 16 lb	70
Medicine ball Russian twist	1-2	50 sec	15 sec	14 lb, 16 lb	164
Medicine ball squat and jump	1-2	50 sec	15 sec	14 lb, 16 lb	71
POD 7					
Exercise	**Sets**	**Reps/time**	**Rest**	**Wt**	**Page #**
Resistance band shoulder press	1-2	20 reps	15 sec	Moderate/heavy	132
Dumbbell hammer curl	1-2	20 reps	15 sec	15 lb, 20 lb, 25 lb	145
Dumbbell supine triceps extension	1-2	20 reps	15 sec	12 lb, 15 lb, 20 lb	141
POD 8					
Exercise	**Sets**	**Reps/time**	**Rest**	**Wt**	**Page #**
Weighted sled pull and push	1	50 sec	15 sec	90 lb	75
Groiner	1	50 sec	15 sec	BW	51
Kettlebell farmer's walk	1	50 sec	15 sec	16 kg, 18 kg 20 kg	98
POD 9					
Exercise	**Sets**	**Reps/time**	**Rest**	**Wt**	**Page #**
Medicine ball sit-up	1	50 sec	15 sec	BW	164
Medicine ball Russian twist	1	50 sec	15 sec	BW	164
Medicine ball chop	1	50 sec	15 sec	BW	72
POD 10					
Exercise	**Sets**	**Reps/time**	**Rest**	**Wt**	**Page #**
Bicycle	1	50 sec	15 sec	BW	162
Scissors	1	50 sec	15 sec	BW	162
Superman	1	50 sec	15 sec	BW	163

Wt = Weight; BW = Bodyweight

13

Programs for Building Lean Mass

In the context of metabolic training, *lean mass* denotes muscle and any additional tissue that isn't fat. Your goal should be to either gain lean mass or retain it. Let's look more closely at some issues related to lean mass and metabolic training.

Methods for Building Lean Mass

Your lean mass is calculated by subtracting your fat mass from your total bodyweight. Some recommendations suggest that somewhere between 60 and 90 percent of your total bodyweight should be lean mass. If your goal is to increase lean mass, there are some program variables that can be manipulated to help you do so.

• Performing multiple sets of an exercise is associated with 40 percent greater hypertrophy compared to performing one set, in both trained and untrained subjects (Krieger 2010).

• Gains in lean mass can be achieved across a spectrum of loading ranges, meaning that repetitions and the weights associated with them can vary from low to high (Schoenfeld, Grgic, Ogborn, and Krieger 2017). It's important to include both eccentric and concentric actions in gaining lean mass; the lengthening and shortening actions while contracting muscles have shown to be effective in increasing lean mass (Schoenfeld et al. 2017).

• Extending the rest interval between sets will minimize total-body fatigue and allow for greater strength demands to be placed on the muscles.

• Complementing metabolic conditioning with stand-alone resistance-training days may further optimize gains in lean mass. By alternating strength training with metabolic training, not only will there be an increase in training volume, but the combination of lower-intensity, higher-volume workouts with higher-intensity, lower-volume workouts will maximize muscle development.

Exercises that tend to produce the greatest gains in lean mass are free-weight oriented, involve multiple joints, and are ground based. Performing these types of exercises helps you to gain more muscle mass, improve your strength, burn more calories, and improve your intramuscular coordination.

- The following exercises should be considered for incorporation into both metabolic conditioning and resistance training:
  - *Squats.* Front, back, and overhead
  - *Presses.* Barbell and dumbbell bench, incline, and overhead
  - *Lunges.* Barbell and dumbbell front, side, and reverse
  - *Pulls.* Clean- and snatch-grip pulls from variable heights

Guidelines and Goals for Building Lean Mass

As you plan your workouts and overall program to achieve your goal of building lean mass, we suggest following these guidelines to maximize your efforts:

- *Set realistic goals.* There are a few factors that can influence the addition and retention of lean mass. These factors include genetics, sex, and age. Genetically, some people can add muscle more quickly and more easily than others. Men can gain more strength and add more lean mass compared to women on account of having higher levels of testosterone. Age also influences the amount of lean mass that can also be gained. A younger adult will make greater gains than an older person, when all other factors are equal.

- *Focus on progress.* Trust that giving your best effort consistently will yield progress. Keep in mind that there will be setbacks along the way, and sometimes your gains will only be marginal, which is fine. It's also perfectly fine not to worry about progress and simply to enjoy a workout.

- *Measure.* As described earlier in the chapter, there are several methods for measuring lean mass. There are also normative data you can use to measure yourself against others. Assessing and measuring progress is fundamental to goal setting.

- *Specific*: Setting time-sensitive goals is a great way to stay focused and to give your training a sense of urgency. Both short- and long-term specific goals can play an important part in your training program.

For example, you could set a goal of gaining x amount of lean mass in y amount of time and then break that long-term goal into shorter-term segments. Or perhaps you might set a goal of completing five total workouts per week, or 20 workouts for the month. The workouts included in this chapter offer the appropriate frequency, intensity, duration, and exercise types to maximize lean-mass improvements.

The pods in the following exercise programs are a combination of three or more exercises performed with short rest periods between them for either a set number of repetitions or a prescribed amount of time.

Lean Mass Program 1A: Beginner

WARM-UP					
Exercise	Sets	Reps/time	Rest	Wt	Page #
March/walk	1	20 sec	10 sec	BW	N/A
Push-up	1	20 sec	10 sec	BW	112
March/walk	1	20 sec	10 sec	BW	N/A
Mountain climbers	1	20 sec	10 sec	BW	49
March/walk	1	20 sec	10 sec	BW	N/A
Burpee	1	20 sec	10 sec	BW	50
March/walk	1	20 sec	10 sec	BW	N/A
Single-leg squat (each leg)	1	20 sec	10 sec	BW	52
March/walk	1	20 sec	10 sec	BW	N/A
Jumping jacks	1	20 sec	10 sec	BW	48
LOWER BODY					
Exercise	Sets	Reps/time	Rest	Wt	Page #
Dumbbell squat	1	8-12 reps	15 sec	12 lb, 15 lb, 20 lb	80
Kettlebell deadlift	1	8-12 reps	15 sec	10 kg, 12 kg, 14 kg	94
Medicine ball overhead box step-up	1	8-12 reps	15 sec	8 lb, 10 lb, 12 lb	87
Dumbbell front lunge	1	8-12 reps	15 sec	8 lb, 10 lb, 12 lb	87
Kettlebell straight-leg deadlift	1	8-12 reps	15 sec	8 kg, 10 kg, 12 kg	95
Medicine ball overhead squat	1	8-12 reps	15 sec	8 lb, 10 lb, 12 lb	85
Dumbbell split squat	1	8-12 reps	15 sec	10 lb, 12 lb, 15 lb	82
Kettlebell goblet squat	1	8-12 reps	15 sec	8 kg, 10 kg, 12 kg	81
Medicine ball overhead lunge	1	8-12 reps	15 sec	8 lb, 10 lb, 12 lb	89
Dumbbell lateral lunge	1	8-12 reps	15 sec	8 lb, 10 lb, 12 lb	90
Kettlebell overhead lunge	1	8-12 reps	15 sec	6 kg, 8 kg, 10 kg	88
Medicine ball overhead backward lunge	1	8-12 reps	15 sec	8 lb, 10 lb, 12 lb	93
UPPER BODY					
Exercise	Sets	Reps/time	Rest	Wt	Page #
Dumbbell alt-arm bench press	1	8-12 reps	15 sec	10 lb, 12 lb, 15 lb	123
Kettlebell one-arm row	1	8-12 reps	15 sec	8 kg, 10 kg, 12 kg	129
Resistance band upright row	1	8-12 reps	15 sec	Light	135
Dumbbell bent-over raise	1	8-12 reps	15 sec	5 lb, 8 lb, 10 lb	140
Kettlebell alt-arm biceps curl	1	8-12 reps	15 sec	4 kg, 6 kg, 8 kg	144
Dumbbell one-arm triceps extension	1	8-12 reps	15 sec	5 lb, 8 lb, 10 lb	142
Suspension elevated push-up	1	8-12 reps	15 sec	BW	113
Dumbbell one-arm row	1	8-12 reps	15 sec	12 lb, 15 lb, 20 lb	129
Kettlebell shoulder press	1	8-12 reps	15 sec	4 kg, 6 kg, 8 kg	131
Resistance band Y	1	8-12 reps	15 sec	Light	116
Dumbbell concentration curl	1	8-12 reps	15 sec	8 lb, 10 lb, 12 lb	146
Kettlebell overhead triceps extension	1	8-12 reps	15 sec	6 kg, 8 kg, 10 kg	120

(continued)

Lean Mass Program 1A: Beginner *(continued)*

CORE					
Exercise	**Sets**	**Reps/time**	**Rest**	**Wt**	**Page #**
Abdominal reach	1	20 reps	15 sec	BW	157
Scissors	1	30 sec	15 sec	BW	162
Front plank	1	30 sec	15 sec	BW	159
Side plank: right	1	30 sec	15 sec	BW	160
Side plank: left	1	30 sec	15 sec	BW	160
Superman	1	30 sec	15 sec	BW	163

Wt = Weight; BW = Bodyweight

Lean Mass Program 1B: Intermediate

WARM-UP					
Exercise	**Sets**	**Reps/time**	**Rest**	**Wt**	**Page #**
Jog in place/jump rope	1	30 sec	10 sec	BW	N/A
Push-up	1	30 sec	10 sec	BW	112
Jog in place/jump rope	1	30 sec	10 sec	BW	N/A
Mountain climbers	1	30 sec	10 sec	BW	49
Jog in place/jump rope	1	30 sec	10 sec	BW	N/A
Burpee	1	30 sec	10 sec	BW	50
Jog in place/jump rope	1	30 sec	10 sec	BW	N/A
Single-leg squat (each leg)	1	30 sec	10 sec	BW	52
Jog in place/jump rope	1	30 sec	10 sec	BW	N/A
Jumping jacks	1	30 sec	10 sec	BW	48
LOWER BODY					
Exercise	**Sets**	**Reps/time**	**Rest**	**Wt**	**Page #**
Dumbbell squat	1-2	8-15 reps	15 sec	15 lb, 20 lb, 25 lb	80
Kettlebell deadlift	1-2	8-15 reps	15 sec	12 kg, 14 kg, 16 kg	94
Medicine ball overhead box step-up	1-2	8-15 reps	15 sec	10 lb, 12 lb, 14 lb	87
Dumbbell front lunge	1-2	8-15 reps	15 sec	10 lb, 12 lb, 15 lb	87
Kettlebell straight-leg deadlift	1-2	8-15 reps	15 sec	12 kg, 14 kg, 16 kg	95
Medicine ball overhead squat	1-2	8-15 reps	15 sec	10 lb, 12 lb, 14 lb	85
Dumbbell split squat	1-2	8-15 reps	15 sec	12 lb, 15 lb, 20 lb	82
Kettlebell goblet squat	1-2	8-15 reps	15 sec	10 kg, 12 kg, 14 kg	81
Medicine ball overhead lunge	1-2	8-15 reps	15 sec	10 lb, 12 lb, 14 lb	89
Dumbbell lateral lunge	1-2	8-15 reps	15 sec	10 lb, 12 lb, 15 lb	90
Kettlebell overhead lunge	1-2	8-15 reps	15 sec	8 kg, 10 kg, 12 kg	88
Medicine ball overhead backward lunge	1-2	8-15 reps	15 sec	10 lb, 12 lb, 14 lb	93

UPPER BODY					
Exercise	Sets	Reps/time	Rest	Wt	Page #
Dumbbell alt-arm bench press	1-2	8-15 reps	15 sec	12 lb, 15 lb, 20 lb	123
Kettlebell one-arm row	1-2	8-15 reps	15 sec	10 kg, 12 kg, 14 kg	129
Resistance band upright row	1-2	8-15 reps	15 sec	Moderate	135
Dumbbell bent-over raise	1-2	8-15 reps	15 sec	8 lb, 10 lb, 12 lb	140
Kettlebell alt-arm biceps curl	1-2	8-15 reps	15 sec	6 kg, 8 kg, 10 kg	144
Dumbbell one-arm triceps extension	1-2	8-15 reps	15 sec	8 lb, 10 lb, 12 lb	142
Suspension elevated push-up	1-2	8-15 reps	15 sec	BW	113
Dumbbell one-arm row	1-2	8-15 reps	15 sec	15 lb, 20 lb, 25 lb	129
Kettlebell shoulder press	1-2	8-15 reps	15 sec	6 kg, 8 kg, 10 kg	131
Resistance band Y	1-2	8-15 reps	15 sec	Moderate	116
Dumbbell concentration curl	1-2	8-15 reps	15 sec	12 lb, 15 lb, 20 lb	146
Kettlebell overhead triceps extension	1-2	8-15 reps	15 sec	10 kg, 12 kg, 14 kg	120
CORE					
Exercise	Sets	Reps/time	Rest	Wt	Page #
Front plank	1	40 sec	15 sec	BW	159
Side plank: right	1	40 sec	15 sec	BW	160
Side plank: left	1	40 sec	15 sec	BW	160
Opposite-shoulder-to-knee crunch	1	30 reps	15 sec	BW	158
Scissors	1	40 sec	15 sec	BW	162
Bicycle	1	40 sec	15 sec	BW	162
Birddog	1	40 sec	15 sec	BW	161
Weighted abdominal crunch	1	30 reps	15 sec	5-10 lb	155
Weighted abdominal reach	1	30 reps	15 sec	5-10 lb	157

Wt = Weight; BW = Bodyweight

Lean Mass Program 1C: Advanced

WARM-UP					
Exercise	Sets	Reps/time	Rest	Wt	Page #
Jog in place/jump rope	1	40 sec	10 sec	BW	N/A
Push-up	1	40 sec	10 sec	BW	112
Jog in place/jump rope	1	40 sec	10 sec	BW	N/A
Mountain climbers	1	40 sec	10 sec	BW	49
Jog in place/jump rope	1	40 sec	10 sec	BW	N/A
Burpee	1	40 sec	10 sec	BW	50
Jog in place/jump rope	1	40 sec	10 sec	BW	N/A
Single-leg squat (each leg)	1	40 sec	10 sec	BW	52
Jog in place/jump rope	1	40 sec	10 sec	BW	N/A
Jumping jacks	1	40 sec	10 sec	BW	48

(continued)

Lean Mass Program 1C: Advanced *(continued)*

LOWER BODY					
Exercise	Sets	Reps/time	Rest	Wt	Page #
Dumbbell squat	1-2	8-15 reps	15 sec	20 lb, 25 lb, 30 lb	80
Kettlebell deadlift	1-2	8-15 reps	15 sec	14 kg, 16 kg, 18 kg	94
Medicine ball overhead box step-up	1-2	8-15 reps	15 sec	12 lb, 14 lb, 16 lb	87
Dumbbell front lunge	1-2	8-15 reps	15 sec	12 lb, 15 lb, 20 lb	87
Kettlebell straight-leg deadlift	1-2	8-15 reps	15 sec	14 kg, 16 kg, 18 kg	95
Medicine ball overhead squat	1-2	8-15 reps	15 sec	12 lb, 14 lb, 16 lb	85
Dumbbell split squat	1-2	8-15 reps	15 sec	15 lb, 20 lb, 25 lb	82
Kettlebell goblet squat	1-2	8-15 reps	15 sec	12 kg, 14 kg, 16 kg,	81
Medicine ball overhead lunge	1-2	8-15 reps	15 sec	12 lb, 14 lb, 16 lb	89
Dumbbell lateral lunge	1-2	8-15 reps	15 sec	12 lb, 15 lb, 20 lb	90
Kettlebell overhead lunge	1-2	8-15 reps	15 sec	10 kg, 12 kg, 14 kg	88
Medicine ball overhead backward lunge	1-2	8-15 reps	15 sec	12 lb, 14 lb, 16 lb	93

UPPER BODY					
Exercise	Sets	Reps/time	Rest	Wt	Page #
Dumbbell alt-arm bench press	1-2	8-15 reps	15 sec	15 lb, 20 lb, 25 lb	123
Kettlebell one-arm row	1-2	8-15 reps	15 sec	12 kg, 14 kg, 16 kg,	129
Resistance band upright row	1-2	8-15 reps	15 sec	Heavy	135
Dumbbell bent-over raise	1-2	8-15 reps	15 sec	10 lb, 12 lb, 14 lb	140
Kettlebell alt-arm biceps curl	1-2	8-15 reps	15 sec	8 kg, 10 kg, 12 kg	144
Dumbbell one-arm triceps extension	1-2	8-15 reps	15 sec	10 lb, 12 lb, 15 lb	142
Suspension elevated push-up	1-2	8-15 reps	15 sec	BW	113
Dumbbell one-arm row	1-2	8-15 reps	15 sec	20 lb, 25 lb, 30 lb	129
Kettlebell shoulder press	1-2	8-15 reps	15 sec	8 kg, 10 kg, 12 kg	131
Resistance band Y	1-2	8-15 reps	15 sec	Heavy	116
Dumbbell concentration curl	1-2	8-15 reps	15 sec	15 lb, 20 lb, 25 lb	146
Kettlebell overhead triceps extension	1-2	8-15 reps	15 sec	12 kg, 14 kg, 16 kg	120

CORE					
Exercise	Sets	Reps/time	Rest	Wt	Page #
Front plank	1	50 sec	15 sec	BW	159
Side plank: right	1	50 sec	15 sec	BW	160
Side plank: left	1	50 sec	15 sec	BW	160
Opposite-shoulder-to-knee crunch	1	40 reps	15 sec	BW	158
Scissors	1	50 sec	15 sec	BW	162
Bicycle	1	50 sec	15 sec	BW	162
Birddog	1	50 sec	15 sec	BW	161
Weighted abdominal crunch	1	40 reps	15 sec	5-10 lb	155
Weighted abdominal reach	1	40 reps	15 sec	5-10 lb	157

Wt = Weight; BW = Bodyweight

Lean Mass Program 2A: Beginner

WARM-UP					
Exercise	Sets	Reps/time	Rest	Wt	Page #
March/walk	1	20 sec	10 sec	BW	N/A
Single-leg squat (each leg)	1	20 sec	10 sec	BW	52
March/walk	1	20 sec	10 sec	BW	N/A
Jumping jacks	1	20 sec	10 sec	BW	48
March/walk	1	20 sec	10 sec	BW	N/A
Push-up	1	20 sec	10 sec	BW	112
March/walk	1	20 sec	10 sec	BW	N/A
Mountain climbers	1	20 sec	10 sec	BW	49
March/walk	1	20 sec	10 sec	BW	N/A
Burpee	1	20 sec	10 sec	BW	50
LOWER BODY					
Exercise	Sets	Reps/time	Rest	Wt	Page #
Kettlebell overhead squat	1	8-12 reps	15 sec	6 kg, 8 kg, 10 kg	83
Resistance band pull-through	1	8-12 reps	15 sec	Moderate	65
Dumbbell backward lunge	1	8-12 reps	15 sec	8 lb, 10 lb, 12 lb	92
Suspension one-leg squat	1	8-12 reps	15 sec	BW	103
Dumbbell one-leg straight-leg deadlift	1	8-12 reps	15 sec	8 lb, 10 lb, 12 lb	97
Resistance band overhead squat	1	8-12 reps	15 sec	Light	84
Dumbbell squat	1	8-12 reps	15 sec	12 lb, 15 lb, 20 lb	80
Kettlebell deadlift	1	8-12 reps	15 sec	10 kg, 12 kg, 14 kg	94
Medicine ball overhead lateral lunge	1	8-12 reps	15 sec	8 lb, 10 lb, 12 lb	91
Dumbbell front lunge	1	8-12 reps	15 sec	8 lb, 10 lb, 12 lb	87
Suspension backward lunge	1	8-12 reps	15 sec	BW	105
Suspension leg curl	1	8-12 reps	15 sec	BW	106
UPPER BODY					
Exercise	Sets	Reps/time	Rest	Wt	Page #
Dumbbell alt-arm incline press	1	8-12 reps	15 sec	8 lb, 10 lb, 12 lb	125
Suspension row	1	8-12 reps	15 sec	BW	135
Dumbbell lateral raise	1	8-12 reps	15 sec	5 lb, 8 lb, 10 lb	137
Resistance band T	1	8-12 reps	15 sec	Light	118
Suspension biceps curl	1	8-12 reps	15 sec	BW	121
Resistance band triceps pushdown	1	8-12 reps	15 sec	Light	149
Kettlebell pullover	1	8-12 reps	15 sec	8 kg, 10 kg, 12 kg	128
Resistance band upright row	1	8-12 reps	15 sec	Moderate	135
Dumbbell shoulder press	1	8-12 reps	15 sec	8 lb, 10 lb, 12 lb	131
Dumbbell front raise	1	8-12 reps	15 sec	5 lb, 8 lb, 10 lb	138
Resistance band hammer curl	1	8-12 reps	15 sec	Light	145
Suspension triceps extension	1	8-12 reps	15 sec	BW	119

(continued)

Lean Mass Program 2A: Beginner *(continued)*

CORE					
Exercise	Sets	Reps/time	Rest	Wt	Page #
Abdominal curl-up	1	20 reps	15 sec	BW	156
Abdominal crunch: legs up	1	30 sec	15 sec	BW	155
Abdominal reach: legs up	1	30 sec	15 sec	BW	157
Opposite-shoulder-to-knee crunch	1	30 sec	15 sec	BW	158
Scissors	1	30 sec	15 sec	BW	162
Birddog	1	30 sec	15 sec	BW	161

Wt = Weight; BW = Bodyweight

Lean Mass Program 2B: Intermediate

WARM-UP					
Exercise	Sets	Reps/time	Rest	Wt	Page #
Jog in place/jump rope	1	30 sec	10 sec	BW	N/A
Single-leg squat (each leg)	1	30 sec	10 sec	BW	52
Jog in place/jump rope	1	30 sec	10 sec	BW	N/A
Jumping jacks	1	30 sec	10 sec	BW	48
Jog in place/jump rope	1	30 sec	10 sec	BW	N/A
Push-up	1	30 sec	10 sec	BW	112
Jog in place/jump rope	1	30 sec	10 sec	BW	N/A
Mountain climbers	1	30 sec	10 sec	BW	49
Jog in place/jump rope	1	30 sec	10 sec	BW	N/A
Burpee	1	30 sec	10 sec	BW	50
LOWER BODY					
Exercise	Sets	Reps/time	Rest	Wt	Page #
Kettlebell overhead squat	1-2	8-15 reps	15 sec	8 kg, 10 kg, 12 kg	83
Resistance band pull-through	1-2	8-15 reps	15 sec	Moderate/heavy	65
Dumbbell backward lunge	1-2	8-15 reps	15 sec	10 lb, 12 lb, 15 lb	92
Suspension one-leg squat	1-2	8-15 reps	15 sec	BW	103
Dumbbell one-leg straight-leg deadlift	1-2	8-15 reps	15 sec	12 lb, 15 lb, 20 lb	97
Resistance band overhead squat	1-2	8-15 reps	15 sec	Moderate	84
Suspension one-leg squat	1-2	8-15 reps	15 sec	BW	103
Kettlebell deadlift	1-2	8-15 reps	15 sec	14 kg, 16 kg, 18 kg	94
Medicine ball overhead lateral lunge	1-2	8-15 reps	15 sec	10 lb, 12 lb, 14 lb	91
Kettlebell overhead lunge	1-2	8-15 reps	15 sec	8 kg, 10 kg, 12 kg	88
Dumbbell backward lunge	1-2	8-15 reps	15 sec	12 lb, 15 lb, 20 lb	92
Suspension leg curl	1-2	8-15 reps	15 sec	BW	106

UPPER BODY					
Exercise	Sets	Reps/time	Rest	Wt	Page #
Dumbbell alt-arm incline press	1-2	8-15 reps	15 sec	12 lb, 15 lb, 20 lb	125
Suspension row	1-2	8-15 reps	15 sec	BW	135
Dumbbell lateral raise	1-2	8-15 reps	15 sec	8 lb, 10 lb, 12 lb	137
Resistance band T	1-2	8-15 reps	15 sec	Moderate	118
Suspension biceps curl	1-2	8-15 reps	15 sec	BW	121
Resistance band triceps pushdown	1-2	8-15 reps	15 sec	Moderate	149
Kettlebell pullover	1-2	8-15 reps	15 sec	12 kg, 14 kg, 16 kg	128
Dumbbell renegade row	1-2	8-15 reps	15 sec	15 lb, 20 lb, 25 lb	130
Kettlebell shoulder press	1-2	8-15 reps	15 sec	6 kg, 8 kg, 10 kg	131
Suspension reverse fly	1-2	8-15 reps	15 sec	BW	127
Dumbbell hammer curl	1-2	8-15 reps	15 sec	12 lb, 15 lb, 20 lb	145
Suspension triceps extension	1-2	8-15 reps	15 sec	BW	119
CORE					
Exercise	Sets	Reps/time	Rest	Wt	Page #
Weighted abdominal crunch	1	30 reps	15 sec	5-10 lb	155
Weighted abdominal reach	1	30 reps	15 sec	5-10 lb	157
Opposite-shoulder-to-knee crunch	1	30 reps	15 sec	BW	158
Scissors	1	40 sec	15 sec	BW	162
Bicycle	1	40 sec	15 sec	BW	162
Front plank	1	40 sec	15 sec	BW	159
Side plank: right	1	40 sec	15 sec	BW	160
Side plank: left	1	40 sec	15 sec	BW	160
Superman	1	40 sec	15 sec	BW	163

Wt = Weight; BW = Bodyweight

Lean Mass Program 2C: Advanced

WARM-UP					
Exercise	Sets	Reps/time	Rest	Wt	Page #
Jog in place/jump rope	1	40 sec	10 sec	BW	N/A
Single-leg squat (each leg)	1	40 sec	10 sec	BW	52
Jog in place/jump rope	1	40 sec	10 sec	BW	N/A
Jumping jacks	1	40 sec	10 sec	BW	48
Jog in place/jump rope	1	40 sec	10 sec	BW	N/A
Push-up	1	40 sec	10 sec	BW	112
Jog in place/jump rope	1	40 sec	10 sec	BW	N/A
Mountain climbers	1	40 sec	10 sec	BW	49
Jog in place/jump rope	1	40 sec	10 sec	BW	N/A
Burpee	1	40 sec	10 sec	BW	50

(continued)

Lean Mass Program 2C: Advanced *(continued)*

LOWER BODY					
Exercise	**Sets**	**Reps/time**	**Rest**	**Wt**	**Page #**
Kettlebell overhead squat	1-2	8-15 reps	15 sec	12 kg, 14 kg, 16 kg	83
Resistance band pull-through	1-2	8-15 reps	15 sec	Heavy	65
Dumbbell backward lunge	1-2	8-15 reps	15 sec	15 lb, 20 lb, 25 lb	92
Suspension one-leg squat	1-2	8-15 reps	15 sec	BW	103
Dumbbell one-leg straight-leg deadlift	1-2	8-15 reps	15 sec	20 lb, 25 lb, 30 lb	97
Resistance band overhead squat	1-2	8-15 reps	15 sec	Heavy	84
Suspension one-leg squat	1-2	8-15 reps	15 sec	BW	103
Kettlebell deadlift	1-2	8-15 reps	15 sec	18 kg, 20 kg, 22 kg	94
Medicine ball overhead lateral lunge	1-2	8-15 reps	15 sec	14 lb, 16 lb, 18 lb	91
Kettlebell overhead lunge	1-2	8-15 reps	15 sec	10 kg, 12 kg, 14 kg	88
Dumbbell backward lunge	1-2	8-15 reps	15 sec	15 lb, 20 lb, 25 lb	92
Suspension leg curl	1-2	8-15 reps	15 sec	BW	106
UPPER BODY					
Exercise	**Sets**	**Reps/time**	**Rest**	**Wt**	**Page #**
Dumbbell alt-arm incline press	1-2	8-15 reps	15 sec	20 lb, 25 lb, 30 lb	125
Suspension row	1-2	8-15 reps	15 sec	BW	135
Dumbbell lateral raise	1-2	8-15 reps	15 sec	10 lb, 12 lb, 15 lb	137
Resistance band T	1-2	8-15 reps	15 sec	Moderate	118
Suspension biceps curl	1-2	8-15 reps	15 sec	BW	121
Resistance band triceps pushdown	1-2	8-15 reps	15 sec	Moderate/heavy	149
Kettlebell pullover	1-2	8-15 reps	15 sec	16 kg, 18 kg, 20 kg	128
Dumbbell renegade row	1-2	8-15 reps	15 sec	20 lb, 25 lb, 30 lb	130
Kettlebell shoulder press	1-2	8-15 reps	15 sec	8 kg, 10 kg, 12 kg	131
Suspension reverse fly	1-2	8-15 reps	15 sec	BW	127
Dumbbell hammer curl	1-2	8-15 reps	15 sec	15 lb, 20 lb, 25 lb	145
Suspension triceps extension	1-2	8-15 reps	15 sec	BW	119
CORE					
Exercise	**Sets**	**Reps/time**	**Rest**	**Wt**	**Page #**
Weighted abdominal crunch	1	40 reps	15 sec	5-10 lb	155
Weighted abdominal reach	1	40 reps	15 sec	5-10 lb	157
Opposite-shoulder-to-knee crunch	1	40 reps	15 sec	BW	158
Scissors	1	50 reps	15 sec	BW	162
Bicycle	1	50 reps	15 sec	BW	162
Front plank	1	50 reps	15 sec	BW	159
Side plank: right	1	50 reps	15 sec	BW	160
Side plank: left	1	50 reps	15 sec	BW	160
Superman	1	50 reps	15 sec	BW	163

Wt = Weight: BW = Bodyweight

Lean Mass Program 3A: Beginner

Note: Each exercise in a pod should be completed before moving to the next pod. A pod is a combination of three or more exercises performed with short rest periods between them for either a set number of repetitions or a prescribed amount of time.

WARM-UP					
Exercise	Sets	Reps/time	Rest	Wt	Page #
March/walk	1	20 sec	10 sec	BW	N/A
Single-leg squat (each leg)	1	20 sec	10 sec	BW	52
March/walk	1	20 sec	10 sec	BW	N/A
Mountain climbers	1	20 sec	10 sec	BW	49
March/walk	1	20 sec	10 sec	BW	N/A
Jumping jacks	1	20 sec	10 sec	BW	48
March/walk	1	20 sec	10 sec	BW	N/A
Burpee	1	20 sec	10 sec	BW	50
March/walk	1	20 sec	10 sec	BW	N/A
Push-up	1	20 sec	10 sec	BW	112
POD 1					
Exercise	Sets	Reps/time	Rest	Wt	Page #
Dumbbell squat	1	12 reps	15 sec	12 lb, 15 lb, 20 lb	80
Dumbbell overhead squat	1	12 reps	15 sec	10 lb, 12 lb, 15 lb	83
Dumbbell goblet squat	1	12 reps	15 sec	10 lb, 12 lb, 15 lb	81
POD 2					
Exercise	Sets	Reps/time	Rest	Wt	Page #
Dumbbell bench press	1	12 reps	15 sec	12 lb, 15 lb, 20 lb	122
Dumbbell renegade row	1	12 reps	15 sec	10 lb, 12 lb, 15 lb	130
Push-up	1	12 reps	15 sec	BW	112
POD 3					
Exercise	Sets	Reps/time	Rest	Wt	Page #
Heavy rope two-arm slams	1	30 sec	15 sec	Rope	169
Heavy rope alt-arm slams	1	30 sec	15 sec	Rope	170
Heavy rope scissors	1	30 sec	15 sec	Rope	171
POD 4					
Exercise	Sets	Reps/time	Rest	Wt	Page #
Dumbbell front lunge	1	12 reps	15 sec	8 lb, 10 lb, 12 lb	87
Dumbbell lateral lunge	1	12 reps	15 sec	8 lb, 10 lb, 12 lb	90
Dumbbell backward lunge	1	12 reps	15 sec	8 lb, 10 lb, 12 lb	92
POD 5					
Exercise	Sets	Reps/time	Rest	Wt	Page #
Dumbbell shoulder press	1	12 reps	15 sec	8 lb, 10 lb, 12 lb	131
Dumbbell upright row	1	12 reps	15 sec	8 lb, 10 lb, 12 lb	134
Dumbbell front raise	1	12 reps	15 sec	5 lb, 8 lb, 10 lb	138
POD 6					
Exercise	Sets	Reps/time	Rest	Wt	Page #
Medicine ball slam	1	30 sec	15 sec	8 lb, 10 lb, 12 lb	66
Medicine ball side slam	1	30 sec	15 sec	8 lb, 10 lb, 12 lb	67
Medicine ball overhead squat	1	30 sec	15 sec	8 lb, 10 lb, 12 lb	85

(continued)

Lean Mass Program 3A: Beginner *(continued)*

POD 7					
Exercise	Sets	Reps/time	Rest	Wt	Page #
Weighted sled push	1	30 sec	15 sec	45 lb	74
Weighted sled pull	1	30 sec	15 sec	45 lb	75
Weighted sled drag	1	30 sec	15 sec	45 lb	76
POD 8					
Exercise	Sets	Reps/time	Rest	Wt	Page #
Dumbbell hammer curl	1	12 reps	15 sec	10 lb, 12 lb, 15 lb	145
Dumbbell triceps kickback	1	12 reps	15 sec	8 lb, 10 lb, 12 lb	143
Dumbbell bent-over raise	1	12 reps	15 sec	5 lb, 8 lb, 10 lb	140
POD 9					
Exercise	Sets	Reps/time	Rest	Wt	Page #
Abdominal reach	1	30 sec	15 sec	BW	157
Bicycle	1	30 sec	15 sec	BW	162
Birddog	1	30 sec	15 sec	BW	161
POD 10					
Exercise	Sets	Reps/time	Rest	Wt	Page #
Abdominal crunch	1	30 sec	15 sec	BW	155
Scissors	1	30 sec	15 sec	BW	162
Opposite-shoulder-to-knee crunch	1	30 sec	15 sec	BW	158

Wt = Weight; BW = Bodyweight

Lean Mass Program 3B: Intermediate

Note: Each exercise in a pod should be completed before moving to the next pod. A pod is a combination of three or more exercises performed with short rest periods between them for either a set number of repetitions or a prescribed amount of time.

WARM-UP					
Exercise	Sets	Reps/time	Rest	Wt	Page #
Jog in place/jump rope	1	30 sec	10 sec	BW	N/A
Single-leg squat (each leg)	1	30 sec	10 sec	BW	52
Jog in place/jump rope	1	30 sec	10 sec	BW	N/A
Mountain climbers	1	30 sec	10 sec	BW	49
Jog in place/jump rope	1	30 sec	10 sec	BW	N/A
Jumping jacks	1	30 sec	10 sec	BW	48
Jog in place/jump rope	1	30 sec	10 sec	BW	N/A
Burpee	1	30 sec	10 sec	BW	50
Jog in place/jump rope	1	30 sec	10 sec	BW	N/A
Push-up	1	30 sec	10 sec	BW	112

POD 1					
Exercise	Sets	Reps/time	Rest	Wt	Page #
Dumbbell squat	1-2	12 reps	15 sec	15 lb, 20 lb, 25 lb	80
Dumbbell overhead squat	1-2	12 reps	15 sec	15 lb, 20 lb, 25 lb	83
Dumbbell goblet squat	1-2	12 reps	15 sec	15 lb, 20 lb, 25 lb	81

POD 2					
Exercise	Sets	Reps/time	Rest	Wt	Page #
Dumbbell bench press	1-2	12 reps	15 sec	20 lb, 25 lb, 30 lb	122
Dumbbell renegade row	1-2	12 reps	15 sec	15 lb, 20 lb, 25 lb	130
Push-up	1-2	12 reps	15 sec	BW	112

POD 3					
Exercise	Sets	Reps/time	Rest	Wt	Page #
Heavy rope two-arm slams	1-2	40 sec	15 sec	Rope	169
Heavy rope alt-arm slams	1-2	40 sec	15 sec	Rope	170
Heavy rope scissors	1-2	40 sec	15 sec	Rope	171

POD 4					
Exercise	Sets	Reps/time	Rest	Wt	Page #
Dumbbell front lunge	1-2	12 reps	15 sec	15 lb, 20 lb, 25 lb	87
Dumbbell lateral lunge	1-2	12 reps	15 sec	15 lb, 20 lb, 25 lb	90
Dumbbell backward lunge	1-2	12 reps	15 sec	15 lb, 20 lb, 25 lb	92

POD 5					
Exercise	Sets	Reps/time	Rest	Wt	Page #
Dumbbell shoulder press	1-2	12 reps	15 sec	15 lb, 20 lb, 25 lb	131
Dumbbell upright row	1-2	12 reps	15 sec	15 lb, 20 lb, 25 lb	134
Dumbbell front raise	1-2	12 reps	15 sec	8 lb, 10 lb, 12 lb	138

POD 6					
Exercise	Sets	Reps/time	Rest	Wt	Page #
Medicine ball slam	1-2	40 sec	15 sec	12 lb, 14 lb, 16 lb	66
Medicine ball side slam	1-2	40 sec	15 sec	12 lb, 14 lb, 16 lb	67
Medicine ball overhead squat	1-2	40 sec	15 sec	10 lb, 12 lb, 14 lb	85

POD 7					
Exercise	Sets	Reps/time	Rest	Wt	Page #
Weighted sled push	1-2	40 sec	15 sec	70 lb	74
Weighted sled pull and push: 1 inch rope	1-2	40 sec	15 sec	70 lb	75
Weighted sled drag	1-2	40 sec	15 sec	70 lb	76

POD 8					
Exercise	Sets	Reps/time	Rest	Wt	Page #
Dumbbell hammer curl	2	12 reps	15 sec	15 lb, 20 lb, 25 lb	145
Dumbbell triceps kickback	2	12 reps	15 sec	12 lb, 15 lb, 20 lb	143
Dumbbell bent-over raise	2	12 reps	15 sec	8 lb, 10 lb, 12 lb	140

(continued)

Lean Mass Program 3B: Intermediate *(continued)*

POD 9					
Exercise	Sets	Reps/time	Rest	Wt	Page #
Abdominal reach	2	40 sec	15 sec	5-10 lb	157
Bicycle	2	40 sec	15 sec	BW	162
Birddog	2	40 sec	15 sec	BW	161
POD 10					
Exercise	Sets	Reps/time	Rest	Wt	Page #
Abdominal crunch	2	40 sec	15 sec	5-10 lb	155
Scissors	2	40 sec	15 sec	BW	162
Opposite-shoulder-to-knee crunch	2	40 sec	15 sec	BW	158

Wt = Weight; BW = Bodyweight

Lean Mass Program 3C: Advanced

Note: Each exercise in a pod should be completed before moving to the next pod. A pod is a combination of three or more exercises performed with short rest periods between them for either a set number of repetitions or a prescribed amount of time.

WARM-UP					
Exercise	Sets	Reps/time	Rest	Wt	Page #
Jog in place/jump rope	1	40 sec	10 sec	BW	N/A
Single-leg squat (each leg)	1	40 sec	10 sec	BW	52
Jog in place/jump rope	1	40 sec	10 sec	BW	N/A
Mountain climbers	1	40 sec	10 sec	BW	49
Jog in place/jump rope	1	40 sec	10 sec	BW	N/A
Jumping jacks	1	40 sec	10 sec	BW	48
Jog in place/jump rope	1	40 sec	10 sec	BW	N/A
Burpee	1	40 sec	10 sec	BW	50
Jog in place/jump rope	1	40 sec	10 sec	BW	N/A
Push-up	1	40 sec	10 sec	BW	112
POD 1					
Exercise	Sets	Reps/time	Rest	Wt	Page #
Dumbbell squat	2	12-15 reps	15 sec	20 lb, 25 lb, 30 lb	80
Dumbbell overhead squat	2	12-15 reps	15 sec	20 lb, 25 lb, 30 lb	83
Dumbbell goblet squat	2	12-15 reps	15 sec	20 lb, 25 lb, 30 lb	81
POD 2					
Exercise	Sets	Reps/time	Rest	Wt	Page #
Dumbbell bench press	2	12-15 reps	15 sec	25 lb, 30 lb, 35 lb	122
Dumbbell renegade row	2	12-15 reps	15 sec	20 lb, 25 lb, 30 lb	130
Push-up	2	12-15 reps	15 sec	BW	112

POD 3					
Exercise	**Sets**	**Reps/time**	**Rest**	**Wt**	**Page #**
Heavy rope two-arm slams	2	50 sec	15 sec	Rope	169
Heavy rope alt-arm slams	2	50 sec	15 sec	Rope	170
Heavy rope scissors	2	50 sec	15 sec	Rope	171
POD 4					
Exercise	**Sets**	**Reps/time**	**Rest**	**Wt**	**Page #**
Dumbbell front lunge	2	12-15 reps	15 sec	20 lb, 25 lb, 30 lb	87
Dumbbell lateral lunge	2	12-15 reps	15 sec	20 lb, 25 lb, 30 lb	90
Dumbbell backward lunge	2	12-15 reps	15 sec	20 lb, 25 lb, 30 lb	92
POD 5					
Exercise	**Sets**	**Reps/time**	**Rest**	**Wt**	**Page #**
Dumbbell shoulder press	2	12-15 reps	15 sec	20 lb, 25 lb, 30 lb	131
Dumbbell upright row	2	12-15 reps	15 sec	20 lb, 25 lb, 30 lb	134
Dumbbell front raise	2	12-15 reps	15 sec	10 lb, 12 lb, 15 lb	138
POD 6					
Exercise	**Sets**	**Reps/time**	**Rest**	**Wt**	**Page #**
Medicine ball slam	2	50 sec	15 sec	14 lb, 16 lb, 18 lb	66
Medicine ball side slam	2	50 sec	15 sec	14 lb, 16 lb, 18 lb	67
Medicine ball overhead squat	2	50 sec	15 sec	12 lb, 14 lb, 16 lb	85
POD 7					
Exercise	**Sets**	**Reps/time**	**Rest**	**Wt**	**Page #**
Weighted sled push	2	50 sec	15 sec	90 lb	74
Weighted sled pull	2	50 sec	15 sec	90 lb	75
Weighted sled drag	2	50 sec	15 sec	90 lb	76
POD 8					
Exercise	**Sets**	**Reps/time**	**Rest**	**Wt**	**Page #**
Dumbbell hammer curl	2	12-15 reps	15 sec	20 lb, 25 lb, 30 lb	145
Dumbbell triceps kickback	2	12-15 reps	15 sec	15 lb, 20 lb, 25 lb	143
Dumbbell bent-over raise	2	12-15 reps	15 sec	10 lb, 12 lb, 15 lb	140
POD 9					
Exercise	**Sets**	**Reps/time**	**Rest**	**Wt**	**Page #**
Abdominal reach	2	50 sec	15 sec	5-10 lb	157
Bicycle	2	50 sec	15 sec	BW	162
Birddog	2	50 sec	15 sec	BW	161
POD 10					
Exercise	**Sets**	**Reps/time**	**Rest**	**Wt**	**Page #**
Abdominal crunch	2	50 sec	15 sec	5-10 lb	155
Scissors	2	50 sec	15 sec	BW	162
Opposite-shoulder-to-knee crunch	2	50 sec	15 sec	BW	158

Wt = Weight; BW = Bodyweight

Lean Mass Program 4A: Beginner

Note: Each exercise in a pod should be completed before moving to the next pod. A pod is a combination of three or more exercises performed with short rest periods between them for either a set number of repetitions or a prescribed amount of time.

WARM-UP					
Exercise	Sets	Reps/time	Rest	Wt	Page #
Mountain climbers	1	20 sec	10 sec	BW	49
Walk in place/march	1	20 sec	10 sec	BW	N/A
Jumping jacks	1	20 sec	10 sec	BW	48
Walk in place/march	1	20 sec	10 sec	BW	N/A
Burpee	1	20 sec	10 sec	BW	50
Walk in place/march	1	20 sec	10 sec	BW	N/A
Push-up	1	20 sec	10 sec	BW	112
Walk in place/march	1	20 sec	10 sec	BW	N/A
Single-leg squat (each leg)	1	20 sec	10 sec	BW	52
Walk in place/march	1	20 sec	10 sec	BW	N/A

POD 1					
Exercise	Sets	Reps/time	Rest	Wt	Page #
Dumbbell squat	1	12 reps	15 sec	12 lb, 15 lb, 20 lb	80
Push-up	1	12 reps	15 sec	BW	112
Dumbbell bench press	1	12 reps	15 sec	12 lb, 15 lb, 20 lb	122

POD 2					
Exercise	Sets	Reps/time	Rest	Wt	Page #
Kettlebell two-hand swing	1	12 reps	15 sec	8 kg, 10 kg, 12 kg	62
Dumbbell upright row	1	12 reps	15 sec	10 lb, 12 lb, 15 lb	134
Suspension row	1	12 reps	15 sec	BW	135

POD 3					
Exercise	Sets	Reps/time	Rest	Wt	Page #
Kettlebell goblet squat	1	12 reps	15 sec	12 lb, 15 lb, 20 lb	81
Dumbbell bench press	1	12 reps	15 sec	8 lb, 10 lb, 12 lb	122
Dumbbell shoulder press	1	12 reps	15 sec	8 lb, 10 lb, 12 lb	131

POD 4					
Exercise	Sets	Reps/time	Rest	Wt	Page #
Heavy rope two-hand slams	1	40 sec	15 sec	Rope	169
Heavy rope alt-arm slams	1	40 sec	15 sec	Rope	170
Heavy rope scissors	1	40 sec	15 sec	Rope	171

POD 5					
Exercise	Sets	Reps/time	Rest	Wt	Page #
Dumbbell straight-leg deadlift	1	12 reps	15 sec	12 lb, 15 lb, 20 lb	95
Dumbbell renegade row	1	12 reps	15 sec	10 lb, 12 lb, 15 lb	130
Kettlebell upright row	1	12 reps	15 sec	6 kg, 8 kg, 10 kg	134

POD 6					
Exercise	Sets	Reps/time	Rest	Wt	Page #
Dumbbell front lunge	1	12 reps	15 sec	8 lb, 10 lb, 12 lb	87
Dumbbell shoulder press	1	12 reps	15 sec	8 lb, 10 lb, 12 lb	131
Dumbbell alt-arm biceps curl	1	12 reps	15 sec	8 lb, 10 lb, 12 lb	144

POD 7					
Exercise	Sets	Reps/time	Rest	Wt	Page #
Dumbbell lateral lunge	1	12 reps	15 sec	8 lb, 10 lb, 12 lb	90
Dumbbell bent-over raise	1	12 reps	15 sec	5 lb, 8 lb, 10 lb	140
Kettlebell overhead triceps extension	1	12 reps	15 sec	6 kg, 8 kg, 10 kg	120

POD 8					
Exercise	Sets	Reps/time	Rest	Wt	Page #
Dumbbell backward lunge	1	12 reps	15 sec	8 lb, 10 lb, 12 lb	92
Dumbbell hammer curl	1	12 reps	15 sec	8 lb, 10 lb, 12 lb	145
Dumbbell triceps kickback	1	12 reps	15 sec	8 lb, 10 lb, 12 lb	143

POD 9					
Exercise	Sets	Reps/time	Rest	Wt	Page #
Weighted sled push	1	30 sec	15 sec	45 lb	74
Weighted sled pull and push	1	30 sec	15 sec	45 lb	75
Farmer's walk	1	30 sec	15 sec	45 lb	98

POD 10					
Exercise	Sets	Reps/time	Rest	Wt	Page #
Front plank	1	30 sec	15 sec	BW	159
Side plank: right	1	30 sec	15 sec	BW	160
Side plank: left	1	30 sec	15 sec	BW	160

POD 11					
Exercise	Sets	Reps/time	Rest	Wt	Page #
Birddog	1	30 sec	15 sec	BW	161
Superman	1	30 sec	15 sec	BW	163
Scissors	1	30 sec	15 sec	BW	162

Wt = Weight; BW = Bodyweight

Lean Mass Program 4B: Intermediate

Note: Each exercise in a pod should be completed before moving to the next pod. A pod is a combination of three or more exercises performed with short rest periods between them for either a set number of repetitions or a prescribed amount of time.

WARM-UP					
Exercise	Sets	Reps/time	Rest	Wt	Page #
Mountain climbers	1	30 sec	10 sec	BW	49
Jog in place/jump rope	1	30 sec	10 sec	BW	N/A
Jumping jacks	1	30 sec	10 sec	BW	48
Jog in place/jump rope	1	30 sec	10 sec	BW	N/A
Burpee	1	30 sec	10 sec	BW	50
Jog in place/jump rope	1	30 sec	10 sec	BW	N/A
Push-up	1	30 sec	10 sec	BW	112
Jog in place/jump rope	1	30 sec	10 sec	BW	N/A
Single-leg squat (each leg)	1	30 sec	10 sec	BW	52
Jog in place/jump rope	1	30 sec	10 sec	BW	N/A

(continued)

POD 1					
Exercise	**Sets**	**Reps/time**	**Rest**	**Wt**	**Page #**
Dumbbell squat	1-2	12 reps	15 sec	15 lb, 20 lb, 25 lb	80
Push-up	1-2	12 reps	15 sec	BW	112
Dumbbell bench press	1-2	12 reps	15 sec	15 lb, 20 lb, 25 lb	122

POD 2					
Exercise	**Sets**	**Reps/time**	**Rest**	**Wt**	**Page #**
Kettlebell two-hand swing	1-2	12 reps	15 sec	10 kg, 12 kg, 14 kg	62
Dumbbell upright row	1-2	12 reps	15 sec	15 lb, 20 lb, 25 lb	134
Suspension row	1-2	12 reps	15 sec	BW	135

POD 3					
Exercise	**Sets**	**Reps/time**	**Rest**	**Wt**	**Page #**
Kettlebell goblet squat	1-2	12 reps	15 sec	15 lb, 20 lb, 25 lb	81
Dumbbell bench press	1-2	12 reps	15 sec	15 lb, 20 lb, 25 lb	122
Dumbbell shoulder press	1-2	12 reps	15 sec	12 lb, 15 lb, 20 lb	131

POD 4					
Exercise	**Sets**	**Reps/time**	**Rest**	**Wt**	**Page #**
Heavy rope kneeling two-arm slams	1	40 sec	15 sec	Rope	175
Heavy rope kneeling alt-arm slams	1	40 sec	15 sec	Rope	176
Heavy rope kneeling scissors	1	40 sec	15 sec	Rope	176

POD 5					
Exercise	**Sets**	**Reps/time**	**Rest**	**Wt**	**Page #**
Dumbbell straight-leg deadlift	1-2	12 reps	15 sec	15 lb, 20 lb, 25 lb	95
Dumbbell renegade row	1-2	12 reps	15 sec	15 lb, 20 lb, 25 lb	130
Kettlebell upright row	1-2	12 reps	15 sec	12 kg, 14 kg, 16 kg	134

POD 6					
Exercise	**Sets**	**Reps/time**	**Rest**	**Wt**	**Page #**
Dumbbell front lunge	1-2	12 reps	15 sec	12 lb, 15 lb, 20 lb	87
Dumbbell shoulder press	1-2	12 reps	15 sec	12 lb, 15 lb, 20 lb	131
Dumbbell alt-arm biceps curl	1-2	12 reps	15 sec	15 lb, 20 lb, 25 lb	144

POD 7					
Exercise	**Sets**	**Reps/time**	**Rest**	**Wt**	**Page #**
Dumbbell lateral lunge	1-2	12 reps	15 sec	12 lb, 15 lb, 20 lb	90
Dumbbell bent-over raise	1-2	12 reps	15 sec	8 lb, 10 lb, 12 lb	140
Kettlebell overhead triceps extension	1-2	12 reps	15 sec	8 kg, 10 kg, 12 kg	120

POD 8					
Exercise	**Sets**	**Reps/time**	**Rest**	**Wt**	**Page #**
Dumbbell backward lunge	1-2	12 reps	15 sec	10 lb, 12 lb, 15 lb	92
Dumbbell hammer curl	1-2	12 reps	15 sec	15 lb, 20 lb, 25 lb	145
Dumbbell triceps kickback	1-2	12 reps	15 sec	12 lb, 15 lb, 20 lb	143

POD 9					
Exercise	**Sets**	**Reps/time**	**Rest**	**Wt**	**Page #**
Weighted sled push	1	40 sec	15 sec	70 lb	74
Weighted sled pull and push: 1 in. rope	1	40 sec	15 sec	70 lb	75
Farmer's walk	1	40 sec	15 sec	70 1b	98

POD 10					
Exercise	Sets	Reps/time	Rest	Wt	Page #
Front plank	2	40 sec	15 sec	BW	159
Side plank: right	2	40 sec	15 sec	BW	160
Side plank: left	2	40 sec	15 sec	BW	160

POD 11					
Exercise	Sets	Reps/time	Rest	Wt	Page #
Suspension hip and knee tuck	2	40 sec	15 sec	BW	165
Superman	2	40 sec	15 sec	BW	163
Scissors	2	40 sec	15 sec	BW	162

Wt = Weight; BW = Bodyweight

Lean Mass Program 4C: Advanced

Note: Each exercise in a pod should be completed before moving to the next pod. A pod is a combination of three or more exercises performed with short rest periods between them for either a set number of repetitions or a prescribed amount of time.

WARM-UP					
Exercise	Sets	Reps/time	Rest	Wt	Page #
Mountain climbers	1	40 sec	10 sec	BW	49
Jog in place/jump rope	1	40 sec	10 sec	BW	N/A
Jumping jacks	1	40 sec	10 sec	BW	48
Jog in place/jump rope	1	40 sec	10 sec	BW	N/A
Burpee	1	40 sec	10 sec	BW	50
Jog in place/jump rope	1	40 sec	10 sec	BW	N/A
Push-up	1	40 sec	10 sec	BW	112
Jog in place/jump rope	1	40 sec	10 sec	BW	N/A
Single-leg squat (each leg)	1	40 sec	10 sec	BW	52
Jog in place/jump rope	1	40 sec	10 sec	BW	N/A

POD 1					
Exercise	Sets	Reps/time	Rest	Wt	Page #
Dumbbell squat	1-2	12-15 reps	15 sec	20 lb, 25 lb, 30 lb	80
Push-up	1-2	12-15 reps	15 sec	BW	112
Dumbbell bench press	1-2	12-15 reps	15 sec	20 lb, 25 lb, 30 lb	122

POD 2					
Exercise	Sets	Reps/time	Rest	Wt	Page #
Kettlebell two-hand swing	1-2	12-15 reps	15 sec	12 kg, 14 kg, 16 kg	62
Dumbbell upright row	1-2	12-15 reps	15 sec	20 lb, 25 lb, 30 lb	134
Suspension row	1-2	12-15 reps	15 sec	BW	135

POD 3					
Exercise	Sets	Reps/time	Rest	Wt	Page #
Kettlebell goblet squat	1-2	12-15 reps	15 sec	20 lb, 25 lb, 30 lb	81
Dumbbell bench press	1-2	12-15 reps	15 sec	20 lb, 25 lb, 30 lb	122
Dumbbell shoulder press	1-2	12-15 reps	15 sec	15 lb, 20 lb, 25 lb	131

(continued)

Lean Mass Program 4C: Advanced (continued)

POD 4					
Exercise	Sets	Reps/time	Rest	Wt	Page #
Heavy rope kneeling two-arm slams	1	50 sec	15 sec	Rope	175
Heavy rope kneeling alt-arm slams	1	50 sec	15 sec	Rope	176
Heavy rope kneeling scissors	1	50 sec	15 sec	Rope	171
POD 5					
Exercise	Sets	Reps/time	Rest	Wt	Page #
Dumbbell straight-leg deadlift	1-2	12-15 reps	15 sec	20 lb, 25 lb, 30 lb	95
Dumbbell renegade row	1-2	12-15 reps	15 sec	20 lb, 25 lb, 30 lb	130
Kettlebell upright row	1-2	12-15 reps	15 sec	14 kg, 16 kg, 18 kg	134
POD 6					
Exercise	Sets	Reps/time	Rest	Wt	Page #
Dumbbell front lunge	1-2	12-15 reps	15 sec	15 lb, 20 lb, 25 lb	87
Dumbbell shoulder press	1-2	12-15 reps	15 sec	15 lb, 20 lb, 25 lb	131
Dumbbell alt-arm biceps curl	1-2	12-15 reps	15 sec	20 lb, 25 lb, 30 lb	144
POD 7					
Exercise	Sets	Reps/time	Rest	Wt	Page #
Dumbbell lateral lunge	1-2	12-15 reps	15 sec	15 lb, 20 lb, 25 lb	90
Dumbbell bent-over raise	1-2	12-15 reps	15 sec	10 lb, 12 lb, 15 lb	140
Kettlebell overhead triceps extension	1-2	12-15 reps	15 sec	14 kg, 16 kg, 18 kg	120
POD 8					
Exercise	Sets	Reps/time	Rest	Wt	Page #
Dumbbell backward lunge	1-2	12-15 reps	15 sec	15 lb, 20 lb, 25 lb	92
Dumbbell hammer curl	1-2	12-15 reps	15 sec	20 lb, 25 lb, 30 lb	145
Dumbbell triceps kickback	1-2	12-15 reps	15 sec	12 lb, 15 lb, 20 lb	143
POD 9					
Exercise	Sets	Reps/time	Rest	Wt	Page #
Weighted sled push	1	50 sec	15 sec	90 lb	74
Weighted sled pull and push: 1 in. rope	1	50 sec	15 sec	90 lb	75
Farmer's walk	1	50 sec	15 sec	16 kg, 18 kg, 20 kg	98
POD 10					
Exercise	Sets	Reps/time	Rest	Wt	Page #
Front plank	2	50 sec	15 sec	BW	159
Side plank: right	2	50 sec	15 sec	BW	160
Side plank: left	2	50 sec	15 sec	BW	160
POD 11					
Exercise	Sets	Reps/time	Rest	Wt	Page #
Suspension pike	2	50 sec	15 sec	BW	166
Superman	2	50 sec	15 sec	BW	163
Scissors	2	50 sec	15 sec	BW	162

Wt = Weight; BW = Bodyweight

14

Programs for Building Muscular Strength and Power

Strength and power are interrelated and interdependent, to a degree. When performing resistance-training exercises, improving strength and power is typically the goal. There are many resistance-training exercises and techniques in this book that will help you improve your levels of strength and power. Aside from the performance-related applications of strength and power, making gains in these areas can make your activities of daily living more comfortable and attainable. Think about carrying groceries up a flight of stairs, doing yard work, or moving furniture. The more strength and power you develop, the easier it will be to do these activities.

Strength is defined as the ability to exert force (McBride 2016), and is often demonstrated by the amount of weight a person can lift. It is most often demonstrated at relatively slow speeds. Activities requiring high levels of strength include lifting heavy objects off the ground, performing weighted lunges, and performing pull-ups with additional weight.

Power is a direct function of force and velocity. Power is often demonstrated by the speed at which force is applied. Unlike demonstrations of strength, demonstrations of power are performed at relatively high speeds. Activities requiring high levels of power include throwing a disc, performing a vertical jump, or sprinting a short distance.

As you perform strength and power training, the body undergoes the following adaptations:

- Muscle fibers get larger (referred to as hypertrophy).
- Positive changes take place in cellular physiology as it responds to anaerobic metabolism.
- Bone density increases, as does strength in tendons, ligaments, and cartilage.

- In the immediate term, strength and power training results in increased heart rate, systolic blood pressure, stroke volume, blood flow to active muscles, and ventilation.
- Performance improvements can be observed in strength, power, muscle endurance, body composition, flexibility, aerobic capacity, and motor performance, such as sprint speed, running economy, and kicking and throwing mechanics (French 2016).

Methods for Building Strength and Power

Methods that are used to train strength and power include, but are not limited to, the following:

- Undulating set and repetition schemes such as high reps-low weight on one day and low reps-high weight on the second day
- Training strength and power two to six days per week
- Training strength and power on alternating days
- Implementing contrasting training methods, such as a high-resistance exercise followed by a lower-resistance exercise that utilizes a similar movement pattern, such as pairing squats and box jumps
- Over time (several weeks), moving training focus from high to low repetitions and adjusting load accordingly (example: two weeks each of the following repetition ranges: 10-12, 6-8, and 4-6, for a total of six weeks of training)
- Accommodated resistance using resistance bands and chains. Resistance bands can be used to supplement traditional strength-training movements. Chains allow for a gradual increase in the amount of applied resistance. Regardless of loading parameters, there should be a well-established foundation in exercise technique before attempting to implement these methods.
- Tire flipping, log lifting, and farmer's walk, with focus on strength and power.

All resistance exercises are designed to improve strength and power. However, some exercises are better suited to progress in these areas than others . Table 14.1 provides examples of exercises that effectively target strength and power.

Table 14.1 Examples of Strength and Power Exercises

Strength exercises	Power exercises
Squat	Power clean and variations
Bench press	Medicine ball pass
Lunge and variations	Split squat jump
Pull-up	Plyometric exercises
Fixed isolated resistance-training machines	Medicine ball throws and tosses
Dumbbell rowing and pulling	Snatch and variations
Most bodyweight calisthenics	Barbell jerk and overhead pressing variations

Guidelines and Goals of Strength and Power Training

There are many factors involved in designing a program focusing on strength and power. While there is no one perfect approach, the following general recommendations will help you develop strength and power through metabolic training:

- Power exercises before strength exercises
- Multijoint movements before single-joint exercises
- Ground-based exercises before isolated exercises
- Fatigue management through logical arrangement of exercises
- Alternating between upper- and lower-body movements
- Rest intervals just long enough to recover for the next set or exercise but no longer
- Avoidance of exhaustive efforts—especially when using strength and power methods—because of their taxing nature
- A longer rest interval—up to two to three minutes—between circuits to mitigate fatigue and allow recovery between efforts

The pods in the following exercise programs are a combination of three or more exercises performed with short rest periods between them for either a set number of repetitions or a prescribed amount of time.

Strength and Power Program 1A: Beginner

WARM-UP					
Exercise	Sets	Reps/time	Rest	Wt	Page #
March/walk	1	20 sec	10 sec	BW	N/A
Jumping jacks	1	20 sec	10 sec	BW	48
March/walk	1	20 sec	10 sec	BW	N/A
Single-leg squat (each leg)	1	20 sec	10 sec	BW	52
March/walk	1	20 sec	10 sec	BW	N/A
Push-up	1	20 sec	10 sec	BW	112
March/walk	1	20 sec	10 sec	BW	N/A
Mountain climbers	1	20 sec	10 sec	BW	49
March/walk	1	20 sec	10 sec	BW	N/A
Burpee	1	20 sec	10 sec	BW	50

(continued)

Strength and Power Program 1A: Beginner *(continued)*

LOWER BODY					
Exercise	Sets	Reps/time	Rest	Wt	Page #
Kettlebell two-hand swing	1	5-8 reps	30 sec	10 kg, 12 kg, 14 kg	62
Kettlebell one-arm clean	1	5-8 reps	30 sec	6 kg, 8 kg, 10 kg	63
Kettlebell deadlift	1	5-8 reps	30 sec	14 kg, 16 kg, 18 kg	94
Kettlebell overhead squat	1	5-8 reps	30 sec	6 kg, 8 kg, 10 kg	83
Kettlebell goblet squat	1	5-8 reps	30 sec	6 kg, 8 kg, 10 kg	81
Kettlebell straight-leg deadlift	1	5-8 reps	30 sec	10 kg, 12 kg, 14 kg	95
Medicine ball overhead squat	1	5-8 reps	30 sec	10 lb, 12 lb, 14 lb	85
Medicine ball overhead box step-up	1	5-8 reps each leg	30 sec	10 lb, 12 lb, 14 lb	87
Medicine ball overhead lunge	1	5-8 reps each leg	30 sec	10 lb, 12 lb, 14 lb	89
Medicine ball overhead backward lunge	1	5-8 reps each leg	30 sec	10 lb, 12 lb, 14 lb	93
Sandbag farmer's walk	1	30 sec	30 sec	20 lb	99
Sandbag front squat	1	5-8 reps	30 sec	20 lb, 40 lb	82
Suspension leg curl	1	5-8 reps	30 sec	BW	106

UPPER BODY					
Exercise	Sets	Reps/time	Rest	Wt	Page #
Dumbbell bench press	1	5-8 reps	30 sec	12 lb, 15 lb, 20 lb	122
Sandbag row	1	5-8 reps	30 sec	20 lb, 40 lb	136
Sandbag upright row	1	5-8 reps	30 sec	20 lb	136
Suspension reverse fly	1	5-8 reps	30 sec	BW	127
Sandbag biceps curl	1	5-8 reps	30 sec	20 lb	121
Sandbag overhead triceps extension	1	5-8 reps	30 sec	20 lb	120
Dumbbell incline press	1	5-8 reps	30 sec	10 lb, 12 lb, 15 lb	124
Kettlebell one-arm row	1	5-8 reps	30 sec	8 kg, 10 kg, 12 kg	129
Dumbbell shoulder press	1	5-8 reps	30 sec	10 lb, 12 lb, 15 lb	131
Resistance band T	1	5-8 reps	30 sec	Light	118
Dumbbell alt-arm bicep curl	1	5-8 reps	30 sec	10 lb, 12 lb, 15 lb	144
Decline push-up	1	5-8 reps	30 sec	10 lb, 12 lb, 14 lb	151

CORE					
Exercise	Sets	Reps/time	Rest	Wt	Page #
Abdominal crunch	1	20 reps	15 sec	BW	155
Front plank	1	30 sec	15 sec	BW	159
Abdominal reach	1	30 sec	15 sec	BW	157
Side plank: right	1	30 sec	15 sec	BW	160
Bicycle	1	30 sec	15 sec	BW	162
Side plank: left	1	30 sec	15 sec	BW	160
Birddog	1	30 sec	15 sec	BW	161

Wt = Weight; BW = Bodyweight

Strength and Power Program 1B: Intermediate

WARM-UP					
Exercise	Sets	Reps/time	Rest	Wt	Page #
Jog in place/jump rope	1	30 sec	10 sec	BW	N/A
Jumping jacks	1	30 sec	10 sec	BW	48
Jog in place/jump rope	1	30 sec	10 sec	BW	N/A
Single-leg squat (each leg)	1	30 sec	10 sec	BW	52
Jog in place/jump rope	1	30 sec	10 sec	BW	N/A
Push-up	1	30 sec	10 sec	BW	112
Jog in place/jump rope	1	30 sec	10 sec	BW	N/A
Mountain climbers	1	30 sec	10 sec	BW	49
Jog in place/jump rope	1	30 sec	10 sec	BW	N/A
Burpee	1	30 sec	10 sec	BW	50
Jog in place/jump rope	1	30 sec	10 sec	BW	N/A
Single-leg squat (each leg)	1	30 sec	10 sec	BW	52
Jog in place/jump rope	1	30 sec	10 sec	BW	N/A
Jumping jacks	1	30 sec	10 sec	BW	48
LOWER BODY					
Exercise	Sets	Reps/time	Rest	Wt	Page #
Kettlebell one-hand swing	2	5-8 reps	30 sec	10 kg, 12 kg, 14 kg	62
Kettlebell two-arm clean	2	5-8 reps	30 sec	10 kg, 12 kg, 14 kg	64
Kettlebell deadlift	2	5-8 reps	30 sec	18 kg, 20 kg, 22 kg	94
Kettlebell overhead squat	2	5-8 reps	30 sec	10 kg, 12 kg, 14 kg	83
Kettlebell goblet squat	2	5-8 reps	30 sec	10 kg, 12 kg, 14 kg	81
Kettlebell one-leg straight-leg deadlift	2	5-8 reps	30 sec	10 kg, 12 kg, 14 kg	97
Medicine ball overhead squat	2	5-8 reps	30 sec	12 lb, 14 lb, 16 lb	85
Medicine ball overhead box step-up	2	5-8 reps each leg	30 sec	12 lb, 14 lb, 16 lb	87
Medicine ball overhead lunge	2	5-8 reps each leg	30 sec	12 lb, 14 lb, 16 lb	89
Medicine ball overhead backward lunge	2	5-8 reps each leg	30 sec	12 lb, 14 lb, 16 lb	93
Sandbag farmer's walk	2	30 sec	30 sec	20 lb, 40 lb	99
Sandbag front squat	2	5-8 reps	30 sec	40 lb, 60 lb	82
Suspension leg curl	2	8-12 reps	30 sec	BW	106
UPPER BODY					
Exercise	Sets	Reps/time	Rest	Wt	Page #
Dumbbell bench press	2	5-8 reps	30 sec	20 lb, 25 lb, 30 lb	122
Sandbag row	2	5-8 reps	30 sec	40 lb, 60 lb	136
Sandbag upright row	2	5-8 reps	30 sec	40 lb, 60 lb	136
Suspension reverse fly	2	5-8 reps	30 sec	BW	127
Sandbag biceps curl	2	5-8 reps	30 sec	20 lb, 40 lb	121
Sandbag overhead triceps extension	2	5-8 reps	30 sec	20 lb, 40 lb	120
Dumbbell incline press	2	5-8 reps	30 sec	15 lb, 20 lb, 25 lb	124
Kettlebell renegade row	2	5-8 reps	30 sec	12 kg, 14 kg, 16 kg	130
Dumbbell shoulder press	2	5-8 reps	30 sec	15 lb, 20 lb, 25 lb	131
Resistance band T	2	5-8 reps	30 sec	Moderate	118
Dumbbell alt-arm bicep curl	2	5-8 reps	30 sec	15 lb, 20 lb, 25 lb	144
Decline push-up	2	8-12 reps	30 sec	14 lb, 16 lb, 18 lb	151

(continued)

Strength and Power Program 1B: Intermediate *(continued)*

CORE					
Exercise	Sets	Reps/time	Rest	Wt	Page #
Weighted abdominal crunch	1	30 reps	15 sec	5-10 lb	155
Weighted abdominal reach	1	30 reps	15 sec	5-10 lb	157
Front plank	1	40 sec	15 sec	BW	159
Side plank: right	1	40 sec	15 sec	BW	160
Side plank: left	1	40 sec	15 sec	BW	160
Opposite-shoulder-to-knee crunch	1	30 reps	15 sec	BW	158
Scissors	1	40 sec	15 sec	BW	162
Bicycle	1	40 sec	15 sec	BW	162
Superman	1	40 sec	15 sec	BW	163

Wt = Weight; BW = Bodyweight

Strength Power Program 1C: Advanced

WARM-UP					
Exercise	Sets	Reps/time	Rest	Wt	Page #
Jog in place/jump rope	1	40 sec	10 sec	BW	N/A
Jumping jacks	1	40 sec	10 sec	BW	48
Jog in place/jump rope	1	40 sec	10 sec	BW	N/A
Single-leg squat (each leg)	1	40 sec	10 sec	BW	52
Jog in place/jump rope	1	40 sec	10 sec	BW	N/A
Push-up	1	40 sec	10 sec	BW	112
Jog in place/jump rope	1	40 sec	10 sec	BW	N/A
Mountain climbers	1	40 sec	10 sec	BW	49
Jog in place/jump rope	1	40 sec	10 sec	BW	N/A
Burpee	1	40 sec	10 sec	BW	50
Jog in place/jump rope	1	40 sec	10 sec	BW	N/A
Single-leg squat (each leg)	1	40 sec	10 sec	BW	52
Jog in place/jump rope	1	40 sec	10 sec	BW	N/A
Jumping jacks	1	40 sec	10 sec	BW	48

LOWER BODY					
Exercise	Sets	Reps/time	Rest	Wt	Page #
Kettlebell one-hand swing	2	5-8 reps	30 sec	14 lb, 16 lb, 18 lb	62
Kettlebell two-arm clean	2	5-8 reps	30 sec	14 lb, 16 lb, 18 lb	64
Kettlebell deadlift	2	5-8 reps	30 sec	48.5 lb, 52.9 lb, 57.3 lb	94
Kettlebell overhead squat	2	5-8 reps	30 sec	14 lb, 16 lb, 18 lb	83
Kettlebell goblet squat	2	5-8 reps	30 sec	14 lb, 16 lb, 18 lb	81
Kettlebell one-leg straight-leg deadlift	2	5-8 reps	30 sec	14 lb, 16 lb, 18 lb	97
Medicine ball overhead squat	2	5-8 reps	30 sec	16 lb, 18 lb, 20 lb	85
Medicine ball overhead box step-up	2	5-8 reps each leg	30 sec	16 lb, 18 lb, 20 lb	87
Medicine ball overhead lunge	2	5-8 reps each leg	30 sec	16 lb, 18 lb, 20 lb	89
Medicine ball overhead backward lunge	2	5-8 reps each leg	30 sec	16 lb, 18 lb, 20 lb	93
Sandbag farmer's walk	2	30 sec	30 sec	40 lb, 60 lb	99
Sandbag front squat	2	5-8 reps	30 sec	40 lb, 60 lb	82
Suspension leg curl	2	12-15 reps	30 sec	BW	106

UPPER BODY					
Exercise	Sets	Reps/time	Rest	Wt	Page #
Dumbbell bench press	2	5-8 reps	30 sec	30 lb, 35 lb, 40 lb	122
Sandbag row	2	5-8 reps	30 sec	60 lb, 80 lb	136
Sandbag upright row	2	5-8 reps	30 sec	60 lb, 80 lb	134
Suspension reverse fly	2	5-8 reps	30 sec	BW	127
Sandbag biceps curl	2	5-8 reps	30 sec	40 lb, 60 lb	121
Sandbag overhead triceps extension	2	5-8 reps	30 sec	40 lb, 60 lb	120
Dumbbell incline press	2	5-8 reps	30 sec	25 lb, 30 lb, 35 lb	124
Kettlebell renegade row	2	5-8 reps	30 sec	14 kg, 16 kg, 18 kg	130
Dumbbell shoulder press	2	5-8 reps	30 sec	25 lb, 30 lb, 35 lb	131
Resistance band T	2	5-8 reps	30 sec	Moderate	118
Dumbbell alt-arm biceps curl	2	5-8 reps	30 sec	25 lb, 30 lb, 35 lb	144
Decline push-up	2	8-12 reps	30 sec	16 lb, 18 lb, 20 lb	151
CORE					
Exercise	Sets	Reps/time	Rest	Wt	Page #
Weighted abdominal crunch	1	40 reps	15 sec	5-10 lb	155
Weighted abdominal reach	1	40 reps	15 sec	5-10 lb	157
Front plank	1	50 sec	15 sec	BW	159
Side plank: right	1	50 sec	15 sec	BW	160
Side plank: left	1	50 sec	15 sec	BW	160
Opposite-shoulder-to-knee crunch	1	40 reps	15 sec	BW	158
Scissors	1	50 sec	15 sec	BW	162
Bicycle	1	50 sec	15 sec	BW	162
Superman	1	50 sec	15 sec	BW	163

Wt = Weight; BW = Bodyweight

Strength and Power Program 2A: Beginner

WARM-UP					
Exercise	Sets	Reps/time	Rest	Wt	Page #
March/walk	1	20 sec	10 sec	BW	N/A
Single-leg squat (each leg)	1	20 sec	10 sec	BW	52
March/walk	1	20 sec	10 sec	BW	N/A
Mountain climbers	1	20 sec	10 sec	BW	49
March/walk	1	20 sec	10 sec	BW	N/A
Burpee	1	20 sec	10 sec	BW	50
March/walk	1	20 sec	10 sec	BW	N/A
Push-up	1	20 sec	10 sec	BW	112
March/walk	1	20 sec	10 sec	BW	N/A
Jumping jacks	1	20 sec	10 sec	BW	48

(continued)

Strength and Power Program 2A: Beginner (continued)

LOWER BODY

Exercise	Sets	Reps/time	Rest	Wt	Page #
Sandbag hang clean	1	5-8 reps	30 sec	20 lb	57
Sandbag push press	1	5-8 reps	30 sec	20 lb	61
Sandbag deadlift	1	5-8 reps	30 sec	40 lb	95
Sandbag overhead squat	1	5-8 reps	30 sec	20 lb	85
Sandbag overhead lunge	1	5-8 reps	30 sec	20 lb	89
Sandbag straight-leg deadlift	1	5-8 reps	30 sec	20 lb	96
Kettlebell push press	1	5-8 reps	30 sec	6 kg, 8 kg, 10 kg	61
Resistance band overhead squat	1	5-8 reps	30 sec	Light	84
Kettlebell deadlift	1	5-8 reps	30 sec	10 kg, 12 kg, 14 kg	94
Kettlebell overhead lunge	1	5-8 reps each leg	30 sec	6 kg, 8 kg, 10 kg	88
Kettlebell farmer's walk	1	30 sec	30 sec	10 kg, 12 kg, 14 kg	98
Dumbbell split squat	1	5-8 reps each leg	30 sec	10 lb, 12 lb, 15 lb	82
Dumbbell hip thrust	1	5-8 reps	30 sec	Moderate	100

UPPER BODY

Exercise	Sets	Reps/time	Rest	Wt	Page #
Dumbbell bench press	1	5-8 reps	30 sec	12 lb, 15 lb, 20 lb	122
Dumbbell one-arm row	1	5-8 reps each arm	30 sec	12 lb, 15 lb, 20 lb	129
Kettlebell upright row	1	5-8 reps	30 sec	8 kg, 10 kg, 12 kg	134
Dumbbell bent-over raise	1	5-8 reps	30 sec	5 lb, 8 lb, 10 lb	140
Kettlebell alt-arm biceps curl	1	5-8 reps	30 sec	6 kg, 8 kg, 10 kg	144
Suspension triceps extension	1	5-8 reps	30 sec	BW	119
Dumbbell alt-arm incline press	1	5-8 reps	30 sec	10 lb, 12 lb, 15 lb	125
Suspension row	1	5-8 reps	30 sec	BW	135
Kettlebell shoulder press	1	5-8 reps	30 sec	6 kg, 8 kg, 10 kg	131
Resistance band Y	1	5-8 reps	30 sec	Light	116
Suspension biceps curl	1	5-8 reps	30 sec	BW	121
Kettlebell overhead triceps extension	1	5-8 reps	30 sec	8 kg, 10 kg, 12 kg	120

CORE

Exercise	Sets	Reps/time	Rest	Wt	Page #
Abdominal reach	1	20 reps	15 sec	BW	157
Scissors	1	30 sec	15 sec	BW	162
Front plank	1	30 sec	15 sec	BW	159
Side plank: right	1	30 sec	15 sec	BW	160
Side plank: left	1	30 sec	15 sec	BW	160
Bicycle	1	30 sec	15 sec	BW	162
Superman	1	30 sec	15 sec	BW	163

Wt = Weight; BW = Bodyweight

Strength and Power Program 2B: Intermediate

WARM-UP					
Exercise	Sets	Reps/time	Rest	Wt	Page #
Jog in place/jump rope	1	30 sec	10 sec	BW	N/A
Single-leg squat (each leg)	1	30 sec	10 sec	BW	52
Jog in place/jump rope	1	30 sec	10 sec	BW	N/A
Mountain climbers	1	30 sec	10 sec	BW	49
Jog in place/jump rope	1	30 sec	10 sec	BW	N/A
Burpee	1	30 sec	10 sec	BW	50
Jog in place/jump rope	1	30 sec	10 sec	BW	N/A
Push-up	1	30 sec	10 sec	BW	112
Jog in place/jump rope	1	30 sec	10 sec	BW	N/A
Jumping jacks	1	30 sec	10 sec	BW	48
LOWER BODY					
Exercise	Sets	Reps/time	Rest	Wt	Page #
Sandbag hang clean	2	5-8 reps	30 sec	40 lb	57
Sandbag push press	2	5-8 reps	30 sec	40 lb	61
Sandbag deadlift	2	5-8 reps	30 sec	60 lb	95
Sandbag overhead squat	2	5-8 reps	30 sec	40 lb	85
Sandbag overhead lunge	2	5-8 reps	30 sec	40 lb	89
Sandbag straight leg deadlift	2	5-8 reps	30 sec	40 lb	96
Kettlebell push press	2	5-8 reps	30 sec	8 kg, 10 kg, 12 kg	61
Resistance band overhead squat	2	5-8 reps	30 sec	Moderate	84
Kettlebell deadlift	2	5-8 reps	30 sec	12 kg, 14 kg, 16 kg	94
Kettlebell overhead lunge	2	5-8 reps each leg	30 sec	8 kg, 10 kg, 12 kg	88
Kettlebell farmer's walk	2	30 sec	30 sec	12 kg, 14 kg, 16 kg	98
Dumbbell split squat	2	5-8 reps each leg	30 sec	15 lb, 20 lb, 25 lb	82
Dumbbell hip thrust	2	5-8 reps	30 sec	Moderate/heavy	100
UPPER BODY					
Exercise	Sets	Reps/time	Rest	Wt	Page #
Dumbbell bench press	2	5-8 reps	30 sec	20 lb, 25 lb, 30 lb	122
Dumbbell one-arm row	2	5-8 reps each arm	30 sec	20 lb, 25 lb, 30 lb	129
Kettlebell upright row	2	5-8 reps	30 sec	10 kg, 12 kg, 14 kg	134
Dumbbell bent-over raise	2	5-8 reps	30 sec	10 lb, 12 lb, 15 lb	140
Kettlebell alt-arm biceps curl	2	5-8 reps	30 sec	8 kg, 10 kg, 12 kg	144
Suspension triceps extension	2	5-8 reps	30 sec	BW	119
Dumbbell alt-arm incline press	2	5-8 reps	30 sec	15 lb, 20 lb, 25 lb	125
Suspension row	2	5-8 reps	30 sec	BW	135
Kettlebell shoulder press	2	5-8 reps	30 sec	8 kg, 10 kg, 12 kg	131
Resistance band Y	2	5-8 reps	30 sec	Moderate	116
Suspension biceps curl	2	5-8 reps	30 sec	BW	121
Kettlebell overhead triceps extension	2	5-8 reps	30 sec	10 kg, 12 kg, 14 kg	120

(continued)

Strength and Power Program 2B: Intermediate *(continued)*

CORE					
Exercise	Sets	Reps/time	Rest	Wt	Page #
Abdominal reach	1	30 reps	15 sec	BW	157
Scissors	1	40 sec	15 sec	BW	162
Front plank	1	40 sec	15 sec	BW	159
Side plank: right	1	40 sec	15 sec	BW	160
Side plank: left	1	40 sec	15 sec	BW	160
Bicycle	1	40 sec	15 sec	BW	162
Superman	1	40 sec	15 sec	BW	163

Wt = Weight; BW = Bodyweight

Strength and Power Program 2C: Advanced

WARM-UP					
Exercise	Sets	Reps/time	Rest	Wt	Page #
Jog in place/jump rope	1	40 sec	10 sec	BW	N/A
Single-leg squat (each leg)	1	40 sec	10 sec	BW	52
Jog in place/jump rope	1	40 sec	10 sec	BW	N/A
Mountain climbers	1	40 sec	10 sec	BW	49
Jog in place/jump rope	1	40 sec	10 sec	BW	N/A
Burpee	1	40 sec	10 sec	BW	50
Jog in place/jump rope	1	40 sec	10 sec	BW	N/A
Push-up	1	40 sec	10 sec	BW	112
Jog in place/jump rope	1	40 sec	10 sec	BW	N/A
Jumping jacks	1	40 sec	10 sec	BW	48
LOWER BODY					
Exercise	Sets	Reps/time	Rest	Wt	Page #
Sandbag hang clean	2-3	5-8 reps	30 sec	40 lb, 60 lb	57
Sandbag push press	2-3	5-8 reps	30 sec	40 lb, 60 lb	61
Sandbag deadlift	2-3	5-8 reps	30 sec	60 lb, 80 lb	95
Sandbag overhead squat	2-3	5-8 reps	30 sec	40 lb, 60 lb	85
Sandbag overhead lunge	2-3	5-8 reps	30 sec	40 lb, 60 lb	89
Sandbag straight leg deadlift	2-3	5-8 reps	30 sec	40 lb, 60 lb	96
Kettlebell push press	2-3	5-8 reps	30 sec	10 kg, 12 kg, 14 kg	61
Resistance band overhead squat	2-3	5-8 reps	30 sec	Moderate/heavy	84
Kettlebell deadlift	2-3	5-8 reps	30 sec	16 kg, 18 kg, 20 kg	94
Kettlebell overhead lunge	2-3	5-8 reps each leg	30 sec	10 kg, 12 kg, 14 kg	88
Kettlebell farmer's walk	2-3	30 sec	30 sec	16 kg, 18 kg, 20 kg	98
Dumbbell split squat	2-3	5-8 reps each leg	30 sec	25 lb, 30 lb, 35 lb	82
Dumbbell hip thrust	2-3	5-8 reps	30 sec	Heavy	100

UPPER BODY					
Exercise	Sets	Reps/time	Rest	Wt	Page #
Dumbbell bench press	2-3	5-8 reps	30 sec	30 lb, 35 lb, 40 lb	122
Dumbbell one-arm row	2-3	5-8 reps each arm	30 sec	30 lb, 35 lb, 40 lb	129
Kettlebell upright row	2-3	5-8 reps	30 sec	14 lb, 16 lb, 18 lb	134
Dumbbell bent-over raise	2-3	5-8 reps	30 sec	12 lb, 15 lb, 20 lb	140
Kettlebell alt-arm biceps curl	2-3	5-8 reps	30 sec	12 kg, 14 kg, 16 kg	144
Suspension triceps extension	2-3	5-8 reps	30 sec	BW	119
Dumbbell alt-arm incline press	2-3	5-8 reps	30 sec	25 lb, 30 lb, 35 lb	125
Suspension row	2-3	5-8 reps	30 sec	BW	135
Kettlebell shoulder press	2-3	5-8 reps	30 sec	12 kg, 14 kg, 16 kg	131
Resistance band Y	2-3	5-8 reps	30 sec	Moderate	116
Suspension biceps curl	2-3	5-8 reps	30 sec	BW	121
Kettlebell overhead triceps extension	2-3	5-8 reps	30 sec	14 kg, 16 kg, 18 kg	120
CORE					
Exercise	Sets	Reps/time	Rest	Wt	Page #
Front plank	1	50 sec	15 sec	BW	159
Side plank: right	1	50 sec	15 sec	BW	160
Side plank: left	1	50 sec	15 sec	BW	160
Scissors	1	50 sec	15 sec	BW	162
Bicycle	1	50 sec	15 sec	BW	162
Weighted abdominal crunch	1	40 reps	15 sec	5-10 lb	155
Weighted abdominal reach	1	40 reps	15 sec	5-10 lb	157
Opposite-shoulder-to-knee crunch	1	40 reps	15 sec	BW	158
Superman	1	50 sec	15 sec	BW	163

Wt = Weight; BW = Bodyweight

Strength and Power Program 3A: Beginner

Note: Each exercise in a pod should be completed before moving to the next pod.

WARM-UP					
Exercise	Sets	Reps/time	Rest	Wt	Page #
Walk in place/march	1	20 sec	10 sec	BW	N/A
Jumping jacks	1	20 sec	10 sec	BW	48
Walk in place/march	1	20 sec	10 sec	BW	N/A
Push-up	1	20 sec	10 sec	BW	112
Walk in place/march	1	20 sec	10 sec	BW	N/A
Single-leg squat (each leg)	1	20 sec	10 sec	BW	52
Walk in place/march	1	20 sec	10 sec	BW	N/A
Burpee	1	20 sec	10 sec	BW	50
Walk in place/march	1	20 sec	10 sec	BW	N/A
Mountain climbers	1	20 sec	10 sec	BW	49

(continued)

Strength and Power Program 3A: Beginner *(continued)*

POD 1					
Exercise	Sets	Reps/time	Rest	Wt	Page #
Kettlebell one-hand swing	1	5-8 reps	30 sec	6 kg, 8 kg, 10 kg	62
Sandbag overhead squat	1	5-8 reps	30 sec	20 lb	85
Dumbbell squat	1	5-8 reps	30 sec	15 lb, 20 lb, 25 lb	80

POD 2					
Exercise	Sets	Reps/time	Rest	Wt	Page #
Dumbbell alt-arm bench press	1	5-8 reps	30 sec	12 lb, 15 lb, 20 lb	123
Kettlebell renegade row	1	5-8 reps	30 sec	6 kg, 8 kg, 10 kg	130
Suspension push-up	1	8-12 reps	30 sec	BW	113

POD 3					
Exercise	Sets	Reps/time	Rest	Wt	Page #
Heavy rope scissors	1	30 sec	30 sec	Rope	171
Heavy rope jumping jacks	1	30 sec	30 sec	Rope	172
Heavy rope alt-arm slams	1	30 sec	30 sec	Rope	170

POD 4					
Exercise	Sets	Reps/time	Rest	Wt	Page #
Sandbag hang clean	1	5-8 reps	30 sec	20 lb	57
Kettlebell push press	1	5-8 reps	30 sec	6 kg, 8 kg, 10 kg	61
Dumbbell box step-up	1	5 each side	30 sec	12 lb, 15 lb, 20 lb	86

POD 5					
Exercise	Sets	Reps/time	Rest	Wt	Page #
Dumbbell incline press	1	5-8 reps	30 sec	12 lb, 15 lb, 20 lb	124
Dumbbell renegade row	1	5-8 reps	30 sec	10 lb, 12 lb, 15 lb	130
Suspension row	1	8-12 reps	30 sec	BW	135

POD 6					
Exercise	Sets	Reps/time	Rest	Wt	Page #
Medicine ball rotational slam	1	30 sec	30 sec	10 lb, 12 lb	67
Medicine ball upward throw	1	30 sec	30 sec	10 lb, 12 lb	68
Medicine ball squat and jump	1	30 sec	30 sec	10 lb, 12 lb	71

POD 7					
Exercise	Sets	Reps/time	Rest	Wt	Page #
Kettlebell deadlift	1	5-8 reps	30 sec	10 kg, 12 kg, 14 kg	94
Dumbbell front lunge	1	5 each side	30 sec	10 lb, 12 lb, 15 lb	87
Sandbag straight-leg deadlift	1	5-8 reps	30 sec	20 lb	96

POD 8					
Exercise	Sets	Reps/time	Rest	Wt	Page #
Kettlebell shoulder press	1	5-8 reps	30 sec	6 kg, 8 kg, 10 kg	131
Sandbag biceps curl	1	5-8 reps	30 sec	20 lb	121
Dumbbell bent-over raise	1	8-12 reps	30 sec	8 lb, 10 lb, 12 lb	140

POD 9					
Exercise	Sets	Reps/time	Rest	Wt	Page #
Weighted sled drag	1	30 sec	30 sec	45 lb	76
Weighted sled push	1	30 sec	30 sec	45 lb	74
Weighted sled pull and push	1	30 sec	30 sec	45 lb	75

POD 10					
Exercise	Sets	Reps/time	Rest	Wt	Page #
Front plank	1	30 sec	15 sec	BW	159
Weighted abdominal crunch	1	20 reps	15 sec	5-10 lb	155
Birddog	1	30 sec	15 sec	BW	161

Wt = Weight; BW = Bodyweight

Strength and Power Program 3B: Intermediate

Note: Each exercise in a pod should be completed before moving to the next pod.

WARM-UP					
Exercise	Sets	Reps/time	Rest	Wt	Page #
Jog in place/jump rope	1	30 sec	10 sec	BW	N/A
Jumping jacks	1	30 sec	10 sec	BW	48
Jog in place/jump rope	1	30 sec	10 sec	BW	N/A
Push-up	1	30 sec	10 sec	BW	112
Jog in place/jump rope	1	30 sec	10 sec	BW	N/A
Single-leg squat (each leg)	1	30 sec	10 sec	BW	52
Jog in place/jump rope	1	30 sec	10 sec	BW	N/A
Burpee	1	30 sec	10 sec	BW	50
Jog in place/jump rope	1	30 sec	10 sec	BW	N/A
Mountain climbers	1	30 sec	10 sec	BW	49

POD 1					
Exercise	Sets	Reps/time	Rest	Wt	Page #
Kettlebell one-hand swing	2	5-8 reps	30 sec	10 kg, 12 kg, 14 kg	62
Sandbag overhead squat	2	5-8 reps	30 sec	40 lb	85
Dumbbell squat	2	5-8 reps	30 sec	25 lb, 30 lb, 35 lb	80

POD 2					
Exercise	Sets	Reps/time	Rest	Wt	Page #
Dumbbell alt-arm bench press	2	5-8 reps	30 sec	15 lb, 20 lb, 25 lb	123
Kettlebell renegade row	2	5-8 reps	30 sec	10 kg, 12 kg, 14 kg	130
Suspension push-up	2	8-12 reps	30 sec	BW	113

POD 3					
Exercise	Sets	Reps/time	Rest	Wt	Page #
Heavy rope scissors	2	40 sec	30 sec	Rope	171
Heavy rope jumping jacks	2	40 sec	30 sec	Rope	172
Heavy rope alt-arm slam	2	40 sec	30 sec	Rope	170

(continued)

Strength and Power Program 3B: Intermediate *(continued)*

POD 4					
Exercise	Sets	Reps/time	Rest	Wt	Page #
Sandbag hang clean	2	5-8 reps	30 sec	40 lb	57
Kettlebell push press	2	5-8 reps	30 sec	10 kg, 12 kg, 14 kg	61
Dumbbell box step-up	2	5 reps each side	30 sec	15 lb, 20 lb, 25 lb	86

POD 5					
Exercise	Sets	Reps/time	Rest	Wt	Page #
Dumbbell incline press	2	5-8 reps	30 sec	15 lb, 20 lb, 25 lb	124
Dumbbell renegade row	2	5-8 reps	30 sec	15 lb, 20 lb, 25 lb	130
Suspension row	2	8-12 reps	30 sec	BW	135

POD 6					
Exercise	Sets	Reps/time	Rest	Wt	Page #
Medicine ball rotational slam	1	40 sec	30 sec	14 lb, 16 lb	67
Medicine ball upward throw	1	40 sec	30 sec	14 lb, 16 lb	68
Medicine ball squat and jump	1	40 sec	30 sec	14 lb, 16 lb	71

POD 7					
Exercise	Sets	Reps/time	Rest	Wt	Page #
Kettlebell deadlift	2	5-8 reps	30 sec	14 kg, 16 kg, 18 kg	94
Dumbbell front lunge	2	5 reps each side	30 sec	12 lb, 15 lb, 20 lb	87
Sandbag straight-leg deadlift	2	5-8 reps	30 sec	40 lb	96

POD 8					
Exercise	Sets	Reps/time	Rest	Wt	Page #
Kettlebell shoulder press	2	5-8 reps	30 sec	8 kg, 10 kg, 12 kg	131
Sandbag biceps curl	2	5-8 reps	30 sec	40 lb	121
Dumbbell bent-over raise	2	8-12 reps	30 sec	10 lb, 12 lb, 15 lb	140

POD 9					
Exercise	Sets	Reps/time	Rest	Wt	Page #
Weighted sled drag	1	40 sec	30 sec	70 lb	76
Weighted sled push	1	40 sec	30 sec	70 lb	74
Weighted sled pull and push	1	40 sec	30 sec	70 lb	75

POD 10					
Exercise	Sets	Reps/time	Rest	Wt	Page #
Front plank	1	40 sec	15 sec	BW	159
Weighted abdominal crunch	1	30 reps	15 sec	5-10 lb	155
Birddog	1	40 sec	15 sec	BW	161

Wt = Weight; BW = Bodyweight

Strength and Power Program 3C: Advanced

Note: Each exercise in a pod should be completed before moving to the next pod.

WARM-UP					
Exercise	Sets	Reps/time	Rest	Wt	Page #
Jog in place/jump rope	1	40 sec	10 sec	BW	N/A
Jumping jacks	1	40 sec	10 sec	BW	48
Jog in place/jump rope	1	40 sec	10 sec	BW	N/A
Push-up	1	40 sec	10 sec	BW	112
Jog in place/jump rope	1	40 sec	10 sec	BW	N/A
Single-leg squat (each leg)	1	40 sec	10 sec	BW	52
Jog in place/jump rope	1	40 sec	10 sec	BW	N/A
Burpee	1	40 sec	10 sec	BW	50
Jog in place/jump rope	1	40 sec	10 sec	BW	N/A
Mountain climbers	1	40 sec	10 sec	BW	49
POD 1					
Exercise	Sets	Reps/time	Rest	Wt	Page #
Kettlebell one-hand swing	2-3	5-8 reps	30 sec	12 kg, 14 kg, 16 kg	62
Sandbag overhead squat	2-3	5-8 reps	30 sec	40 lb, 60 lb	85
Dumbbell squat	2-3	5-8 reps	30 sec	25 lb, 30 lb, 35 lb	80
POD 2					
Exercise	Sets	Reps/time	Rest	Wt	Page #
Dumbbell alt-arm bench press	2-3	5-8 reps	30 sec	25 lb, 30 lb, 35 lb	123
Kettlebell renegade row	2-3	5-8 reps	30 sec	14 kg, 16 kg, 18 kg	130
Suspension push-up	2-3	12-15 reps	30 sec	BW	113
POD 3					
Exercise	Sets	Reps/time	Rest	Wt	Page #
Heavy rope scissors	2	50 sec	30 sec	Rope	171
Heavy rope jumping jacks	2	50 sec	30 sec	Rope	172
Heavy rope alt-arm slams	2	50 sec	30 sec	Rope	170
POD 4					
Exercise	Sets	Reps/time	Rest	Wt	Page #
Sandbag hang clean	2	5-8 reps	30 sec	40 lb, 60 lb	57
Kettlebell push press	2	5-8 reps	30 sec	12 kg, 14 kg, 16 kg	61
Dumbbell box step-up	2	5 reps each side	30 sec	20 lb, 25 lb, 30 lb	86
POD 5					
Exercise	Sets	Reps/time	Rest	Wt	Page #
Dumbbell incline press	2	5-8 reps	30 sec	20 lb, 25 lb, 30 lb	124
Dumbbell renegade row	2	5-8 reps	30 sec	20 lb, 25 lb, 30 lb	130
Suspension row	2	12-15 reps	30 sec	BW	135

(continued)

Strength and Power Program 3C: Advanced *(continued)*

POD 6					
Exercise	**Sets**	**Reps/time**	**Rest**	**Wt**	**Page #**
Medicine ball rotational slam	1	50 sec	30 sec	16 lb, 18 lb	67
Medicine ball upward throw	1	50 sec	30 sec	16 lb, 18 lb	68
Medicine ball squat and jump	1	50 sec	30 sec	16 lb, 18 lb	71

POD 7					
Exercise	**Sets**	**Reps/time**	**Rest**	**Wt**	**Page #**
Kettlebell deadlift	2	5-8 reps	30 sec	18 kg, 20 kg, 22 kg	94
Dumbbell front lunge	2	5 reps each side	30 sec	20 lb, 25 lb, 30 lb	87
Sandbag straight-leg deadlift	2	5-8 reps	30 sec	40 lb, 60 lb	96

POD 8					
Exercise	**Sets**	**Reps/time**	**Rest**	**Wt**	**Page #**
Kettlebell shoulder press	2	5-8 reps	30 sec	10 kg, 12 kg, 14 kg	131
Sandbag biceps curl	2	5-8 reps	30 sec	40 lb, 60 lb	121
Dumbbell bent-over raise	2	12-15 reps	30 sec	12 lb, 15 lb, 20 lb	140

POD 9					
Exercise	**Sets**	**Reps/time**	**Rest**	**Wt**	**Page #**
Weighted sled drag	1	50 sec	30 sec	90 lb	76
Weighted sled push	1	50 sec	30 sec	90 lb	74
Weighted sled pull and push	1	50 sec	30 sec	90 lb	75

POD 10					
Exercise	**Sets**	**Reps/time**	**Rest**	**Wt**	**Page #**
Front plank	1	50 sec	15 sec	BW	159
Weighted abdominal crunch	1	40 reps	15 sec	BW	155
Birddog	1	50 sec	15 sec	BW	161

Wt = Weight; BW = Bodyweight

Strength and Power Program 4A: Beginner

Note: Each exercise in a pod should be completed before moving to the next pod.

WARM-UP					
Exercise	**Sets**	**Reps/time**	**Rest**	**Wt**	**Page #**
March/walk	1	20 sec	10 sec	BW	N/A
Jumping jacks	1	20 sec	10 sec	BW	48
March/walk	1	20 sec	10 sec	BW	N/A
Push-up	1	20 sec	10 sec	BW	112
March/walk	1	20 sec	10 sec	BW	N/A
Single-leg squat (each leg)	1	20 sec	10 sec	BW	52
March/walk	1	20 sec	10 sec	BW	N/A
Burpee	1	20 sec	10 sec	BW	50
March/walk	1	20 sec	10 sec	BW	N/A
Mountain climbers	1	20 sec	10 sec	BW	49

POD 1

Exercise	Sets	Reps/time	Rest	Wt	Page #
Kettlebell one-arm clean	1	5-8 reps	30 sec	6 kg, 8 kg, 10 kg	63
Sandbag deadlift	1	5-8 reps	30 sec	40 lb	95
Dumbbell one-arm snatch	1	5-8 reps	30 sec	10 lb, 12 lb, 15 lb	58

POD 2

Exercise	Sets	Reps/time	Rest	Wt	Page #
Dumbbell bench press	1	5-8 reps	30 sec	15 lb, 20 lb, 25 lb	122
Sandbag row	1	5-8 reps	30 sec	40 lb	136
Suspension fly	1	5-8 reps	30 sec	BW	127

POD 3

Exercise	Sets	Reps/time	Rest	Wt	Page #
Heavy rope two-arm unbalanced slams	1	30 sec	30 sec	Rope	177
Heavy rope alt-arm unbalanced slams	1	30 sec	30 sec	Rope	177
Heavy rope two-arm slams	1	30 sec	30 sec	Rope	169

POD 4

Exercise	Sets	Reps/time	Rest	Wt	Page #
Sandbag push press	1	5-8 reps	30 sec	20 lb	61
Kettlebell two-hand swing	1	5-8 reps	30 sec	10 kg, 12 kg, 14 kg	62
Dumbbell lateral lunge	1	5 reps each side	30 sec	12 lb, 15 lb, 20 lb	90

POD 5

Exercise	Sets	Reps/time	Rest	Wt	Page #
Dumbbell alt-arm incline press	1	5-8 reps	30 sec	12 lb, 15 lb, 20 lb	125
Sandbag row	1	5-8 reps	30 sec	40 lb	136
Suspension row	1	5-8 reps	30 sec	BW	135

POD 6

Exercise	Sets	Reps/time	Rest	Wt	Page #
Medicine ball chop	1	30 sec	30 sec	10 lb, 12 lb	72
Medicine ball side chop	1	30 sec	30 sec	10 lb, 12 lb	73
Medicine ball rotational slam	1	30 sec	30 sec	10 lb, 12 lb	67

POD 7

Exercise	Sets	Reps/time	Rest	Wt	Page #
Sandbag front squat	1	5-8 reps	30 sec	20 lb	82
Medicine ball overhead lunge	1	5 reps each side	30 sec	10 lb, 12 lb	89
Dumbbell one-leg straight-leg deadlift	1	5-8 reps	30 sec	10 lb, 12 lb, 15 lb	97

POD 8

Exercise	Sets	Reps/time	Rest	Wt	Page #
Dumbbell push press	1	5-8 reps	30 sec	10 lb, 12 lb, 15 lb	60
Suspension biceps curl	1	5-8 reps	30 sec	BW	121
Suspension reverse fly	1	5-8 reps	30 sec	BW	127

(continued)

Strength and Power Program 4A: Beginner *(continued)*

POD 9					
Exercise	Sets	Reps/time	Rest	Wt	Page #
Sandbag farmer's walk	1	30 sec	30 sec	20 lb	99
Weighted sled push	1	30 sec	30 sec	45 lb	74
Kettlebell farmer's walk	1	30 sec	30 sec	10 kg, 12 kg, 14 kg	98
POD 10					
Exercise	Sets	Reps/time	Rest	Wt	Page #
Abdominal reach	1	20 reps	15 sec	BW	157
Side plank: left	1	30 sec	15 sec	BW	160
Side plank: right	1	30 sec	15 sec	BW	160

Wt = Weight; BW = Bodyweight

Strength and Power Program 4B: Intermediate

Note: Each exercise in a pod should be completed before moving to the next pod.

WARM-UP					
Exercise	Sets	Reps/time	Rest	Wt	Page #
Jog in place/jump rope	1	30 sec	10 sec	BW	N/A
Jumping jacks	1	30 sec	10 sec	BW	48
Jog in place/jump rope	1	30 sec	10 sec	BW	N/A
Push-up	1	30 sec	10 sec	BW	112
Jog in place/jump rope	1	30 sec	10 sec	BW	N/A
Single-leg squat (each leg)	1	30 sec	10 sec	BW	52
Jog in place/jump rope	1	30 sec	10 sec	BW	N/A
Burpee	1	30 sec	10 sec	BW	50
Jog in place/jump rope	1	30 sec	10 sec	BW	N/A
Mountain climbers	1	30 sec	10 sec	BW	49
POD 1					
Exercise	Sets	Reps/time	Rest	Wt	Page #
Kettlebell one-arm clean	2	5-8 reps	30 sec	8 kg, 10 kg, 12 kg	63
Sandbag deadlift	2	5-8 reps	30 sec	40 lb, 60 lb	95
Dumbbell one-arm snatch	2	5-8 reps	30 sec	12 lb, 15 lb, 20 lb	58
POD 2					
Exercise	Sets	Reps/time	Rest	Wt	Page #
Dumbbell bench press	2	5-8 reps	30 sec	25 lb, 30 lb, 35 lb	122
Sandbag row	2	5-8 reps	30 sec	40 lb, 60 lb	136
Suspension fly	2	5-8 reps	30 sec	BW	127
POD 3					
Exercise	Sets	Reps/time	Rest	Wt	Page #
Heavy rope two-arm unbalanced slams	1	40 sec	30 sec	Rope	177
Heavy rope alt-arm unbalanced slams	1	40 sec	30 sec	Rope	177
Heavy rope two-arm slams	1	40 sec	30 sec	Rope	169

POD 4					
Exercise	Sets	Reps/time	Rest	Wt	Page #
Sandbag push press	2	5-8 reps	30 sec	40 lb	61
Kettlebell two-hand swing	2	5-8 reps	30 sec	14 kg, 16 kg, 18 kg	62
Dumbbell lateral lunge	2	5 reps each side	30 sec	15 lb, 20 lb, 25 lb	90

POD 5					
Exercise	Sets	Reps/time	Rest	Wt	Page #
Dumbbell alt-arm incline press	2	5-8 reps	30 sec	15 lb, 20 lb, 25 lb	125
Sandbag row	2	5-8 reps	30 sec	60 lb	136
Suspension row	2	5-8 reps	30 sec	BW	135

POD 6					
Exercise	Sets	Reps/time	Rest	Wt	Page #
Medicine ball chop	1	40 sec	30 sec	14 lb, 16 lb	72
Medicine ball side chop	1	40 sec	30 sec	14 lb, 16 lb	73
Medicine ball rotational slam	1	40 sec	30 sec	14 lb, 16 lb	67

POD 7					
Exercise	Sets	Reps/time	Rest	Wt	Page #
Sandbag front squat	2	5-8 reps	30 sec	40 lb	82
Medicine ball overhead lunge	2	5 reps each side	30 sec	12 lb, 14 lb	89
Dumbbell one-leg straight-leg deadlift	2	5-8 reps	30 sec	12 lb, 15 lb, 20 lb	97

POD 8					
Exercise	Sets	Reps/time	Rest	Wt	Page #
Dumbbell push press	2	5-8 reps	30 sec	15 lb, 20 lb, 25 lb	60
Suspension biceps curl	2	5-8 reps	30 sec	BW	121
Suspension reverse fly	2	5-8 reps	30 sec	BW	127

POD 9					
Exercise	Sets	Reps/time	Rest	Wt	Page #
Sandbag farmer's walk	1	40 sec	30 sec	40 lb	99
Weighted sled push	1	40 sec	30 sec	70 lb	74
Kettlebell farmer's walk	1	40 sec	30 sec	14 kg, 16 kg, 18 kg	98

POD 10					
Exercise	Sets	Reps/time	Rest	Wt	Page #
Suspension hip and knee tuck	2	40 sec	15 sec	BW	165
Side plank: left	2	40 sec	15 sec	BW	160
Side plank: right	2	40 sec	15 sec	BW	160

Wt = Weight; BW = Bodyweight

Strength and Power Program 4C: Advanced

Note: Each exercise in a pod should be completed before moving to the next pod.

WARM-UP					
Exercise	Sets	Reps/time	Rest	Wt	Page #
Jog in place/jump rope	1	40 sec	10 sec	BW	N/A
Jumping jacks	1	40 sec	10 sec	BW	48
Jog in place/jump rope	1	40 sec	10 sec	BW	N/A
Push-up	1	40 sec	10 sec	BW	112
Jog in place/jump rope	1	40 sec	10 sec	BW	N/A
Single-leg squat (each leg)	1	40 sec	10 sec	BW	52
Jog in place/jump rope	1	40 sec	10 sec	BW	N/A
Burpee	1	40 sec	10 sec	BW	50
Jog in place/jump rope	1	40 sec	10 sec	BW	N/A
Mountain climbers	1	40 sec	10 sec	BW	49
POD 1					
Exercise	Sets	Reps/time	Rest	Wt	Page #
Kettlebell one-arm clean	2-3	5-8 reps	30 sec	12 kg, 14 kg, 16 kg	63
Sandbag deadlift	2-3	5-8 reps	30 sec	60 lb, 80 lb	95
Dumbbell one-arm snatch	2-3	5-8 reps	30 sec	15 lb, 20 lb, 25 lb	58
POD 2					
Exercise	Sets	Reps/time	Rest	Wt	Page #
Dumbbell bench press	2-3	5-8 reps	30 sec	30 lb, 35 lb, 40 lb	122
Sandbag row	2-3	5-8 reps	30 sec	60 lb, 80 lb	136
Suspension fly	2-3	5-8 reps	30 sec	BW	127
POD 3					
Exercise	Sets	Reps/time	Rest	Wt	Page #
Heavy rope two-arm unbalanced slams	1	50 sec	30 sec	Rope	177
Heavy rope alt-arm unbalanced slams	1	50 sec	30 sec	Rope	177
Heavy rope two-arm slams	1	50 sec	30 sec	Rope	169
POD 4					
Exercise	Sets	Reps/time	Rest	Wt	Page #
Sandbag push press	2-3	5-8 reps	30 sec	40 lb, 60 lb	61
Kettlebell two-hand swing	2-3	5-8 reps	30 sec	18 kg, 20 kg, 22 kg	62
Dumbbell lateral lunge	2-3	5 reps each side	30 sec	20 lb, 25 lb, 30 lb	90
POD 5					
Exercise	Sets	Reps/time	Rest	Wt	Page #
Dumbbell alt-arm incline press	2-3	5-8 reps	30 sec	20 lb, 25 lb, 30 lb	125
Sandbag row	2-3	5-8 reps	30 sec	60 lb, 80 lb	136
Suspension row	2-3	5-8 reps	30 sec	BW	135

POD 6					
Exercise	Sets	Reps/time	Rest	Wt	Page #
Medicine ball chop	1	50 sec	30 sec	18 lb (8.2 kg), 20 lb (9.1 kg)	72
Medicine ball side chop	1	50 sec	30 sec	18 lb, 20 lb	73
Medicine ball rotational slam	1	50 sec	30 sec	18 lb, 20 lb	67
POD 7					
Exercise	Sets	Reps/time	Rest	Wt	Page #
Sandbag front squat	2-3	5-8 reps	30 sec	40 lb, 60 lb	82
Medicine ball overhead lunge	2-3	5 reps each side	30 sec	16 lb, 18 lb	89
Dumbbell one-leg straight-leg deadlift	2-3	5-8 reps	30 sec	15 lb, 20 lb, 25 lb	97
POD 8					
Exercise	Sets	Reps/time	Rest	Wt	Page #
Dumbbell push press	2-3	5-8 reps	30 sec	20 lb, 25 lb, 30 lb	60
Suspension biceps curl	2-3	5-8 reps	30 sec	BW	121
Suspension reverse fly	2-3	5-8 reps	30 sec	BW	127
POD 9					
Exercise	Sets	Reps/time	Rest	Wt	Page #
Sandbag farmer's walk	1	50 sec	30 sec	40 lb, 60 lb	99
Weighted sled push	1	50 sec	30 sec	90 lb	74
Kettlebell farmer's walk	1	50 sec	30 sec	18 kg, 20 kg, 22 kg	98
POD 10					
Exercise	Sets	Reps/time	Rest	Wt	Page #
Suspension pike	1	50 sec	15 sec	BW	166
Side plank: left	1	50 sec	15 sec	BW	160
Side plank: right	1	50 sec	15 sec	BW	160

Wt = Weight; BW = Bodyweight

15

Programs for Improving Sport Performance

Metabolic conditioning can be used in many different ways to improve sport performance. Because of the wide variety of physical demands in sport, it would stand to reason that programming for sport performance must be accordingly adaptable.

Methods for Improving Sport Performance

Metabolic conditioning for sport performance will complement the three areas of biomechanics, metabolics, and motor patterning. Let's take a closer look at each one of these areas.

Biomechanics

Biomechanics is the method in which the musculoskeletal system interrelates to produce movement, strength, and power. There are key movements and positions in every sport. Those movements and positions should be practiced in the context of the metabolic-conditioning program. There is an infinite number of sport-specific actions to use as examples for biomechanics, but let's look at two in particular: In baseball training, a rotation at the torso could be used to mimic the swing. In basketball training, a two-handed chest pass could be replicated with a medicine ball chest pass.

To further explain this concept, let's look at running and rowing. Running in sport is ubiquitous. The action of running involves loading the hip, knee, and ankle and then extending those same joints. This action is sometimes known as "triple extension (simultaneous extension from the ankle, knee and hip in an explosive movement)." Biomechanically, you can load the hip, knee, and ankle with exercises such as the squat and lunge. Rowing involves extensive lower body and core movement. While the oar is in the water, the muscles of the legs and core must overcome resistance. This action requires a high degree of effort from the muscles of the legs and core. Biomechanically, rowing motions using kettlebells and dumbbells can simulate this sport-specific exercise.

Metabolics

Metabolics is the total energy produced through anabolic, catabolic, and ender-gonic reactions in the body (Herda and Cramer 2016). There are three metabolic pathways: the ATP-PC, lactic-acid, and aerobic pathways. The ATP-PC pathway delivers energy to the muscles during the first 10-30 seconds of exercise, and is associated with explosive movement; the lactic-acid pathway is used from 30 seconds into an exercise session until about two minutes; the aerobic pathway becomes dominant during efforts lasting longer than two minutes. A targeted metabolic-conditioning program can reflect efforts that are used in a particular sport. For instance, the average play in football lasts for about five seconds, with a 20-25-second rest interval. A metabolic-conditioning program could be designed to mirror the same metabolic pathway, with work and rest intervals that mimic actual play. The recommended work-to-rest ratio for a maximally effective met-abolic-training session varies from 1:6 to 1:1. Reductions in the work-to-rest ratio can take place as you adapt to the training.

Motor Patterning

Motor patterning refers to the neural pattern or construct that coordinates muscles to accomplish a movement (French 2016). Highly technical sport skills, such as those in gymnastics, require a high degree of fine motor patterning. By comparison, the motor patterning of walking is much less refined and does not require a high degree of coordination. Performing sport-specific movements with varying loads will reinforce motor patterning—and, consequently, sport-specific skill—by forc-ing the body to complete the same movement under different levels of resistance.

Let's use the baseball swing as an example of motor patterning. Activation of the muscles of the hips and torso allow for a horizontal or near-horizontal rotation while swinging. A simple method to load the torso would be to use a medicine ball toss or cable twist. Loading parameters can be adjusted to account for speed of movement, the amount of resistance, the number of sets and reps, and the length of rest intervals.

Some of the equipment used to target sport-specific actions and metabolic path-ways are barbells, dumbbells, medicine balls, and cable resistance machines. Being flexible and creative will help when creating your sport-specific programming.

Guidelines and Goals

The goals for a sports-performance program should focus on injury prevention and performance enhancement. Emphasis should be placed on achieving desired results in body composition, muscle hypertrophy, strength, endurance, speed, agility, coordination, balance, and power (McBride 2016). The length of exercise efforts should resemble competition conditions, and the movements themselves should be specific to the motor patterns and biomechanics required by a certain sport. Rest intervals can be reduced as metabolic fitness improves.

The pods in the following exercise programs are a combination of three or more exercises performed with short rest periods between them for either a set number of repetitions or a prescribed amount of time.

Sports Performance Program 1A: Beginner

WARM-UP					
Exercise	Sets	Reps/time	Rest	Wt	Page #
Hand walk	1	10 yd (9.1 m)	15 sec	BW	39
Knee-hug lunge	1	10 yd (9.1 m)	15 sec	BW	40
Front lunge with forearm to instep	1	10 yd (9.1 m)	15 sec	BW	41
Lateral lunge: right and left	1	10 yd (9.1 m)	15 sec	BW	42
Backward lunge and twist	1	10 yd (9.1 m)	15 sec	BW	43
High knees	1	20 yd (18.3 m)	15 sec	BW	44
Heel-up	1	20 yd (18.3 m)	15 sec	BW	46
High knees with lower-leg extension	1	20 yd (18.3 m)	15 sec	BW	45
Lateral high knees: right and left	1	20 yd (18.3 m)	15 sec	BW	45
POD 1					
Exercise	Sets	Reps/time	Rest	Wt	Page #
Dumbbell hang clean	1-2	5 reps	30 sec	10 lb, 12 lb, 15 lb	56
Dumbbell one-arm snatch	1-2	5 reps	30 sec	8 lb, 10 lb, 12 lb	58
Dumbbell push press	1-2	5 reps	30 sec	8 lb, 10 lb, 12 lb	60
Dumbbell squat	1-2	12-15 reps	30 sec	10 lb, 12 lb, 15 lb	80
POD 2					
Exercise	Sets	Reps/time	Rest	Wt	Page #
Kettlebell goblet squat	1	12-15 reps	30 sec	6 kg, 8 kg, 10 kg	81
Kettlebell overhead squat	1	12-15 reps	30 sec	6 kg, 8 kg, 10 kg	83
Kettlebell overhead lunge	1	12-15 reps	30 sec	6 kg, 8 kg, 10 kg	88
Kettlebell one-leg straight-leg deadlift	1	12-15 reps	30 sec	6 kg, 8 kg, 10 kg	98
POD 3					
Exercise	Sets	Reps/time	Rest	Wt	Page #
Resistance band standing chest press	1	12-15 reps	30 sec	Light/moderate	147
Sandbag row	1	12-15 reps	30 sec	20 lb	136
Sandbag upright row	1	12-15 reps	30 sec	20 lb	136
Resistance band shoulder press	1	12-15 reps	30 sec	Light	132
POD 4					
Exercise	Sets	Reps/time	Rest	Wt	Page #
Medicine ball slam	1	10 reps	30 sec	10 lb, 12 lb	66
Medicine ball side slam	1	10 reps	30 sec	10 lb, 12 lb	67
Medicine ball upward throw	1	10 reps	30 sec	10 lb, 12 lb	68
Medicine ball backward throw	1	10 reps	30 sec	10 lb, 12 lb	69
POD 5					
Exercise	Sets	Reps/time	Rest	Wt	Page #
Abdominal crunch: legs up	1-2	20 reps	15 sec	BW	155
Abdominal reach: legs up	1-2	20 reps	15 sec	BW	157
Opposite-shoulder-to-knee crunch	1-2	20 reps	15 sec	BW	158
Superman	1-2	30 sec	15 sec	BW	163

Wt = Weight; BW = Bodyweight

Sports Performance Program 1B: Intermediate

WARM-UP					
Exercise	Sets	Reps/time	Rest	Wt	Page #
Hand walk	1	10 yd (9.1 m)	15 sec	BW	39
Knee-hug lunge	1	10 yd (9.1 m)	15 sec	BW	40
Front lunge with forearm to instep	1	10 yd (9.1 m)	15 sec	BW	41
Lateral lunge: right and left	1	10 yd (9.1 m)	15 sec	BW	42
Backward lunge and twist	1	10 yd (9.1 m)	15 sec	BW	43
High knees	1	20 yd (18.3 m)	15 sec	BW	44
Heel-up	1	20 yd (18.3 m)	15 sec	BW	46
High knees with lower-leg extension	1	20 yd (18.3 m)	15 sec	BW	45
Lateral high knees: right and left	1	20 yd (18.3 m)	15 sec	BW	45
POD 1					
Exercise	Sets	Reps/time	Rest	Wt	Page #
Dumbbell hang clean	2	5 reps	30 sec	15 lb, 20 lb, 25 lb	56
Dumbbell one-arm snatch	2	5 reps	30 sec	12 lb, 15 lb, 20 lb	58
Dumbbell push press	2	5 reps	30 sec	12 lb, 15 lb, 20 lb	60
Dumbbell squat	2	12-15 reps	30 sec	20 lb, 25 lb, 30 lb	80
POD 2					
Exercise	Sets	Reps/time	Rest	Wt	Page #
Kettlebell goblet squat	2	12-15 reps	30 sec	10 kg, 12 kg, 14 kg	81
Kettlebell overhead squat	2	12-15 reps	30 sec	10 kg, 12 kg, 14 kg	83
Kettlebell overhead lunge	2	12-15 reps	30 sec	10 kg, 12 kg, 14 kg	88
Kettlebell one-leg straight-leg deadlift	2	12-15 reps	30 sec	10 kg, 12 kg, 14 kg	98
POD 3					
Exercise	Sets	Reps/time	Rest	Wt	Page #
Resistance band standing chest press	2	12-15 reps	30 sec	Moderate/heavy	147
Sandbag row	2	12-15 reps	30 sec	40 lb	136
Sandbag upright row	2	12-15 reps	30 sec	40 lb	136
Resistance band shoulder press	2	12-15 reps	30 sec	Moderate	132
POD 4					
Exercise	Sets	Reps/time	Rest	Wt	Page #
Medicine ball slam	2	15 reps	30 sec	14 lb, 16 lb	66
Medicine ball side slam	2	15 reps	30 sec	14 lb, 16 lb	67
Medicine ball upward throw	2	15 reps	30 sec	14 lb, 16 lb	68
Medicine ball backward throw	2	15 reps	30 sec	14 lb, 16 lb	69
POD 5					
Exercise	Sets	Reps/time	Rest	Wt	Page #
Abdominal crunch: legs up	2	40 reps	15 sec	10 lb	155
Abdominal reach: legs up	2	40 reps	15 sec	10 lb	157
Opposite-shoulder-to-knee crunch	2	40 reps	15 sec	BW	158
Superman	2	40 sec	15 sec	BW	163

Wt = Weight; BW = Bodyweight

Sports Performance Program 1C: Advanced

WARM-UP					
Exercise	Sets	Reps/time	Rest	Wt	Page #
Hand walk	1	10 yd (9.1 m)	15 sec	BW	39
Knee-hug lunge	1	10 yd (9.1 m)	15 sec	BW	40
Front lunge with forearm to instep	1	10 yd (9.1 m)	15 sec	BW	41
Lateral lunge: right and left	1	10 yd (9.1 m)	15 sec	BW	42
Backward lunge and twist	1	10 yd (9.1 m)	15 sec	BW	43
High knees	1	20 yd (18.1 m)	15 sec	BW	44
Heel-up	1	20 yd (18.1 m)	15 sec	BW	46
High knees with lower-leg extension	1	20 yd (18.1 m)	15 sec	BW	45
Lateral high knees: right and left	1	20 yd (18.1 m)	15 sec	BW	45
POD 1					
Exercise	Sets	Reps/time	Rest	Wt	Page #
Dumbbell hang clean	3	5 reps	30 sec	20 lb, 25 lb, 30 lb	56
Dumbbell one-arm snatch	3	5 reps	30 sec	20 lb, 25 lb, 30 lb	58
Dumbbell push press	3	5 reps	30 sec	15 lb, 20 lb, 25 lb	60
Dumbbell squat	3	12-15 reps	30 sec	30 lb, 35 lb, 40 lb	80
POD 2					
Exercise	Sets	Reps/time	Rest	Wt	Page #
Kettlebell goblet squat	2	12-15 reps	30 sec	14 kg16 kg, 18 kg	81
Kettlebell overhead squat	2	12-15 reps	30 sec	14 kg, 16 kg, 18 kg	83
Kettlebell overhead lunge	2	12-15 reps	30 sec	14 kg, 16 kg, 18 kg	88
Kettlebell one-leg straight-leg deadlift	2	12-15 reps	30 sec	12 kg, 14 kg, 16 kg	98
POD 3					
Exercise	Sets	Reps/time	Rest	Wt	Page #
Resistance band standing chest press	2	12-15 reps	30 sec	Heavy	147
Sandbag row	2	12-15 reps	30 sec	60 lb	136
Sandbag upright row	2	12-15 reps	30 sec	60 lb	136
Resistance band shoulder press	2	12-15 reps	30 sec	Moderate/heavy	132
POD 4					
Exercise	Sets	Reps/time	Rest	Wt	Page #
Medicine ball slam	2	15 reps	30 sec	16 lb, 18 lb	66
Medicine ball side slam	2	15 reps	30 sec	16 lb, 18 lb	67
Medicine ball upward throw	2	15 reps	30 sec	16 lb, 18 lb	68
Medicine ball backward throw	2	15 reps	30 sec	16 lb, 18 lb	69
POD 5					
Exercise	Sets	Reps/time	Rest	Wt	Page #
Abdominal crunch: legs up	2	40 reps	15 sec	10 lb	155
Abdominal reach: legs up	2	40 reps	15 sec	10 lb	157
Opposite-shoulder-to-knee crunch	2	40 reps	15 sec	BW	158
Superman	2	50 sec	15 sec	BW	163

Wt = Weight; BW = Bodyweight

Sports Performance Program 2A: Beginner

WARM-UP					
Exercise	Sets	Reps/time	Rest	Wt	Page #
Hand walk	1	10 yd (9.1 m)	15 sec	BW	39
Knee-hug lunge	1	10 yd (9.1 m)	15 sec	BW	40
Front lunge with forearm to instep	1	10 yd (9.1 m)	15 sec	BW	41
Lateral lunge: right and left	1	10 yd (9.1 m)	15 sec	BW	42
Backward lunge and twist	1	10 yd (9.1 m)	15 sec	BW	43
High knees	1	20 yd (18.1 m)	15 sec	BW	44
Heel-up	1	20 yd (18.1 m)	15 sec	BW	46
High knees with lower-leg extension	1	20 yd (18.1 m)	15 sec	BW	45
Lateral high knees: right and left	1	20 yd (18.1 m)	15 sec	BW	45
POD 1					
Exercise	Sets	Reps/time	Rest	Wt	Page #
Sandbag hang clean	2	5 reps	30 sec	20 lb	57
Sandbag push press	2	5 reps	30 sec	20 lb	61
Sandbag deadlift	2	12 reps	30 sec	40 lb	95
Sandbag straight-leg deadlift	2	12 reps	30 sec	20 lb	96
POD 2					
Exercise	Sets	Reps/time	Rest	Wt	Page #
Dumbbell front lunge	1	12 reps per side	30 sec	8 lb, 10 lb, 12 lb	87
Dumbbell lateral lunge	1	12 reps per side	30 sec	8 lb, 10 lb, 12 lb	90
Dumbbell backward lunge	1	12 reps per side	30 sec	8 lb, 10 lb, 12 lb	92
Dumbbell straight-leg deadlift	1	12 reps	30 sec	8 lb, 10 lb, 12 lb	95
POD 3					
Exercise	Sets	Reps/time	Rest	Wt	Page #
Kettlebell pullover	1	12 reps	30 sec	8 kg, 10 kg, 12 kg	128
Kettlebell one-arm row	1	12 reps	30 sec	8 kg, 10 kg, 12 kg	129
Kettlebell shoulder press	1	12 reps	30 sec	6 kg, 8 kg, 10 kg	131
Kettlebell upright row	1	12 reps	30 sec	8 kg, 10 kg, 12 kg	134
POD 4					
Exercise	Sets	Reps/time	Rest	Wt	Page #
Heavy rope two-arm slams	1	30 sec	30 sec	Rope	169
Heavy rope two-hand shuffle slams	1	30 sec	30 sec	Rope	174
Heavy rope two-hand backpedal slams	1	30 sec	30 sec	Rope	174
Heavy rope two-arm unbalanced slams	1	30 sec	30 sec	Rope	177
POD 5					
Exercise	Sets	Reps/time	Rest	Wt	Page #
Front plank	1	30 sec	15 sec	BW	159
Side plank: right	1	30 sec	15 sec	BW	160
Side plank: left	1	30 sec	15 sec	BW	160
Scissors	1	30 sec	15 sec	BW	162

Wt = Weight; BW = Bodyweight

Sports Performance Program 2B: Intermediate

WARM-UP					
Exercise	**Sets**	**Reps/time**	**Rest**	**Wt**	**Page #**
Hand walk	1	10 yd (9.1 m)	15 sec	BW	39
Knee-hug lunge	1	10 yd (9.1 m)	15 sec	BW	40
Front lunge with forearm to instep	1	10 yd (9.1 m)	15 sec	BW	41
Lateral lunge with right and left	1	10 yd (9.1 m)	15 sec	BW	42
Backward lunge and twist	1	10 yd (9.1 m)	15 sec	BW	43
High knees	1	20 yd (18.1 m)	15 sec	BW	44
Heel-up	1	20 yd (18.1 m)	15 sec	BW	46
High knees with lower-leg extension	1	20 yd (18.1 m)	15 sec	BW	45
Lateral high knees: right and left	1	20 yd (18.1 m)	15 sec	BW	45
POD 1					
Exercise	**Sets**	**Reps/time**	**Rest**	**Wt**	**Page #**
Sandbag hang clean	2	5 reps	30 sec	40 lb, 60 lb	57
Sandbag push press	2	5 reps	30 sec	40 lb, 60 lb	61
Sandbag deadlift	2	12 reps	30 sec	40 lb, 60 lb	95
Sandbag straight-leg deadlift	2	12 reps	30 sec	40 lb, 60 lb	96
POD 2					
Exercise	**Sets**	**Reps/time**	**Rest**	**Wt**	**Page #**
Dumbbell front lunge	2	12 reps per side	30 sec	12 lb, 15 lb, 20 lb	87
Dumbbell lateral lunge	2	12 reps per side	30 sec	12 lb, 15 lb, 20 lb	90
Dumbbell backward lunge	2	12 reps per side	30 sec	12 lb, 15 lb, 20 lb	92
Dumbbell one-leg straight-leg deadlift	2	12 reps	30 sec	12 lb, 15 lb, 20 lb	97
POD 3					
Exercise	**Sets**	**Reps/time**	**Rest**	**Wt**	**Page #**
Kettlebell pullover	2	12 reps	30 sec	12 kg, 14 kg, 16 kg	128
Kettlebell renegade row	2	12 reps	30 sec	12 kg, 14 kg, 16 kg	130
Kettlebell shoulder press	2	12 reps	30 sec	8 kg, 10 kg, 12 kg	131
Kettlebell upright row	2	12 reps	30 sec	12 kg, 14 kg, 16 kg	134
POD 4					
Exercise	**Sets**	**Reps/time**	**Rest**	**Wt**	**Page #**
Heavy rope two-arm slams	1	40 sec	30 sec	Rope	169
Heavy rope two-hand shuffle slams	1	40 sec	30 sec	Rope	174
Heavy rope two-hand backpedal slams	1	40 sec	30 sec	Rope	174
Heavy rope two-arm unbalanced slams	1	40 sec	30 sec	Rope	177
POD 5					
Exercise	**Sets**	**Reps/time**	**Rest**	**Wt**	**Page #**
Front plank	2	40 sec	15 sec	BW	159
Side plank: right	2	40 sec	15 sec	BW	160
Side plank: left	2	40 sec	15 sec	BW	160
Scissors	2	40 sec	15 sec	BW	162

Wt = Weight; BW = Bodyweight

Sports Performance Program 2C: Advanced

WARM-UP					
Exercise	Sets	Reps/time	Rest	Wt	Page #
Hand walk	1	10 yd (9.1 m)	15 sec	BW	39
Knee-hug lunge	1	10 yd (9.1 m)	15 sec	BW	40
Front lunge/forearm to instep	1	10 yd (9.1 m)	15 sec	BW	41
Lateral lunge: right and left	1	10 yd (9.1 m)	15 sec	BW	42
Backward lunge and twist	1	10 yd (9.1 m)	15 sec	BW	43
High knees	1	20 yd (18.1 m)	15 sec	BW	44
Heel-up	1	20 yd (18.1 m)	15 sec	BW	46
High knees with lower-leg extension	1	20 yd (18.1 m)	15 sec	BW	45
Lateral high knees: right and left	1	20 yd (18.1 m)	15 sec	BW	45
POD 1					
Exercise	Sets	Reps/time	Rest	Wt	Page #
Sandbag hang clean	2-3	5 reps	30 sec	60 lb, 80 lb	57
Sandbag push press	2-3	5 reps	30 sec	60 lb, 80 lb	61
Sandbag deadlift	2-3	12 reps	30 sec	60 lb, 80 lb	95
Sandbag straight-leg deadlift	2-3	12 reps	30 sec	60 lb, 80 lb	96
POD 2					
Exercise	Sets	Reps/time	Rest	Wt	Page #
Dumbbell front lunge	2-3	12 reps per side	30 sec	15 lb, 20 lb, 25 lb	87
Dumbbell lateral lunge	2-3	12 reps per side	30 sec	15 lb, 20 lb, 25 lb	90
Dumbbell backward lunge	2-3	12 reps per side	30 sec	15 lb, 20 lb, 25 lb	92
Dumbbell one-leg straight leg deadlift	2-3	12 reps	30 sec	15 lb, 20 lb, 25 lb	97
POD 3					
Exercise	Sets	Reps/time	Rest	Wt	Page #
Kettlebell pullover	2-3	12 reps	30 sec	16 kg, 18 kg, 20 kg	128
Kettlebell renegade row	2-3	12 reps	30 sec	16 kg, 18 kg, 20 kg	130
Kettlebell shoulder press	2-3	12 reps	30 sec	12 kg, 14 kg, 16 kg	131
Kettlebell upright row	2-3	12 reps	30 sec	16 kg, 18 kg, 20 kg	134
POD 4					
Exercise	Sets	Reps/time	Rest	Wt	Page #
Heavy rope two-arm slams	1	50 sec	30 sec	Rope	169
Heavy rope two-hand shuffle slams	1	50 sec	30 sec	Rope	174
Heavy rope two-hand backpedal slams	1	50 sec	30 sec	Rope	174
Heavy rope two-arm unbalanced slams	1	50 sec	30 sec	Rope	177
POD 5					
Exercise	Sets	Reps/time	Rest	Wt	Page #
Front plank	2	50 sec	15 sec	BW	159
Side plank: right	2	50 sec	15 sec	BW	160
Side plank: left	2	50 sec	15 sec	BW	160
Scissors	2	50 sec	15 sec	BW	162

Wt = Weight; BW = Bodyweight

Sports Performance Program 3A: Beginner

WARM-UP					
Exercise	**Sets**	**Reps/time**	**Rest**	**Wt**	**Page #**
Hand walk	1	10 yd (9.1 m)	15 sec	BW	39
Knee-hug lunge	1	10 yd (9.1 m)	15 sec	BW	40
Front lunge/forearm to instep	1	10 yd (9.1 m)	15 sec	BW	41
Lateral lunge: right and left	1	10 yd (9.1 m)	15 sec	BW	42
Backward lunge and twist	1	10 yd (9.1 m)	15 sec	BW	43
High knees	1	20 yd (18.1 m)	15 sec	BW	44
Heel-up	1	20 yd (18.1 m)	15 sec	BW	46
High knees with foreleg extension	1	20 yd (18.1 m)	15 sec	BW	45
Lateral high knees: right and left	1	20 yd (18.1 m)	15 sec	BW	45
POD 1					
Exercise	**Sets**	**Reps/time**	**Rest**	**Wt**	**Page #**
Kettlebell one-arm clean	1-2	5 reps each arm	30 sec	6 kg, 8 kg, 10 kg	63
Kettlebell two-hand swing	2	12 reps	30 sec	8 kg, 10 kg, 12 kg	62
Kettlebell deadlift	2	12 reps	30 sec	12 kg, 14 kg, 16 kg	94
Kettlebell straight-leg deadlift	2	12 reps	30 sec	8 kg, 10 kg, 12 kg	95
POD 2					
Exercise	**Sets**	**Reps/time**	**Rest**	**Wt**	**Page #**
Sandbag front squat	2	12 reps	30 sec	20 lb, 40 lb	82
Sandbag overhead squat	2	12 reps	30 sec	20 lb	85
Sandbag overhead lunge	2	6 reps each leg	30 sec	20 lb	89
Sandbag straight-leg deadlift	2	12 reps	30 sec	20 lb, 40 lb	96
POD 3					
Exercise	**Sets**	**Reps/time**	**Rest**	**Wt**	**Page #**
Dumbbell bench press	2	12 reps	30 sec	10 lb, 12 lb, 15 lb	122
Dumbbell one-arm row	2	12 reps	30 sec	10 lb, 12 lb, 15 lb	129
Dumbbell alt-arm biceps curl	2	12 reps	30 sec	8 lb, 10 lb, 12 lb	144
Dumbbell supine triceps extension	2	12 reps	30 sec	8 lb, 10 lb, 12 lb	141
POD 4					
Exercise	**Sets**	**Reps/time**	**Rest**	**Wt**	**Page #**
Weighted sled push	1	30 sec	30 sec	45 lb	74
Weighted sled pull and push	1	30 sec	30 sec	45 lb	75
Weighted sled drag	1	30 sec	30 sec	45 lb	76
Sandbag farmer's walk	1	30 sec	30 sec	20 lb	99
POD 5					
Exercise	**Sets**	**Reps/time**	**Rest**	**Wt**	**Page #**
Abdominal crunch: legs up	1-2	20 reps	15 sec	BW	155
Abdominal reach: legs up	1-2	20 reps	15 sec	BW	157
Opposite-shoulder-to-knee crunch	1-2	20 reps	15 sec	BW	158
Birddog	1-2	10 reps each side	15 sec	BW	161

Wt = Weight; BW = Bodyweight

Sports Performance Program 3B: Intermediate

WARM-UP					
Exercise	**Sets**	**Reps/time**	**Rest**	**Wt**	**Page #**
Hand walk	1	10 yd (9.1 m)	15 sec	BW	39
Knee-hug lunge	1	10 yd (9.1 m)	15 sec	BW	40
Front lunge with forearm to instep	1	10 yd (9.1 m)	15 sec	BW	41
Lateral lunge: right and left	1	10 yd (9.1 m)	15 sec	BW	42
Backward lunge and twist	1	10 yd (9.1 m)	15 sec	BW	43
High knees	1	20 yd (18.1 m)	15 sec	BW	44
Heel-up	1	20 yd (18.1 m)	15 sec	BW	46
High knees with lower-leg extension	1	20 yd (18.1 m)	15 sec	BW	45
Lateral high knees: right and left	1	20 yd (18.1 m)	15 sec	BW	45
POD 1					
Exercise	**Sets**	**Reps/time**	**Rest**	**Wt**	**Page #**
Kettlebell two-arm clean	2	5 reps each arm	30 sec	10 kg, 12 kg, 14 kg	64
Kettlebell one-hand swing	2	12 reps	30 sec	10 kg, 12 kg, 14 kg	62
Kettlebell deadlift	2	12 reps	30 sec	16 kg, 18 kg, 20 kg	94
Kettlebell one-leg straight-leg deadlift	2	12 reps	30 sec	12 kg, 14 kg, 16 kg	98
POD 2					
Exercise	**Sets**	**Reps/time**	**Rest**	**Wt**	**Page #**
Sandbag front squat	2	12 reps	30 sec	40 lb, 60 lb	82
Sandbag overhead squat	2	12 reps	30 sec	40 lb, 60 lb	85
Sandbag overhead lunge	2	6 reps each leg	30 sec	40 lb, 60 lb	89
Sandbag straight-leg deadlift	2	12 reps	30 sec	40 lb, 60 lb	96
POD 3					
Exercise	**Sets**	**Reps/time**	**Rest**	**Wt**	**Page #**
Dumbbell alt-arm bench press	2	12 reps	30 sec	15 lb, 20 lb, 25 lb	123
Dumbbell renegade row	2	12 reps	30 sec	15 lb, 20 lb, 25 lb	130
Dumbbell alt-arm biceps curl	2	12 reps	30 sec	12 lb, 15 lb, 20 lb	144
Dumbbell supine triceps extension	2	12 reps	30 sec	12 lb, 15 lb, 20 lb	141
POD 4					
Exercise	**Sets**	**Reps/time**	**Rest**	**Wt**	**Page #**
Weighted sled push	1	30 sec	30 sec	70 lb	74
Weighted sled pull and push	1	30 sec	30 sec	70 lb	75
Weighted sled drag	1	30 sec	30 sec	70 lb	76
Sandbag farmer's walk	1	30 sec	30 sec	40 lb	99
POD 5					
Exercise	**Sets**	**Reps/time**	**Rest**	**Wt**	**Page #**
Weighted abdominal crunch: legs up	2	30 reps	15 sec	10 lb	155
Weighted abdominal reach: legs up	2	30 reps	15 sec	10 lb	157
Opposite-shoulder-to-knee crunch	2	30 reps	15 sec	BW	158
Birddog	2	15 reps each side	15 sec	BW	161

Wt = Weight; BW = Bodyweight

Sports Performance Program 3C: Advanced

WARM-UP					
Exercise	Sets	Reps/time	Rest	Wt	Page #
Hand walk	1	10 yd (9.1 m)	15 sec	BW	39
Knee-hug lunge	1	10 yd (9.1 m)	15 sec	BW	40
Front lunge with forearm to instep	1	10 yd (9.1 m)	15 sec	BW	41
Lateral lunge: right and left	1	10 yd (9.1 m)	15 sec	BW	42
Backward lunge and twist	1	10 yd (9.1 m)	15 sec	BW	43
High knees	1	20 yd (18.1 m)	15 sec	BW	44
Heel-up	1	20 yd (18.1 m)	15 sec	BW	46
High knees with lower-leg extension	1	20 yd (18.1 m)	15 sec	BW	45
Lateral high knees: right and left	1	20 yd (18.1 m)	15 sec	BW	45

POD 1					
Exercise	Sets	Reps/time	Rest	Wt	Page #
Kettlebell two-arm clean	3	5 reps each arm	30 sec	14 kg, 16 kg, 18 kg	64
Kettlebell one-hand swing	3	12 reps	30 sec	14 kg, 16 kg, 18 kg	62
Kettlebell deadlift	3	12 reps	30 sec	20 kg, 22 kg, 24 kg	94
Kettlebell one-leg straight-leg deadlift	3	12 reps	30 sec	16 kg, 18 kg, 20 kg	98

POD 2					
Exercise	Sets	Reps/time	Rest	Wt	Page #
Sandbag front squat	3	12 reps	30 sec	60 lb, 80 lb	82
Sandbag overhead squat	3	12 reps	30 sec	60 lb	85
Sandbag overhead lunge	3	6 reps each leg	30 sec	60 lb	89
Sandbag straight-leg deadlift	3	12 reps	30 sec	60 lb, 80 lb	96

POD 3					
Exercise	Sets	Reps/time	Rest	Wt	Page #
Dumbbell alt-arm bench press	3	12 reps	30 sec	25 lb, 30 lb, 35 lb	123
Dumbbell renegade row	3	12 reps	30 sec	25 lb, 30 lb, 35 lb	130
Dumbbell alt-arm biceps curl	3	12 reps	30 sec	20 lb, 25 lb, 30 lb	144
Dumbbell supine triceps extension	3	12 reps	30 sec	15 lb, 20 lb, 25 lb	141

POD 4					
Exercise	Sets	Reps/time	Rest	Wt	Page #
Weighted sled push	1	40 sec	30 sec	90 lb	74
Weighted sled pull and push	1	40 sec	30 sec	90 lb	75
Weighted sled drag	1	40 sec	30 sec	90 lb	76
Sandbag farmer's walk	1	40 sec	30 sec	60 lb, 80 lb	99

POD 5					
Exercise	Sets	Reps/time	Rest	Wt	Page #
Weighted abdominal crunch: legs up	2	40 reps	15 sec	10 lb	155
Weighted reach: legs up	2	40 reps	15 sec	10 lb	157
Opposite-shoulder-to-knee crunch	2	40 reps	15 sec	BW	158
Birddog	2	20 reps each side	15 sec	BW	161

Wt = Weight; BW = Bodyweight

Sports Performance Program 4A: Beginner

WARM-UP					
Exercise	Sets	Reps/time	Rest	Wt	Page #
Hand walk	1	10 yd (9.1 m)	15 sec	BW	39
Knee-hug lunge	1	10 yd (9.1 m)	15 sec	BW	40
Front lunge/forearm to instep	1	10 yd (9.1 m)	15 sec	BW	41
Lateral lunge: right and left	1	10 yd (9.1 m)	15 sec	BW	42
Backward lunge and twist	1	10 yd (9.1 m)	15 sec	BW	43
High knees	1	20 yd (18.1 m)	15 sec	BW	44
Heel-up	1	20 yd (18.1 m)	15 sec	BW	46
High knees with lower-leg extension	1	20 yd (18.1 m)	15 sec	BW	45
Lateral high knees: right and left	1	20 yd (18.1 m)	15 sec	BW	45
POD 1					
Exercise	Sets	Reps/time	Rest	Wt	Page #
Dumbbell hang clean	1-2	5 reps	30 sec	10 lb, 12 lb, 15 lb	56
Kettlebell one-arm snatch	1-2	5 reps	30 sec	6 kg, 8 kg, 10 kg	59
Sandbag push press	1-2	5 reps	30 sec	20 lb	61
Kettlebell one-leg straight-leg deadlift	1-2	12 reps each leg	30 sec	6 kg, 8 kg, 10 kg	98
POD 2					
Exercise	Sets	Reps/time	Rest	Wt	Page #
Dumbbell squat	1	12 reps	30 sec	12 lb, 15 lb, 20 lb	80
Kettlebell overhead lunge	1	12 reps	30 sec	6 kg, 8 kg, 10 kg	88
Medicine ball overhead backward lunge	1	6 reps each leg	30 sec	8 lb, 10 lb	93
Sandbag front squat	1	12 reps	30 sec	20 lb	82
POD 3					
Exercise	Sets	Reps/time	Rest	Wt	Page #
Resistance band standing chest press	1	12 reps	30 sec	Moderate	147
Resistance band standing row	1	12 reps	30 sec	Moderate	148
Kettlebell alt-arm biceps curl	1	12 reps	30 sec	4 kg, 6 kg, 8 kg	144
Kettlebell overhead triceps extension	1	12 reps	30 sec	6 kg, 8 kg, 10 kg	120
POD 4					
Exercise	Sets	Reps/time	Rest	Wt	Page #
Medicine ball burpee	1	50 sec	30 sec	10 lb	70
Medicine ball squat and jump	1	50 sec	30 sec	10 lb	71
Medicine ball chop	1	50 sec	30 sec	10 lb	72
Medicine ball side chop	1	50 sec	30 sec	10 lb	73
POD 5					
Exercise	Sets	Reps/time	Rest	Wt	Page #
Scissors	1	30 sec	15 sec	BW	162
Bicycle	1	30 sec	15 sec	BW	162
Side plank: right	1	30 sec	15 sec	BW	160
Side plank: left	1	30 sec	15 sec	BW	160

Wt = Weight; BW = Bodyweight

Sports Performance Program 4B: Intermediate

WARM-UP					
Exercise	**Sets**	**Reps/time**	**Rest**	**Wt**	**Page #**
Hand walk	1	10 yd (9.1 m)	15 sec	BW	39
Knee-hug lunge	1	10 yd (9.1 m)	15 sec	BW	40
Front lunge with forearm to instep	1	10 yd (9.1 m)	15 sec	BW	41
Lateral lunge: right and left	1	10 yd (9.1 m)	15 sec	BW	42
Backward lunge and twist	1	10 yd (9.1 m)	15 sec	BW	43
High knees	1	20 yd (18.1 m)	15 sec	BW	44
Heel-ups	1	20 yd (18.1 m)	15 sec	BW	46
High knees with lower-leg extension	1	20 yd (18.1 m)	15 sec	BW	45
Lateral high knees: right and left	1	20 yd (18.1 m)	15 sec	BW	45
POD 1					
Exercise	**Sets**	**Reps/time**	**Rest**	**Wt**	**Page #**
Dumbbell hang clean	2	5 reps	30 sec	15 lb, 20 lb, 25 lb	56
Kettlebell one-arm snatch	2	5 reps	30 sec	10 kg, 12 kg, 14 kg	59
Sandbag push press	2	5 reps	30 sec	40 lb	61
Kettlebell one-leg straight-leg deadlift	2	12 per each leg	30 sec	10 kg, 12 kg, 14 kg	98
POD 2					
Exercise	**Sets**	**Reps/time**	**Rest**	**Wt**	**Page #**
Dumbbell squat	2	12 reps	30 sec	20 lb, 25 lb, 30 lb	80
Kettlebell overhead lunge	2	12 reps	30 sec	10 kg, 12 kg, 14 kg	88
Medicine ball overhead backward lunge	2	6 per each leg	30 sec	12 lb, 14 lb	93
Sandbag front squat	2	12 reps	30 sec	40 lb	82
POD 3					
Exercise	**Sets**	**Reps/time**	**Rest**	**Wt**	**Page #**
Resistance band standing chest press	2	12 reps	30 sec	Moderate/heavy	147
Resistance band standing row	2	12 reps	30 sec	Moderate/heavy	148
Kettlebell alt-arm biceps curl	2	12 reps	30 sec	8 kg, 10 kg, 12 kg	144
Kettlebell overhead triceps extension	2	12 reps	30 sec	8 kg, 10 kg, 12 kg	120
POD 4					
Exercise	**Sets**	**Reps/time**	**Rest**	**Wt**	**Page #**
Medicine ball burpee	1	40 sec	30 sec	12 lb	70
Medicine ball squat and jump	1	40 sec	30 sec	12 lb	71
Medicine ball chop	1	40 sec	30 sec	12 lb	72
Medicine ball side chop	1	40 sec	30 sec	12 lb	73
POD 5					
Exercise	**Sets**	**Reps/time**	**Rest**	**Wt**	**Page #**
Scissors	2	40 sec	15 sec	BW	162
Suspension hip and knee tuck	2	40 sec	15 sec	BW	165
Side plank: right	2	40 sec	15 sec	BW	160
Side plank: left	2	40 sec	15 sec	BW	160

Wt = Weight; BW = Bodyweight

Sports Performance Program 4C: Advanced

WARM-UP					
Exercise	**Sets**	**Reps/time**	**Rest**	**Wt**	**Page #**
Hand walk	1	10 yd (9.1 m)	15 sec	BW	39
Knee-hug lunge	1	10 yd (9.1 m)	15 sec	BW	40
Front lunge with forearm to instep	1	10 yd (9.1 m)	15 sec	BW	41
Lateral lunge: right and left	1	10 yd (9.1 m)	15 sec	BW	42
Backward lunge and twist	1	10 yd (9.1 m)	15 sec	BW	43
High knees	1	20 yd (18.1 m)	15 sec	BW	44
Heel-ups	1	20 yd (18.1 m)	15 sec	BW	46
High knees with lower-leg extension	1	20 yd (18.1 m)	15 sec	BW	45
Lateral high knees: right and left	1	20 yd (18.1 m)	15 sec	BW	45
POD 1					
Exercise	**Sets**	**Reps/time**	**Rest**	**Wt**	**Page #**
Dumbbell hang clean	2-3	5 reps	30 sec	25 lb, 30 lb, 35 lb	56
Kettlebell one-arm snatch	2-3	5 reps	30 sec	14 kg, 16 kg, 18 kg	59
Sandbag push press	2-3	5 reps	30 sec	60 lb	61
Kettlebell one-leg straight-leg deadlift	2-3	12 reps each leg	30 sec	14 kg, 16 kg, 18 kg	98
POD 2					
Exercise	**Sets**	**Reps/time**	**Rest**	**Wt**	**Page #**
Dumbbell squat	2	12 reps	30 sec	30 lb, 35 lb, 40 lb	80
Kettlebell overhead lunge	2	12 reps	30 sec	14 kg, 16 kg, 18 kg	88
Medicine ball overhead backward lunge	2	6 reps each leg	30 sec	16 lb, 18 lb	93
Sandbag front squat	2	12 reps	30 sec	60 lb	82
POD 3					
Exercise	**Sets**	**Reps/time**	**Rest**	**Wt**	**Page #**
Resistance band standing chest press	2	12 reps	30 sec	Heavy	147
Resistance band standing row	2	12 reps	30 sec	Heavy	135
Kettlebell alt-arm biceps curl	2	12 reps	30 sec	12 kg, 14 kg, 16 kg	144
Kettlebell overhead triceps extension	2	12 reps	30 sec	12 kg, 14 kg, 16 kg	120
POD 4					
Exercise	**Sets**	**Reps/time**	**Rest**	**Wt**	**Page #**
Medicine ball burpee	1	50 sec	30 sec	14 lb	70
Medicine ball squat and jump	1	50 sec	30 sec	14 lb	71
Medicine ball chop	1	50 sec	30 sec	14 lb	72
Medicine ball side chop	1	50 sec	30 sec	14 lb	73
POD 5					
Exercise	**Sets**	**Reps/time**	**Rest**	**Wt**	**Page #**
Suspension pike	2	50 sec	15 sec	BW	166
Bicycle	2	50 sec	15 sec	BW	162
Side plank: right	2	50 sec	15 sec	BW	160
Side plank: left	2	50 sec	15 sec	BW	160

Wt = Weight; BW = Bodyweight

Appendix

Metric Equivalents for Weighted Equipment

For weights not listed here, you can calculate conversions using this equivalent: 1 kilogram = 2.2 pounds (roughly 2 lb) and 1 pound = 0.45 kilogram (roughly half a kilogram).

Table 1   Common Dumbbell Pound Increments Converted to Kilogram

5 lb	2.3 kg
8 lb	3.6 kg
10 lb	4.5 kg
12 lb	5.4 kg
15 lb	6.8 kg
20 lb	9.1 kg
25 lb	11.3 kg
30 lb	13.6 kg
35 lb	15.9 kg
40 lb	18.1 kg

Table 2   Common Kettlebell Kilogram Increments Converted to Pounds

4 kg	8.8 lb
6 kg	13.2 lb
6.4 kg	14 lb
7.3 kg	16 lb
8 kg	17.6 lb
8.2 kg	18 lb
10 kg	22.0 lb
12 kg	26.5 lb
14 kg	30.9 lb
16 kg	35.3 lb
18 kg	39.7 lb
20 kg	44.1 lb
22 kg	48.5 lb
24 kg	52.9 lb
26 kg	57.3 lb

Table 3 Common Medicine Ball Pound Increments Converted to Kilogram

8 lb	3.6 kg
10 lb	4.5 kg
12 lb	5.4 kg
14 lb	6.4 kg
16 lb	7.3 kg
18 lb	8.2 kg
20 lb	9.1 kg

Table 4 Common Sandbag Pound Increments Converted to Kilogram

20 lb	9.1 kg
40 lb	18.1 kg
60 lb	27.2 kg
80 lb	36.3 kg

Table 5 Common Weight Pound Increments Converted to Kilogram

45 lb	20.4 kg
70 lb	31.8 kg
90 lb	40.8 kg

References

Chapter 1

Cissik, J., and J. Dawes. 2015. *Maximum Interval Training.* Champaign, IL: Human Kinetics.

Nuñez, T.P., T.A. Fabiano, N.M. Beltz, C.M. Mermier, T.A. Moriarty, R.C. Nava, T. A. VanDusseldorp, and L. Kravitz, *J Exerc Sci Fit.* 2020 Jan; 18(1): 14–20

Laursen, P. and M. Buchheit, eds. 2019. *Science and Application of High-Intensity Interval Training.* Champaign, IL: Human Kinetics.

Chapter 2

Borsheim, E., and R. Bahr. 2003. "Effect of Exercise Intensity, Duration and Mode of Post-Exercise Oxygen Consumption." *Sports Medicine* 33:1037-60.

Herda, T.J., and J.T. Cramer. 2016. "Bioenergetics of Exercise and Training." In *Essentials of Strength Training and Conditioning*, 4th ed., edited by G. G. Haff and N. T. Triplett, 43-63. Champaign, IL: Human Kinetics.

French, D. 2016. "Adaptations to Anaerobic Training Programs." In *Essentials of Strength Training and Conditioning*, 4th ed., edited by G. G. Haff and N. T. Triplett, 87-113. Champaign, IL: Human Kinetics.

Statler, T., and A. Dubois. 2016. "Psychology of Athletic Preparation and Performance." In *Essentials of Strength Training and Conditioning*, 4th ed., edited by G. G. Haff and N. T. Triplett, 155-174. Champaign, IL: Human Kinetics.

Chapter 3

Beardsley, C., and B. Contreras. 2014. "The Role of Kettlebells in Strength and Conditioning. *Strength and Conditioning Journal* 36 (3):64-70.

Cotter, S. 2022. *Kettlebell Training.* Champaign, IL: Human Kinetics.

Berryman, J.W. 2012. "Motion and Rest: Galen on Exercise and Health." *The Lancet* 380 (9838): 210-11.

Cissik, J., and J. Dawes. 2015. *Maximum Interval Training.* Champaign, IL: Human Kinetics.

Faigenbaum, A.D., and M. Mediate. 2006. "Effects of Medicine Ball Training on Fitness Performance of High-School Physical Education Students." *Physical Educator* 63: 160-68.

Faigenbaum, A.D., J. Kang, A. Farrell, N.A. Ratamess, N. Ellis, I. Vought, and J. Bush. 2018. "Acute Cardiometabolic Responses to Medicine Ball Exercise in Children." *Medicine and Science in Sports and Exercise* 50(5S): 527.

Ford, E. 1955. "The *De Arte Gymnastica* of Mecuriale." *Australian Journal of Physiotherapy* 1 (1): 30-32.

Haff, G.G., D. Berninger, and S. Caulfield. 2016. "Exercise Techniques for Alternative Modes and Nontraditional Implement Training." In *Essentials of Strength Training and Conditioning*, 4th ed., edited by G.G. Haff and N.T. Triplett, 409-438. Champaign, IL: Human Kinetics.

Hagberg, L.A., B. Lindahl, L. Nyberg, and M. L. Hellénius. 2009. "Importance of Enjoyment When Promoting Physical Exercise." *Scandinavian Journal of Medicine and Science in Sports* 19 (5): 740-47.

Harrison, J.S. 2011. "Bodyweight Training: A Return to Basics." *Strength and Conditioning Journal* \32 (2): 86-89.

Harrison, J.S., B. Schoenfeld, and M.L. Schoenfeld. 2011. "Applications of Kettlebells in Exercise Program Design." *Strength and Conditioning Journal* 33 (6): 86-89.

Herda, T.J., and J.T. Cramer. 2016. "Bioenergetics of Exercise and Training." In *Essentials of Strength Training and Conditioning*, 4th ed., edited by G.G. Haff and N.T. Triplett, 43-63. Champaign, IL: Human Kinetics.

Jay, K., D. Frisch, K. Hansen, M.K. Zebis, C.H. Andersen, O.S. Mortensen, and L.L. Andersen. 2011. "Kettlebell Training for Muscular Skeletal and Cardiovascular Health: A Randomized Controlled Trial." *Scand J Work, Environ Health* 37:196-203.

Lake, J.P., and M.A. Lauder. 2012. "Kettlebell Swing Training Improves Maximal and Explosive Strength." *Journal of Strength and Conditioning Research* 26:2228-33.

Manocchia, P., D.K. Spierer, A.K. Lufkin, J. Minichiello, and J. Castro. 2013. "Transfer of Kettlebell Strength Training to Strength, Power and Endurance." *Journal of Strength and Conditioning Research* 27:477-84.

Otto, W.H., III, J.W. Coburn, L.E. Brown, and B.A. Spiering. 2012. "Effects of Weight Training vs. Kettlebell Training on Vertical Jump, Strength and Body Composition." *Journal of Strength and Conditioning Research* 26:1199-1202.

Page, P., and T.S. Ellenbecker. 2020. *Resistance Band Training.* Champaign, IL: Human Kinetics.

Ratamess, N.A., and Izquierdo, M. 2008. "Neuromuscular Adaptations to Training." In *The Olympic Textbook of Medicine in Sport*, edited by M.P. Schwellnus, 67-78. Hoboken, NJ: Wiley.

Roberts, R.J. 2020. "The Long History of the Medicine Ball." Physical Culture Study. Last modified January 29, 2020. https://physicalculturestudy.com/2020/01/29/the-long-history-of-the-medicine-ball.

Sheppard, J.M., and N.T. Triplett. 2016. "Program Design for Resistance Training." In *Essentials of Strength Training and Conditioning*, 4th ed., edited by G.G. Haff and N.T. Triplett, 439-469. Champaign, IL: Human Kinetics.

Todd, J. 2003. "The Strength Builders: A History of Barbells, Dumbbells and Indian Clubs." *The International Journal of the History of Sport* 20 (1): 65-90.

Vincent, J., L. Traywick, and L. Washburn. 2013. *Increasing Physical Activity as We Age: Strength Training with Medicine Balls.* Fayetteville: University of Arkansas Division of Agriculture Research and Extension.

Chapter 4

Bompa, T.O., and G.G. Haff. 2009. *Periodization: Theory and Methodology of Training,* Champaign, IL: Human Kinetics, 1-424.

Bondarchuk, A.P. 1988. Constructing a Training System. *Track Tech* 102: 254-269.

Bondarchuk, A.P. 1994. The Role and Sequence of Using Different Training-Load Intensities. *Fit Sport Rev Inter* 29:202-204.

Foster, C. 1998. Monitoring Training in Athletes with Reference to Overtraining Syndrome. *Med Sci Sports Exerc* 30: 1164-1168.

Haff, G. 2016. "Bioenergetics of Exercise and Training." In *Essentials of Strength Training and Conditioning,* 4th ed., edited by G.G. Haff and N.T. Triplett, 583-604. Champaign, IL: Human Kinetics.

Issurin, V.B. 2008. *Block Periodization: Breakthrough in Sports Training.* Muskegon, MI: Ultimate Athlete Concepts, 1-213

Stone, M.H., H.S. O'Bryant, J. J. Garhammer, J. L. McMillan, and R. Rozenek. 1982. A Theoretical Model for Strength Training. *NSCA J* 4:36-39.

Stone, M.H., M.E. Stone, and W.A. Sands. 2007. "Modes in Resistance Training." In *Principals and Practice of Resistance Training,* 241-287. Champaign, IL: Human Kinetics.

Zatsiorsky, V.M. and W.J. Kraemer. 2006. *Science and Practice of Strength Training.,* 2nd ed., Champaign, IL: Human Kinetics, 3-14; 89–108.

Chapter 11

Riebe, D., J.K. Ehrman, G. Liguori, and M. Migal. 2018. "General Principles for Exercise Prescription." In *ACSM's Guidelines for Exercise Testing and Prescription,* 10th ed., by American College of Sports Medicine. Philadelphia: Wolters Kluwer.

Chapter 12

Purdom, T., L. Kravitz, K. Dokladny, C. Mermier. 2018. "Understanding the Factors That Effect Maximal Fat Oxidation." *Journal of International Society of Sports Nutrition* 15 (1).

Bircher, S., and B. Knechtle. 2004. "Relationship Between Fat Oxidation and Lactate Threshold in Athletes and Obese Women and Men. *Journal of Sports Science and Medicine.* 3 (3): 174-81.

Boutcher, S. 2010. "High Intensity Intermittent Exercise and Fat Loss." *Journal of Obesity* 868305.

Chapter 13

Krieger, J.W. 2010. "Single Versus Multiple Sets of Resistance Exercise for Muscle Hypertrophy." *Journal of Strength and Conditioning Research* 24 (4): 1150-1159.

Schoenfeld, B., B.J. Grgic, J. Ogborn, and J.W. Krieger. 2017a. "Strength and Hypertrophy Adaptations between Low- vs. High-Load Resistance Training: A Systematic Review and Meta-Analysis." *Journal of Strength and Conditioning Research* 31 (12):3508-3523.

Schoenfeld, B., B.J. Ogborn, D.I. Vigotsky, and A.D. Franchi. 2017b. "Hypertrophic Effects of Concentric vs. Eccentric Muscle Actions: A Systematic Review and Meta-Analysis." *Journal of Strength and Conditioning Research* 31 (9): 2599-2608.

Chapter 14

French, D. 2016. "Adaptations to Anaerobic Training Programs." In *Essentials of Strength Training and Conditioning,* 4th ed., edited by G.G. Haff and N.T. Triplett, 87-113. Champaign, IL: Human Kinetics.

McBride, J.M. 2016. "Biomechanics of Resistance Exercise." In *Essentials of Strength Training and Conditioning,* 4th ed., edited by G. G. Haff and N. T. Triplett, 19-42 Champaign, IL: Human Kinetics.

Chapter 15

McBride, J.M. 2016. "Biomechanics of Resistance Exercise." In *Essentials of Strength Training and Conditioning,* 4th ed., edited by G.G. Haff and N.T. Triplett, 19-42. Champaign, IL: Human Kinetics.

Herda, T.J., and J.T. Cramer. 2016. "Bioenergetics of Exercise and Training." In *Essentials of Strength Training and Conditioning,* 4th ed., edited by G.G. Haff and N.T. Triplett, 43-64. Champaign, IL: Human Kinetics.

French, D. 2016. "Adaptations to Anaerobic Training Programs." In *Essentials of Strength Training and Conditioning,* 4th ed., edited by G.G. Haff and N.T. Triplett, 87-113. Champaign, IL: Human Kinetics.

Statler, T., and V. Brown. 2016. "Facility, Policies, Procedures and Legal Issues." In *Essentials of Strength Training and Conditioning,* 4th ed., edited by G.G. Haff and N.T. Triplett, 641-656. Champaign, IL: Human Kinetics.

About the Authors

John Graham, MS, ACSM EP-C, CSCS*D, RSCC*E, FNSCA, has enjoyed an accomplished 40-year career in the health, fitness, and strength and conditioning industry. He has served in many roles with the National Strength and Conditioning Association (NSCA), including as the board vice president, secretary/treasurer, and chair for the certification committee, conference committee chair, and nominations committee. He has also held leadership positions with American Council on Exercise (ACE) and Medical Fitness Association (MFA). From 2012 to 2015, he was a member of the industry advisory panel for the American Council on Exercise (ACE). He currently serves as associate editor of NSCA's *Strength and Conditioning Journal.*

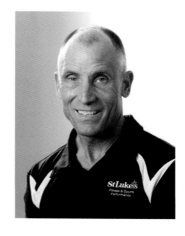

Graham is a senior network administrator in lifestyle health and wellness, medical fitness, fitness and sports performance at St. Luke's University Health Network in Pennsylvania and New Jersey, and he is a senior contributor at SportsEdTV. Graham has authored or contributed to local, regional, and national peer-reviewed and popular publications on health, fitness, sports conditioning, and chronic conditions and disorders prevention and management. He has given local, regional, national, and international presentations—including at Perform Better, NSCA, ACSM, and MFA.

His contributions to fitness and sports performance have resulted in recognition by many organizations, including ACE, MFA, National Multiple Sclerosis Society, and NSCA. He has served as an adjunct professor at Cedar Crest College, The College of New Jersey, and DeSales University.

Michael Barnes, Med, CSCS*D, NSCA-CPT*D, brings over 25 years of experience to the strength and conditioning and fitness industry. He is the president and owner of Infinity Personal Training and Fitness in Colorado Springs, Colorado. His previous experience includes working in Division I athletics, working in the National Football League with the San Francisco 49ers, and serving as the director of education for the National Strength and Conditioning Association (NSCA).

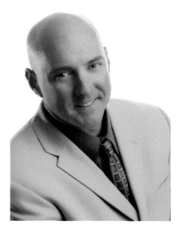

Barnes is an author, speaker, subject matter expert, industry consultant, and practitioner. He holds three of the most respected professional certifications in the industry as well as a master's degree in exercise science.

Barnes has presented to coaches, athletes, and fitness enthusiasts with organizations such as Major League Baseball, NSCA, USA Triathlon, USA Rugby, the World Class Athlete Program of the U.S. Army, NCAA, U.S. Ski and Snowboard Association, USA Judo, and the U.S. Association of Deaf and Blind Athletes. He has traveled the world to educate, train, and interact with leaders in the fitness industry in Japan, Australia, Puerto Rico, Bermuda, Greece, and Denmark.

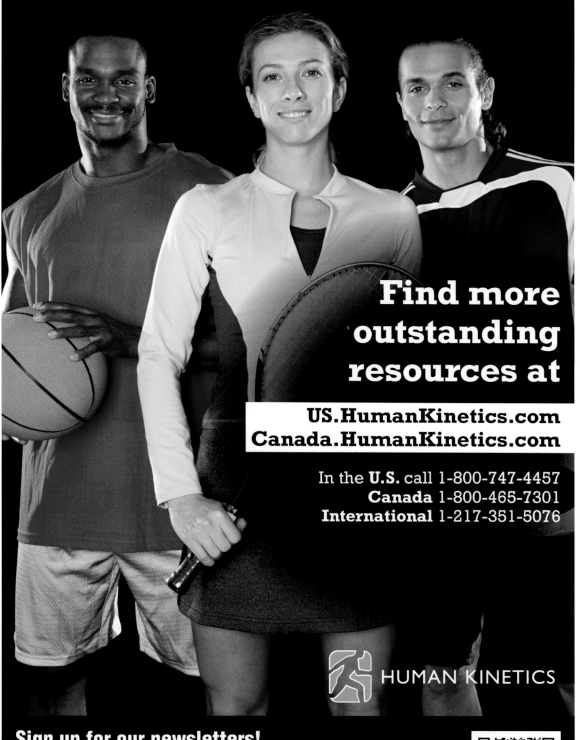

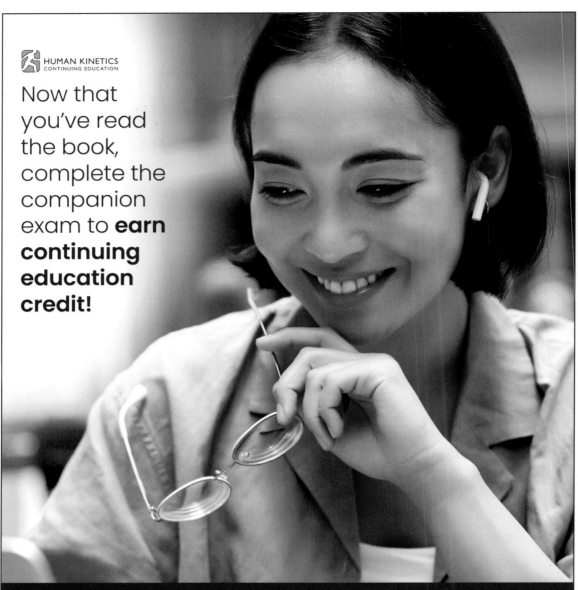
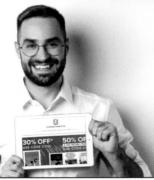